2

# The Heart of Listening

*A Visionary Approach to*
*Craniosacral Work*

**Anatomy, Technique, Transcendence**

**2**

# The Heart of Listening

*A Visionary Approach to*
*Craniosacral Work*

**Anatomy, Technique, Transcendence**

**Hugh Milne**

Book
Secret language of the body

*North Atlantic Books, Berkeley, California*

*The osteopathic, shamanistic, and visionary practices
set forth in this book should not be considered as an
exclusive method of treatment. The appropriate medical or
psychotherapeutic authorities should be consulted for the
diagnosis and treatment of any medical or psychological
condition.*

*The osteopathic, shamanistic, and visionary practices
as described in this book are best considered as an adjunct
to orthodox medical or psychotherapeutic treatments.
This book is designed to be used as a training manual by
licensed health care providers, to enhance their understanding of, and competence in, complementary healing
practices.*

Published by
  North Atlantic Books
  P.O. Box 12327
  Berkeley, California 94712

Cover art *Body, Mind, Spirit* © copyright 1985 by Alex Grey
Line art by Jamey Garbett and © copyright Nielsen/Garbett
1995, except for art listed below
Line art on pages xvi, xvii, 8, 10, 66, 84, 96, 120, 132, 138,
148, 157, 162, 168, 170, 176, 188, 190, reprinted with per-
mission of Georg Thieme Verlag
Photography by Hugh Milne
Cover and book design by Marti Spiegelman
Typesetting and production by Catherine E. Campaigne

Printed in the United States of America

*The Heart of Listening* is sponsored by the Society for the
Study of Native Arts and Sciences, a nonprofit educational
corporation whose goals are to develop an educational and
cross-cultural perspective linking various scientific, social,
and artistic fields; to nurture a holistic view of arts, sciences,
humanities, and healing; and to publish and distribute literature on the relationship of mind, body, and nature.

North Atlantic Books' publications are available through
most bookstores. For further information, visit our website
at www.northatlanticbooks.com or call 800-733-3000.

ISBN-13 (Volume 2): 978-1-55643-280-4

Library of Congress Cataloging-in-Publication Data
Milne, Hugh.
    The heart of listening : a visionary approach to cranio-
sacral work / Hugh Milne.
      v.  <   > cm.
    Includes bibliographical references and index.
    Contents: v. 1. Origins, destination points, unfold-
ment. v. 2. Anatomy, technique, transcendence.
      ISBN 1–55643–279–8 (v. 1 : pbk. : alk. paper). — ISBN
1-55643-280-1 (v. 2 : pbk. : alk. paper)
    1. Craniosacral therapy.  I. Title.
RZ399.C73M54   1998b
615.8'9—dc21                                          98-15082
                                                          CIP

9  10  11  12  13  MALLOY  18  17  16  15  14

# Permissions

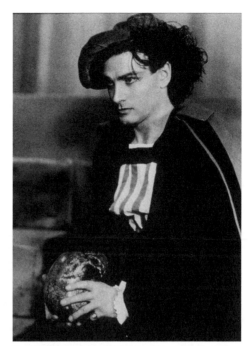

# Dedication

*To my father Sandy,
who first showed me
how to reinterpret
statements, symptoms,
and gestures according
to a deeper reality.*

*To my mother Joycelyn,
who first showed me
intuitive perception and
who lived the
compassionate heart.*

*And to all Teachers.*

# Acknowledgements

*This book existed in manuscript form for three years, and was used as a handbook by hundreds of students all over the world. During that time I repeatedly appealed for comments, criticism, feedback of any kind. Not a soul responded until one day Marti Spiegelman said "I would like to help you," and she really did. She provided absolutely invaluable help with the flow, content and psychic weight of this book. A woman of many talents, she has also set the page layouts, and overseen the artwork and the typesetting. To this book she is midwife.*

*Jodie Arey began a seemingly endless amount of transcribing, letter writing and literary research with irrepressible and infectious good humor. Courtney Childs and Dove Grace completed her work with aptitude. Brian Lyke spent many hours footnoting, with astonishing aptitude and focus. Rabia Erduman helped with the soul-centers, Craig Carr with the Windows To The Sky points, and David Schanakar always came through with the Taoist truth. Trent Cornell provided invaluable help with the dynamics of transference. Wojciech Tarnowski was prompt and diligent with my requests for help with dental research, and Angeles Arrien defined "visionary" for me in the way I understood it, but no dictionary defined it.*

*Julie Chertow, Teresa Gaffin, Sabine Grandke, Kim Luchau, Reiko Miyamoto, Mark Nilsson and Marti Spiegelman all posed patiently and good-humoredly for the technique photographs. Gary Russell, of GMR in Monterey, was extremely helpful with photo refinement and reproduction.*

*Anne Hoff provided exactly the right mixture of alertness, enquiry, and understanding for the initial editing. Catherine Campaigne did a heroic job of combining last-minute updates and changes with typesetting, and did so with unfailing warmth and goodwill. She was a joy to work with.*

*My heartfelt thanks to you all.*

# The Heart

*"Heart" has four words in it:*

- *Ear*
- *Hear*
- *Heat*
- *Art*

*The "Heart of Listening" requires us to have not only an ear, but to hear with our whole being; it is energy work, and the heat in a healer's hands is a potent form of energy. Working with real, whole human beings is a hot-blooded endeavor that is, above all things else, an art.*

*Perception is the visual, external component of intuition, and insight is the contemplative, internal component of intuition. It is "in-sight"; it is the internal seeing of self and other. A visionary is someone who trusts what they perceive outside and what they sense inside, and values both equally. Many people can hold the parts, many people can hold the whole, but very few people can hold the parts and the whole. This book presents a visionary approach to craniosacral work.*

*I hope that it will show you a way inside, a way outside, and a way to combine the two.*

# Table of Contents

# Preface

Over the years, many therapists have asked me if I can teach them what happens when I give them a session. This book is an attempt to write about it, detailing a visionary approach to an art more commonly presented in strictly technical terms. It is designed to offer an alternative approach to the emergent healer who wishes to develop her skill.

For me, working with people's heads is spiritual practice. It is based upon a profound respect for the individual, imbued with reverence and overlain with a sense of awe. For others, working with the head is simply a mechanical art. This does not make it ineffective. Rumi, the Persian mystic, notes that "there are hundreds of different ways to kneel and kiss the ground."[1]

What is now popularly known as "craniosacral work," like any art, can be practiced many different ways. Some osteopaths practice "cranial osteopathy" as a technical skill that focuses on treating symptoms in ten- to twenty-minute sessions. Many chiropractors practice "craniology" with great mechanical and tactile aptitude in similarly brief visits. Both chiropractors and osteopaths tend to base their work upon the mechanical models of bone movement they were educated in. Gifted bodyworkers use craniosacral work as an adjunct to their hour-long sessions. They tend to interpret what they do in terms of balance, gravity, muscle tonus, and fascial length. Massage therapists may employ a few craniosacral techniques at the end of each session. Exceptionally gifted with tactile sensitivity, they tend to let their hands tell them what to do. Christian healers touch the head while "laying on hands"; they treat by praying. Psychics use craniosacral work as a way to access deep realms of the spirit during "psychic healing." Working through visionary perception, they see what is wrong with the head. In "past life regression," therapists use craniosacral touch to help induct people into sensitive realms of experience. They work in altered states of consciousness, using their extraordinary sensitivity to the body's electrical field, or chi.

My sessions encompass aspects of each approach mentioned above; appropriately used, each has its value and its contribution to healing. The sessions begin with an intuitive reading, which focuses on perceiving what really troubles the client, his strengths and weaknesses, and how he can access his potential. From that point, the session may be wholly devoted to sitting together, or may turn upon harnessing the initial perception in order to touch the client more accurately at deeper levels.

To honor womankind and the essentially feminine nature of visionary craniosacral work, I have made references to the healer "she" and the client "he." I hope this will help dull the feelings of exclusion that can result from the traditional use of exclusively male pronouns.

Many students told me that they experienced the first edition of this book as a little too large to transport without inflicting damage to cover or contents. For this reason the second edition has been printed both in hardback and softback: the hardback as one volume, the softback split into two, more manageable, volumes. There are no content differences between softcover and hardcover, and the only changes from the first edition are a number of corrections to the drawings, and minor corrections to the Windows To The Sky. Otherwise the text, and the message, is unchanged.

*Hugh Milne, Big Sur, California, February 7, 1998*

# The Best Listener of All

*An intelligence officer is nothing if he has lost his will to listen, and George Smiley – plump, troubled, cuckolded, unassuming, indefatigable George, forever polishing his spectacles on the lining of his tie, puffing to himself and sighing in his perrenial distraction – was the best listener of all.*

*I shall remember all my life the compelling power of his patience. Smiley was listening as only Smiley can, eyes half closed, chins sunk into his neck. I thought I was telling him everything I knew. Perhaps he thought I was too, though I doubt it, for he understood far better than I the levels of self-deception that are the means of our survival. Despite the disturbing tendency of his questions, I was beginning to feel a great need to talk to him.*

*Smiley could listen with his hooded, sleepy eyes; he could listen by the very inclination of his tubby body, by his stillness and his understanding smile. He could listen because with one exception, which was Ann, his wife, he expected nothing of his fellow souls, criticized nothing, condoned the worst of you long before you had revealed it. He could listen better than a microphone because his mind lit at once upon the essentials; he seemed able to spot them before he knew where they were leading.*

*The surest knowledge we have of one another comes from instinct.*

*– extracts from* The Secret Pilgrim *by John le Carré*

# Introduction

This is a book about healing. It represents the distillation not only of the author's own studies and practice, but also those of his father and grandfather. This comes through in Hugh's work, and in his teaching. It shows in this book. *The Heart of Listening* also illuminates the unknowable, which to me is always intriguing.

I find the amount of information, and the way it is interwoven, to be fascinating. My experience of working with this book is that it is one of the few works that combines the physical with the emotional and the spiritual. It has enriched what I have learned first-hand as a student in Hugh's classes.

Visionary craniosacral work is valuable for those of us who do bodywork because it fits with, and deepens, what we are already doing. It improves the results of our efforts. Whether we use it with our existing work, or do pure cranial sessions, it allows us to access more profound levels of healing.

Hugh has been the third pivotal teacher in my life. My own evolution as a healer began with my father, when I experienced the healing power of his hands. When one of his children had an ache or a pain, he would massage the painful place. He could always take the pain away. This was my first exposure to healing.

A movie-set designer, he taught me about the processes required to makes thoughts become reality. He was a designer of fantasy, and he loved it. (In fact he did the set designs for "Fantasia" and many other Walt Disney movies, including "Around the World in Eighty Days.") He taught me about structures, the strengths and qualities of materials, and how pulleys and gears work. The greatest thing that he taught me was that if you really wanted to figure something out, you had to "get into it." You had to understand it completely first. I can remember watching him fix things. He would keep them running through their actions, watching them until he understood how they were

supposed to work. Reading this book reminds me of his persistence: everything you need in order to understand the intermarriage of energy and cranial bone movement patterns is comprehensively set out here. The reader can really "get into it."

Design has always been my love. My parents, being artists, groomed me for it. I apprenticed with architects and structural engineers for ten years before taking the state board exams. After working as an architect for another ten years, I met Ida Rolf in 1970. I was Al Drucker and Don Johnson's Rolfing model. I would sit at Ida's feet while she taught and held court from her famous rocking chair. In those days it was difficult for me to sit on the floor, and I was in a lot of pain. At one point Ida sensed this, and told Al to work on a particular place in my back, which gave me great relief. I thought to myself, "Wow! This lady can see around corners."

In that moment I knew that she had something I wanted to know, and could teach it to me. That's when I asked her if she would train me to be a Rolfer. It had to do with the magic of proper structure. When I was doing architecture I would become amazed and frustrated by all the pieces it took to make one building. I used to dream of the one-piece structure. After I trained with the Rolf Institute I realized that the body was that one-piece structure. Rolfing was to become my second major teacher.

Hugh's craniosacral work has proved to be a different teaching than Rolfing, but one equally important to me. It doesn't just add another technique to my repertoire, but alters and enhances all that I have learned previously.

One structure I had always wanted to design was a temple. In cranial work I discovered that the "one-piece building" was also the Temple. This was, and is, incredibly exciting, a great mystery. I still don't understand it all, and perhaps I never will. What sets a temple aside from other buildings is a certain almost magical awareness of the sacred space. When I am connected with a client's cranial bones, I feel that I am connected directly into their soul. This work enables me to become a "tender of the temple." The temple is where we become aware of God, of that which never dies and was never born. Cranial work is one way of taking the client into the temple and showing it to them.

For the first few years of cranial work I didn't allow myself to become totally immersed in the cranial bone movements, because I have another trait from my father: always doubting. It took me five years until I was ready to get quiet enough to really feel the specific movements. Now it feels more like a spiritual practice to me than it does work. A session is like holding satsang, never knowing which of us is the teacher.

What I learned in Rolfing was look, listen, roll up my sleeves and get to work. What I've learned in craniosacral work is to go very deep, like the blue whale, and then get very still. From that place of stillness I have learned to feel at an altogether different level. I have been able to feel cranial motion for many years, but I could not extract the information hidden within the cranial structures. I could not language what I was feeling. Visionary craniosacral work enables me to access another part of my brain, a part where I can respond more precisely to what I am seeing and feeling. One day in a cranial class I began to see like Hugh can see (and Ida could see). For the first time I could envision the cranium, and really understood the structure, the dynamics, and what was going on. It has been an incredible revelation to me.

When I do tissue work, I notice time and time again that when I end it by checking in to the sacrum, neck, and sphenoid, it carries the whole body of work deeper. It imprints in a different department in the client's brain. It is like planting a seed properly. Cranial work is akin to taking that seed and putting it deep into the opening created by the tissue work. It is a kind of alchemy,

transforming the previous work. Hugh taught me how to hold a knee and connect with the client's sphenoid. He taught me how to focus, then spread, my intention to specific points in the body (a technique you can read about in this book) in order to create a release. The clients feel it, which amazes me sometimes, and they actually know where I have been. I don't know another way to get their attention quite like that. I have people right after the cranial part of the session saying "God, I want more of that." They don't know what it was, they just know they want to do it again.

When clients are passing through periods of extreme emotional disturbance, there is something about cranial work that really connects them with Self. As soon as we move to the cranial part of the session virtually everybody quiets down, sinks in, and becomes aware that what we are doing is meditating, physically connected meditating. This book is a roadmap for learning to work at these levels.

The techniques described in this book are individual tools that, once you become used to handling them, can open doorways to a greater creativity. Such simple tools can do so much. A versatility emerges, a versatility without dogma. Hugh stresses the importance of seeing and feeling what is happening, and of not adhering to a set way of working. Let what you feel guide you. This approach is very alive, and profoundly healing.

I have found it very easy to receive what Hugh teaches, and it has the effect of making me hungry for more. And I know he has that "more."

Richard Stratman
Certified Rolfer and Architect

# Abbreviations, Nomenclature, and Metric Conversions

## Directions in Space

All directions refer to the body in the anatomical position, as illustrated.

| | |
|---|---|
| Anterior | Toward the front |
| Posterior | Toward the rear |
| Inferior | Below |
| Superior | Above |
| Lateral | Away from the midline |
| Medial | Toward the midline |
| Dorsal | The back |
| Ventral | The front |
| Deep | Away from the surface |
| Superficial | Toward or on the surface |
| Cephalad | Toward the head |
| Caudad | Toward the coccyx |
| Pedad | Toward the feet |

## Abbreviations

| | |
|---|---|
| ACI | Acupuncture Chinese inch |
| AOJ | Atlanto-occipital joint |
| ASS | Anterior superior spines |
| CN | Cranial nerve – e.g., CNV is the fifth cranial nerve |
| COE | Constant-on engram |
| COEX | Area of condensed experience from Stanislav Grof |
| CRI | Cranial rhythmic impulse |
| DDR | Deep-diving reflex |
| GV16 | Governor Vessel 16, Wind Palace |
| GV22 | Governor Vessel 22, Middle of Man |
| IOP | Internal Occipital Protruberance |
| H9 | Heart 9, Little Rushing In |
| LI10 | Large Intestine 10, Arm Three Miles |
| NC | Neurocranium |
| NDE | Near-death experience |
| OBP | Odorant binding protein |
| RIT | Reciprocal innervation technique |
| RTM | Reciprocal tension membrane |
| SAD | Seasonal affective disorder |
| SBJ | Sphenobasilar joint |
| SCM | Sternocleidomastoid |
| SGS | Stomatognathic system |
| ST15 | Stomach 15, Room Screen |
| TLA | Three-letter acronym |
| TW21 | Triple Warmer 21, Ear Gate |
| TMJ | Temporomandibular joint |
| VC | Viscerocranium |

*Directions in space*

*1 Anterior*
*2 Posterior*
*3 Inferior*
*4 Superior*
*5 Lateral*
*6 Medial*
*7 Cephalad*
*8 Caudad*
*9 Pedad*
*10 Transverse Plane (or Section)*
*11 Paramedian or Parasagittal Plane*
*12 Median or Sagittal Plane*
*13 Coronal Plane*

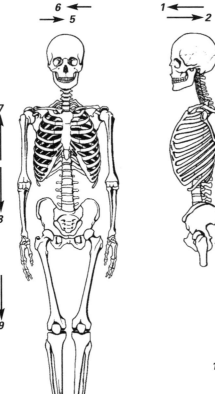
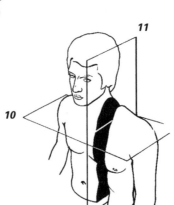
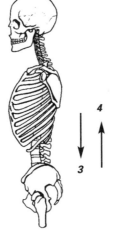
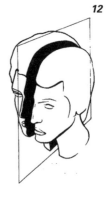
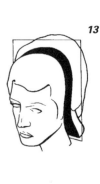

## Motion and Direction Nomenclature

***Flexion*** Increasing the angle of a joint, forward-bending, or movement into the fetal position

***Extension*** Decreasing the angle of a joint, backward-bending, or movement out of the fetal position

***Cranial flexion*** The central reference is the movement of the sphenoid into forward-bending, commonly known as "nose-diving." The movement that all other cranial bones undergo as the sphenoid moves into flexion is also called flexion, even if, strictly speaking, the movement is actually an extension, or backward-bending movement.

***Cranial extension*** The central reference is the backward-bending movement, or extension, of the sphenoid. The movement that all other cranial bones undergo as the sphenoid moves into extension is also called extension.

***Proximal*** Nearest the point of attachment, center of the body, or point of reference

***Distal*** Farthest from the center, from a medial line, or from the trunk

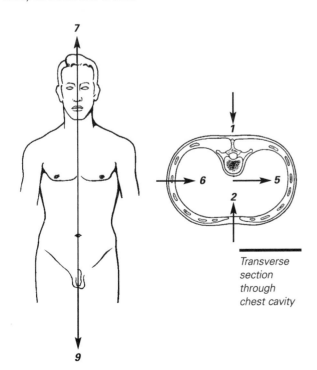

*Transverse
section
through
chest cavity*

***Ipsilateral*** On the same side

***Homolateral movement*** Moving the left arm and left leg together, right arm and right leg together

***Contralateral*** On the opposite side

***Contralateral movement*** Moving the left arm and right leg together, right arm and left leg together

***Homologous movement*** Moving both arms and both legs together

## Spirit, Soul, and Consciousness

As used in this book, the word "spirit" refers to the measurable electrical field of the human body, which begins to shut down at the moment of death.

"Soul" refers to a nonmeasurable presence, sometimes called a body of light, which is not part of the physical body, but rather resides slightly outside or above it, usually above the vertex of the head. Those who have gone through near-death experiences recount seeing the world from a vantage point above, typically from the top-left corner of the room; they are "seeing" from the location of their soul.

"Consciousness" is a form of energy. It refers to the presence of a metacommunicator, or central awareness of self, that can separate itself from the grip of instinctual forces. Consciousness is thus the "watcher on the hill" that knows when we are feeling angry, sexual, sad, or euphoric, and can clearly say so in the midst of experiencing the wash of such feelings. In Sanskrit, consciousness is *drashta*, the looker. When Krishna says that the secret of immortality is "to know that you are the field, and the knower of the field," the knower he is referring to is *drashta*, consciousness.

## Metric Conversions

### Metric to English

| Symbol | Unit | Multiply by | To Find | Symbol |
|--------|------|-------------|---------|--------|
| in | inch | 2.54 | centimeter | cm |
| ft | foot | 30.48 | centimeter | cm |
| yd | yard | 0.91 | meter | m |
| mi | mile | 1.61 | kilometer | km |
| $in^2$ | square inch | 6.45 | square centimeter | $cm^2$ |
| $ft^2$ | square foot | 0.09 | square meter | $m^2$ |
| $mi^2$ | square mile | 0.84 | square kilometer | $km^2$ |
| oz | ounce | 28.35 | gram | g |
| lb | pound | 0.45 | kilogram | kg |
| short ton | (2,000 lbs) | 0.91 | metric ton | t |
| fl oz | fluid ounce | 29.57 | milliliter | ml |
| c | cup | 0.24 | liter | L |
| qt | quart | 0.95 | liter | L |
| gal | gallon | 3.78 | liter | L |
| $ft^3$ | cubic foot | 0.03 | cubic meter | $m^3$ |
| $yd^3$ | cubic yard | 0.76 | cubic meter | $m^3$ |
| F | degrees Fahrenheit | 0.55 (first subtract 32) | degrees Celsius | C |

### English to Metric

| Symbol | Unit | Multiply | To Find | Symbol |
|--------|------|----------|---------|--------|
| cm | centimeter | 0.39 | inch | in |
| cm | centimeter | 0.033 | foot | ft |
| m | meter | 1.09 | yard | yd |
| km | kilometer | 0.62 | mile | mi |
| $cm^2$ | square centimeter | 0.15 | square inch | $in^2$ |
| $m^2$ | square meter | 10.76 | square good | $ft^2$ |
| $m^2$ | square meter | 1.20 | square yard | $yd^2$ |
| $km^2$ | square kilometer | 0.39 | square mile | $mi^2$ |
| ha | hectare | 2.47 | acre | |
| g | gram | 0.035 | ounce | oz |
| kg | kilogram | 2.21 | pounds | lbs |
| t | metric ton | 1.10 | short ton (2,000 lbs) | |
| mL | milliliter | 0.03 | fluid ounce | fl oz |
| L | liter | 4.24 | cup | c |
| L | liter | 1.05 | quart (liquid) | qt |
| L | liter | 0.25 | gallon | gal |
| $m^3$ | cubic meter | 35.32 | cubic foot | $ft^3$ |
| $m^3$ | cubic meter | 1.32 | cubic yard | $yd^3$ |
| C | degrees Celcius | 1.80 (then add 32) | degrees Fahrenheit | F |

## Useful Standards of Reference

n A bar is 14.7 pounds per square inch.

n A centimeter is 0.40 inch.

n An inch is 2.54 centimeters.

n A liter is 1.06 quarts.

n A quart is 0.95 liter.

n A gram is 0.04 ounce.

n A pound is 453.59 grams.

n A kilogram is 2.20 pounds.

n A meter is 1.09 yards.

n A square meter is 10.76 square feet.

n A micron is one millionth of a meter, or $10^{-6}$ meter. (A micron is $\frac{1}{100}$ the thickness of this page. The maximum observed amplitude of the cranial wave is forty microns, just less than half the thickness of this page.) Sensitive human beings can discern the difference to their bite that a 3 micron dental promintory makes – the thickness of a piece of fine dental carbon paper.

n A nanometer is one trillionth of a meter, or $10^{-9}$ meter.

n An angstrom is 0.1 nanometer, or $10^{-12}$ meter.

# ANATOMY AND PHYSIOLOGY

# 16
# An Anatomical Guided Tour through the Cranial Field

To facilitate clear analytic understanding of its component parts, the physical body is divided into the following divisions in craniosacral work: "the mechanism," the neurocranium (which comprises the cranial base and cranial vault), the viscerocranium, the stomatognathic system, and the speed reducers.

## The Mechanism

The phrase "the mechanism" as used in craniosacral work refers to the sum total of the parts that make up the craniosacral system, including the connective membrane of the meningeal and spinal dura. Thus, it includes:

- All 21 cranial bones (this count excludes the 6 auditory ossicles)
- The brain, spinal cord, and cerebrospinal fluid
- All 24 vertebrae
- The sacrum
- The dural membrane system, or reciprocal tension membrane (RTM), which includes the spinal dura

## The Cranial Base

The cranial base is made up of six bones:

- The occiput (1 bone; excluding inter-parietal portion)
- The sphenoid (1 bone; including body, lesser wings, roots of greater wings)
- The ethmoid (1 bone)
- The temporals (2 bones; excluding squamous portion)
- The frontal (1 bone)

## The Cranial Vault

The cranial vault comprises seven bones:

- The frontal (1 bone; excluding the horizontal, or orbito-nasal, portion)
- The parietals (2 bones)
- The interparietal portion of the occipital bone (1)
- The squamous portions of the temporal bones (2)
- The sphenoid, greater wing portions only (1)

## The Viscerocranium

The viscerocranium consists of fifteen bones:

- The ethmoid (1 bone)
- The frontal (1 bone)
- The maxillae (2 bones)
- The zygomae (2 bones)
- The concha (2 bones)
- The lacrimals (2 bones)
- The palatines (2 bones)
- The nasals (2 bones)
- The vomer (1 bone)

## The Stomatognathic System

The stomatognathic system consists of 27 bones:

- The occiput (1 bone)
- The temporals (2 bones)
- The sphenoid (1 bone)
- The maxillae (2 bones)
- The mandible (1 bone)
- The hyoid (1 bone)
- The clavicles (2 bones)
- The scapulae (2 bones)

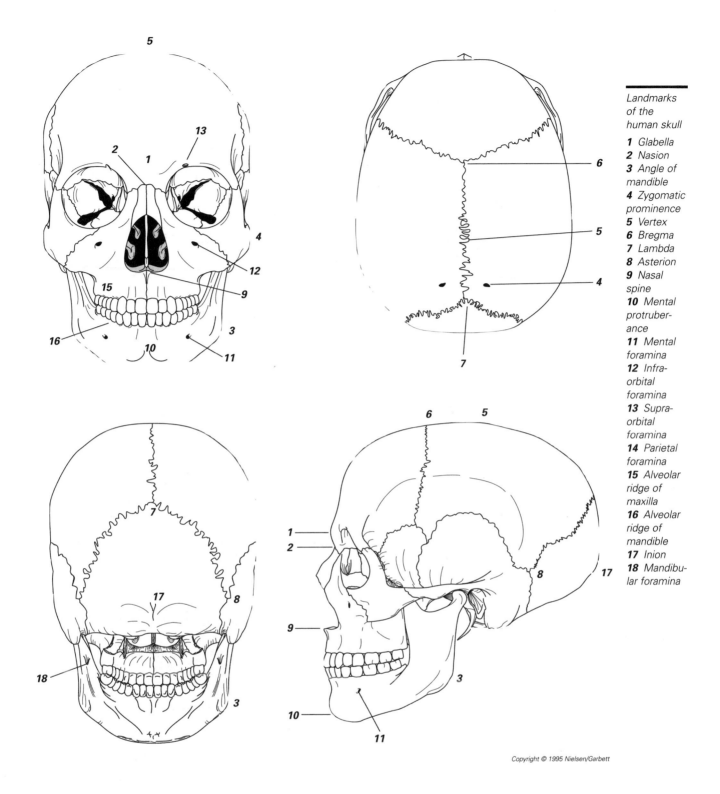

Landmarks
of the
human skull

**1** Glabella
**2** Nasion
**3** Angle of
mandible
**4** Zygomatic
prominence
**5** Vertex
**6** Bregma
**7** Lambda
**8** Asterion
**9** Nasal
spine
**10** Mental
protruber-
ance
**11** Mental
foramina
**12** Infra-
orbital
foramina
**13** Supra-
orbital
foramina
**14** Parietal
foramina
**15** Alveolar
ridge of
maxilla
**16** Alveolar
ridge of
mandible
**17** Inion
**18** Mandibu-
lar foramina

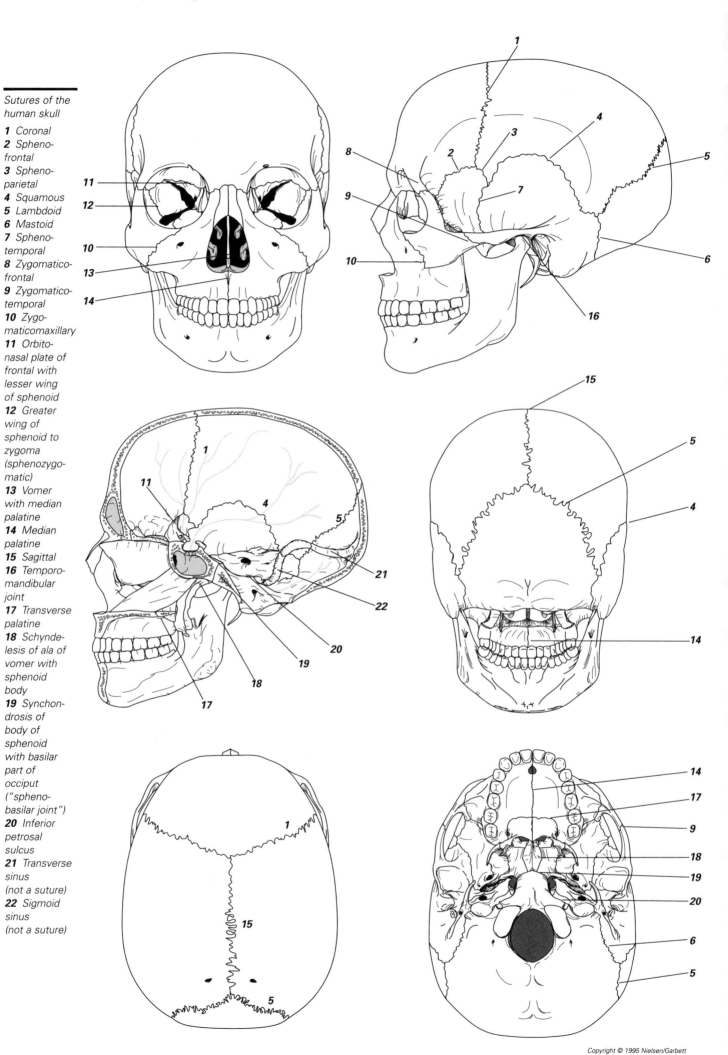

Sutures of the human skull

**1** Coronal
**2** Spheno-frontal
**3** Spheno-parietal
**4** Squamous
**5** Lambdoid
**6** Mastoid
**7** Spheno-temporal
**8** Zygomatico-frontal
**9** Zygomatico-temporal
**10** Zygo-maticomaxillary
**11** Orbito-nasal plate of frontal with lesser wing of sphenoid
**12** Greater wing of sphenoid to zygoma (sphenozygo-matic)
**13** Vomer with median palatine
**14** Median palatine
**15** Sagittal
**16** Temporo-mandibular joint
**17** Transverse palatine
**18** Schynde-lesis of ala of vomer with sphenoid body
**19** Synchon-drosis of body of sphenoid with basilar part of occiput ("spheno-basilar joint")
**20** Inferior petrosal sulcus
**21** Transverse sinus (not a suture)
**22** Sigmoid sinus (not a suture)

- The sternum (1 bone)
- The upper two ribs on each side (4 bones)
- The 7 cervical and first 3 thoracic vertebrae (10 bones)

## The Speed Reducers

The "speed reducers" consist of

- The zygomae (2 bones)
- The palatines (2 bones)
- The vomer (1 bone)

## Landmarks

The basic landmarks of the skull are as follows:

- Nasion (located at the midline of the nasofrontal suture)
- Glabella (located between the eyebrow ridges, at the exit point of the inner eye)
- Bregma (located where the sagittal and coronal sutures meet, the crown soul)
- Pterion (located where the frontal, sphenoid, temporal and parietal bones meet at the temple)
- Asterion (located where the parietal and temporal bones meet the occiput, the acupuncture point Gall Bladder 19)
- Lambda (located where the superior portion of the occiput meets the sagittal suture)

Advanced landmarking includes:

- Obelion (located on the sagittal suture between the parietal foramina, the acupuncture point Governor Vessel 18)
- Gonion (the point of the angle of the mandible, the acupuncture point Stomach 5)
- Opisthion (the acupuncture point Wind Palace, Governor Vessel 16, an ancillary soul center)
- Ear Gate (located where the auricle of the ear meets the superior margin of the temporal portion of the zygomatic arch, the acupuncture point Triple Warmer 21)

The following terms amplify basic anatomical nomenclature:

- Cephalad, or toward the vertex ("cranial" is synonymous)
- Caudad, or toward the "tail"
- Pedad, or toward the feet
- Vector: movement and/or energy directed along a specific angle

## Overview

We developed cranial bones because we wanted to. We lived, ate, procreated, and died, and something in us wanted to understand the process, to have some control over it, to live better and longer.[1,2] We needed neuronal tissue in order to understand, and the neuronal tissue needed a safe, protected space. Because the neuronal tissue kept the wave-like pulsation of its oceanic origins, the protected space had to accommodate this movement. Hence sutures, hence the bony malleability of the thinner cranial bones. Osseous mobility was also essential for birth. This motility has had several advantageous spin-offs, one of which is enhanced protection: a mobile bone absorbs and dissipates shock[3] and inhibits bony fracturing much better than a "fixed" dome of bone.

Movement is also totemistic: we define ourselves – our consciousness and our relationship to our body and soul – by our movement. Until very recently, our very survival lay in a lifestyle of movement – first as a hunter-gatherer, then as the traveling nomadic herdsman, finally in the smaller movements of the farmer. Now our need for movement has found new expression in the freeway, the mountain bike, and the gym.

The reciprocal tension membrane (RTM) helps to dissipate the force of impact, and reduces the chance of damage to the brain itself. The way the head responds to physical trauma is rather like the way a tai chi master responds to assault – by sliding out of the way, by being round and slippery, flexible, and behaving like sea water. In Taoism this is called "the watercourse way" (wu wei wu).

## Wolff's Law

In the seventeenth century, Galilei Galileo (1564–1642) found that the laws of motion could be explained by mathematical principles.[4] He described an immutable relationship between a person's body weight and movement, and his resultant bone shape and density.[5] In his 1892 work, *The Law of Bone Transformation*, Julius Wolff explained that relationship in detail. Wolff noted that:

*Every change in the function of a bone is followed by certain definite changes in internal architecture and external conformation in accordance with mathematical laws.*

That is, bony structures orient themselves in form and mass to best respond to extrinsic forces. This has become known as "Wolff's Law."

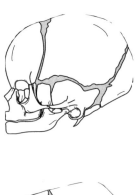
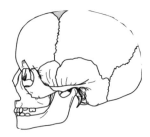
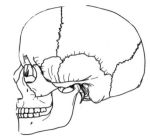
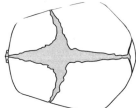
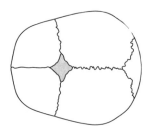
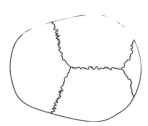

*Develop-
ment of
fontanels
and sutures,
lateral and
superior
views at
birth (left), 2
years (mid-
dle), and 4
years (right)*

Posture, work and play habits, and the ubiqui-
tous effects of gravity provide the main stressor
components to bone. Inside the neurocranium, the
tension within the membrane system and the
weight of the brain exert powerful influences in
determining the shape of the bony structures.

Genetics plays a pivotal role, one which is unaffected by use (computer measurements of skulls
can distinguish the minor genetic signatures of
shape that differentiate human racial types.[6]) Psychological, psychic, and physiological demands further determine bone shape, density, strength, and
pliancy.

The science of "reading" bones is now so specialized that individuals can be identified from
mass graves,[7] and ten-thousand-year-old forearm
bones found in Ethiopia can be definitively classified as belonging to javelin throwers.[8] (They
exhibit the same humeral tuberosity shape as
golfers' arms do today.) A mummified skeleton
found in an Egyptian tomb can be demonstrated to
belong to a male scribe: the exact location, size,
and orientation of muscle and ligament tuberosities in the right hand are only explicable by the
actions of prolonged finger flexion, as in holding a
stylus.[9,10,11]

Bone formation is dramatically affected by the
molding compressions of childbirth, and may be
deformed by forceps impressions. Abnormal spinous processes and facets in the lumbar spine are
seen in African children whose mothers carry them
in slings on their backs while working in the

fields. Cranial bones can develop flat spots from
the pressure of a child's habitual sleeping pattern.
This is especially true while the cranial bones are
thin, single-walled structures, which they are until
the third year of life (diploic bone does not form in
the cranium until the third to fourth year).

Wolff's Law is an important key in understanding both internal and external cranial structures.
The falx and tentorium, for instance, leave sharp,
very well-defined ridges, processes, and pinnacles
within the neurocranium.

In the part of the occipital squama where there
is no membrane system attachment, particularly
inferior to the transverse sinus, the bone is paper-
thin and transparent. This is a good example of
Wolff's Law: the form and mass of the bone determined by its function.

## Joint Law

In an evolutionary sense we have always loved
joints, for joints gave us movement, which was the
source of our survival, our joy, and our identity as
a migratory, hunter-gatherer species. Joints
between cranial bones allow the brain to dance, to
have space and movement. Joints allow the brain
to breathe.

Joints exist according to the demands for movement placed upon them. That is, movement determines the shape of the joint.

This makes sense when you consider that at birth
all of our joints are wholly composed of cartilage,
and that many bones, such as the vertebra,[12] are
composed of distinct parts separated by cartilage.

From birth onward, the infant begins to move.
Sometimes the movement is constrained by swad-

dling clothes – still used in parts of Africa, Mongolia and Russia – sometimes by strollers. But the child *will* move. He begins to master walking, then running, and models his posture after his elders, especially his role models. In countries where sitting cross-legged on the floor is the norm, children grow up with hip and sacroiliac joints up to 30 percent more extensive in surface area than those of children who grow up in "chair cultures." [13]

The shape of the bony sacrum,[14] and its articulations with the ilia and the lumbar spine, for instance, form in response to posture and to habitual, repetitive movements. Motion, at least initially, is not determined by the shape of the bone.

When you take this logic and apply it to the cranium, the architecture of individual sutures begins to make sense. At birth, the sutures are all "open" – that is, possessed of smooth edges, free of any interdigitation; hence the movement of the cranial bones will determine the shape of the sutures, within the parameters set down by genetic coding.[15]

The more movement demanded of a cranial bone, the greater joint surface it will tend to have. The cranial wave, by moving the sutures of the head ten times a minute throughout life, helps keep the cranial sutures open. The quality and direction of the wave as it interfaces with any two cranial bones helps to determine the exact shape of the junction between them.

The larger a sutural surface area, the more elastic tissue is present to permit motion between the adjacent bones. This observation applies to the depth of sutural interlocking, and also to the thickness of the bone itself. A larger suture surface area does not mean the bones are more tightly connected, but rather the reverse – they can move more, and do so in more security. Such heads can dissipate the forces of crashing impacts more successfully than thinner bones and simpler sutures. Hence alpha-male rams, the flock leaders who butt heads with challengers all through the mating season, develop thicker cranial bones, with more deeply interdigitated sutures, than do their occasional challengers.[16] Animals for whom escape and attack velocity is paramount have thinner, lighter cranial bones.[17]

Sutures allow compression and tension forces under impact, reducing the likelihood of fracture, much as intervertebral discs may allow a fifteen-foot (four meter) fall onto the feet without spinal fracture.

The most extensive sutural area in the human cranium is found at the squamous suture, where the temporal bone articulates with the parietal. It needs this large area to accommodate to the many different traumas, large and small, which are transmitted to the temporal bones via the temporomandibular joints.

This helps explain the mechanism through which heavyweight boxers can absorb uppercut punches to their mandible with only the rare occurrence of mandibular fracture.

The motility of the individual bones of the head is permitted by two factors – the presence of the sutures and the slight pliancy of the bones themselves.

Attitude is also important. The more attitudinally relaxed and open a person is, the more mobile his cranial sutures will be. This is a positive-feedback loop: being free and open in the head helps us have free and open attitudes, which helps the head be free and open. I remember when Florence walked into the classroom, eighty years old, a quaint little hair net primly fastened over her bun. I thought to myself, "Well, there is going to be precious little movement in *her* head!" I was to be amazed. She had the cranial motility of a teenager. But then, I got to thinking, here she is in an esoteric activity like a craniosacral class at age eighty, what wonderful openness of attitude,[18] no wonder her sutures are so open.

Remember:

■ Bone form and mass exists according to the stress acting upon it.
■ Joints exist according to the degree of movement they are called upon to provide.
■ Conditioning and consciousness play key roles in determining how much stress and what kind of motion bones and joints are exposed to.

## The Sutures

There are five different layers of cellular tissue in each cranial suture: two osteogenic cell layers, two periosteal layers (called dural layers by some anatomists), and one sutural ligament connective tissue layer.[19,20,21]

Some of the connective tissue is fibrous, some reticular. The collective elasticity of these connective tissues allows most of the cranial bone movement that our fingers detect in craniosacral work. These layers of sutural cells allow for more motility than the pliancy of the bones does, except in the case of exquisitely fine bones like the palatines, the ethmoid, and the vomer. Bone can only grow at the suture, hence when a suture is fixed or absent the brain may not have sufficient room to develop normally.[22]

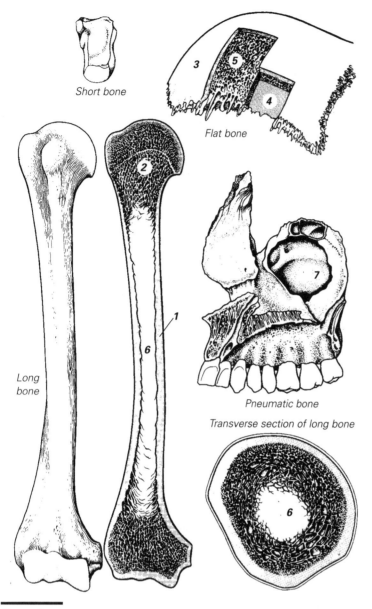

Short bone

Flat bone

Long
bone

Pneumatic bone

Transverse section of long bone

*Types of
bone*

**1** *Compact
or cortical
bone*
**2** *Travecular
or cancellous
bone*
**3** *External
lamina of
cortical bone*
**4** *Internal
lamina of
cortical bone*
**5** *Diploe or
diploic layer
of cancellous
bone*
**6** *Bone
marrow or
medullary
cavity*
**7** *Maxillary
air sinus
(Antrum of
Highmore)
cavity lined
with mucus
membrane*

## Bone

Bone represents the archetype of the indestructible. Myths turning upon the use, sacrifice, fracture, or illness of bones show up in every culture. (In North America we call a close family member a "blood relative." We say that "blood is thicker than water." But in Turkey a close family member is said to be a "bone relative," to stress that the relationship is deeper and more permanent than that of the blood.)

Cranial bones are not solid, they are wet and pliant. Some students have difficulties grasping this – they cannot rid themselves of what they know of dried, medically prepared bones: white, hard, and breakable, like bone china. In fact, living bone is saturated with blood and blood vessels. Living bone is red and pink and white. Living bone is slightly pliant, malleable, and certainly plastic.

Were it like bone china, it would shatter into a thousand pieces the moment you leapt over a fence. Living bone responds within hours to changes in its use, or in the gravitational field that it is subjected to.

If a student sees bone as being brittle, like bone china, he cannot visualize its slight inherent motility.

It is initially impossible for him to visualize the sphenoid (the central bone of the head) as a slightly pliant, ever-changing hologram of consciousness, as part of body, mind, and spirit. To visualize the sphenoid as it responds to cranial touch, he is better served replacing the classical image of bone with a visualization of a plasma field, or a poetic picture – such as a jellyfish pulsating through a kelp bed, or a tired puppy slowly squirming in its basket.

### Bone Pliancy

All bones have pliancy, known as "intraosseous pliability."[23] The human femur will flex one half inch (1.3 centimeters) before breaking at its load limit of eighty-eight hundred pounds (four thousand kilograms). Some cranial bones are exceptionally robust, like the parietals, and do not deflect more than a few microns under the influence of brain expansion and contraction.[24] (They deflect more, to dissipate shock and inhibit bony fracture, under external impact.) Other bones, like the more delicate parts of the sphenoid – the thin-walled body, the lesser wings, and the pterygoid processes – do change shape minutely and meaningfully during each cranial wave. And the exceptionally thin-walled bones like the ethmoid, palatines, and vomer change shape readily and continually, albeit in amounts of motion measured in a few microns.

Sutural elasticity and bone pliancy combine to allow the expansion and contraction of the cranial wave to occur in what appears at first glance to be a dauntingly robust, cohesive cranial structure.

### The Components of Bone

Bone can be considered to comprise seven parts:

■ *An inorganic component* This is made up of bone lime salts, dominated by calcium, the fifth most common inorganic element in the body, composing some 70 percent of each bone in terms of weight.[25] Lesser amounts of sodium and magnesium complete the major inorganic components – 30 percent of the body's sodium is stored in the bones, as is 50 percent of its magnesium. Boron, a trace element found chiefly in green leafy vegetables and fruit, has recently been found to be essential for a bone's ability to use calcium to form bone.[26]

■ *A connective tissue component* The matrix of connective tissues in which the lime salts are embedded makes up the remaining 30 percent of bone weight. This component is strengthened by the presence of proline, hydroxyproline and deoxyproline, three organic compounds that help brace bone by interlacing and cross-bracing its collagenous structure, and make up at least 14 percent of the collagen molecule.[27] The architecture of this collagenous organic component plays a critical part in bony strength and pliancy. This connective tissue is malleable and elastic – that is, it tends to return to its preexisting shape after deformation, all other things being equal. This "two-phase" composite of connective tissue and lime salts is stronger, lighter and more resilient than either of its constituents would be alone.[28]

■ *A functional component* This is the continual movement of the bone, which is both fine (the cranial wave) and gross (respiration and large body movement).

■ *A weight-bearing component* Bone is a weight-bearing tissue that permits locomotion and tool usage.

■ *A production component* Bone also acts as an organ, serving as a blood cell producer.

■ *A warehouse component* Bone acts as an irreplaceable mineral warehouse, a huge reservoir of complex insoluble forms of calcium, sodium, magnesium, and other minerals. Bone is in dynamic equilibrium with the soluble calcium circulating in the blood and the lymph. The body regulates these levels within exacting diurnal parameters of plus or minus 3 percent.[29]

■ *An energetic or spiritual component* Bone represents our foundation, our freedom to move and create, and sometimes also fixity, stiffness, or brittleness in life.

*We* can become ossified. We are much happier when we behave more like joints – loose, flexible, accommodating, pliant. Nothing makes the energetic loading of stiff bones and joints more clear than the immediate effects of a fracture. We "let go of a whole lot of things" and "feel like we have had a breakthrough."

The spirit is a fluctuating electrical field;[30] the piezoelectric charge (or "bioelectric field"), of bones can be measured, and this charge changes markedly under tensile or compressive loading. Since the bioelectric field is life itself, it follows that the injection of cytotoxic (tissue-killing) drugs or high energy ultrasound waves, both capable of killing small sections of bone, results in the complete loss of bioelectricity in the targeted area.[31]

### Bone Loss: Weightlessness, Osteoporosis, and Hip Fractures

Weightlessness provides a wonderful example of the truth of Wolff's Law. In outer space, there is hardly any need for bone to exist at all, and bone recognizes this with a rapidity that is startling.

The early astronauts, chosen from the very elite warrior cadres of their respective countries, were all quite exceptional athletes. Yet even in the single-orbit Gemini spaceflights (and more so in the one- to five-day Apollo flights) loss of bone matrix material and mineral content was found to be both immediate and widespread.

In a longer spaceflight – the Skylab 4 eighty-four-day mission in the early 1970s[32,33] – an average decrease of 3.9 percent in calcaneal (heel bone) density was observed.[34] This data can be collected thanks to the proline and deoxyproline that strengthen the organic component of bone: they are compounds unique to bone, and can be accurately measured in urine when bone breaks down. They are the key indicators that determine the amount of bone loss occurring during a spaceflight.

The most remarkable bone changes due to weightlessness are seen in the rapidly remodeling bones of the spine. This makes sense: no weight bearing, no need for the bone to be there.

Yuri Romanenko, the Russian cosmonaut who, until March 1995,[35] held the space duration record of 326 days,[36] lost a total of 5 percent of his bone calcium and suffered severe architectural loss to his matrix material.[37,38] He was muscularly unable to stand up for two weeks after his return to gravity. Had he stood, he might have suffered immediate and spontaneous femoral neck fracture, similar to what a ninety-year-old can experience falling off a ladder.

### Osteoporosis

After menopause, some women's bones behave much like an astronaut's do in outer space. The degree of calcium loss experienced by a woman in later life is partially determined by her calcium intake from puberty to the age of twenty, when bone mass is at its densest. The calcium in a woman's diet, the amount she absorbs, and the exercise she engages in all set the pattern for bone response after menopause.[39] Most young American women in the present "soda pop" generation have diets that lack adequate calcium, and their postmenopausal osteoporosis will be severe.[40] At present, some women lose up to 5 percent of their bone mass each year in the five years after

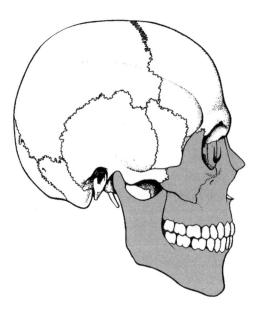

*The neuro-cranium and viscero-cranium (shaded)*

menopause. The loss then slows, but does not cease. Elderly white women, in particular, tend to suffer from osteoporosis. More than 66 percent of those suffering hip fractures from falls are women. While men also suffer from bone loss after middle age, it is less severe than that of women.

Seventh-Day Adventists, who are vegetarians, have a much lower incidence of osteoporosis than their meat-eating peers. Inuit living on a traditional diet eat almost nothing but meat, and also have a high incidence of osteoporosis.[41] Estrogen pills can be highly effective at slowing this loss, but they increase the chance of uterine cancer, the second major cause of death in women. (Uterine cancer is so deadly in part because it is difficult to detect in its early stages, while it is still encapsulated.) The benefits of estrogen therapy are promptly wiped out by smoking, but moderate drinking by postmenopausal women actually raises their estrogen levels. Simply eating more calcium-rich food after menopause will not halt osteoporosis in susceptible women.[42] An extensive Danish study on bone calcium loss in forty-three postmenopausal women receiving two thousand milligrams of calcium supplementation daily found nothing more than a minor positive effect to the arm and leg bones, and no effect to the spine and wrists.

The incidence of hip fractures in men and women has doubled in Britain in the past thirty years. Researchers compared the bone density of 87 women buried between 1729 and 1852 with 294 present-day women;[43,44] the older bones were stronger. For women of similar age, bone loss was found to be significantly greater today; further, premenopausal women today show bone loss, while none was exhibited in the skeletal remains. One reason for these differences is probably the reduced amount of physical exercise that modern women undergo.[45] Many women in the earlier era worked fourteen-hour shifts as silk weavers and walked[46,47] a great deal. Being poor, they had no alternative transportation.

This discussion of bone behavior under differing circumstances is designed to increase your respect for bone's sensitivity and responsiveness. The weight-bearing structures of the skull and the stressed ridges of the reciprocal tension membrane attachment are all affected by our posture, our environment, and our attitudes. They are alive – "living twigs."[48] Touch them and they respond: they know you are there.

## Neurocranium And Viscerocranium

The neurocranium, the part of the skull that encloses the brain, is divided into the cranial base and the cranial vault. The viscerocranium, in turn, provides the bony framework for the face.

### The Neurocranium

**Intrauterine Cranial Development** The cranial base of the infant skull is laid down in cartilage. The cranial vault is laid down by membrane, thrown up and over the rapidly developing hemispheres. A column of bone-building cells (osteoblasts) invests in the membrane or cartilage, developing an "ossification center" (usually marked at birth by a prominent dome or cone shape [an eminence] – such as the frontal eminences, which are often visible throughout life) – and begin growing outward in centrifugal rings, forming new circles of columnar bone cells around the original column.

The fontanels (from the Latin for fountain, so named because you can feel a fountain-like rush of blood with each arterial pulse) exist precisely because cranial vault bones grow in this centrifugal pattern. A gap is left when these circles meet an adjoining bone because the final configuration architecturally required of the bones is not circular (in the parietals, for instance, it is rectangular). Since the bones grow centrifugally, the meeting of four bones that will finally become quadrilateral provides an appreciable aperture to be filled by more "pointed" growth. That aperture is a fontanel.

Fontanels are soft, vulnerable areas that act as tight struts, helping the young cranial bones brace and encompass the cranium. They also help permit and guide major cranial bone circumduction to occur safely during natural childbirth, with its resultant brain molding. The fontanels help control the dural "tent," and act as anchors. The posterior fontanel is closed by the end of the first year, the anterior by the end of the second. The anterior fontanel should not be used as a cranial correction contact until about 18 months of age (like the "no-step" areas on an aircraft wing: no pressure here). But they are wonderful locations to feel the brain move, and sense the fluctuation of the cerebrospinal fluid.

*Birth* As we have seen, at birth every joint in the body is composed of membrane or cartilage, not bone. There is softness everywhere, the body like liquid gold. There is less of a sense of division than at any other time. Many of the cranial bones are subdivided at birth: the occiput in four parts, the temporals in three, the frontal and mandible in two parts each. The atlas is in three parts. The various parts are united by cartilage, floating like icebergs in a sea of ever-moving, responsive dura.

Physiological molding during the birth process ideally slips the parietal bones gently over and external to the frontal and occipital bones. One parietal bone overlaps the other at the sagittal suture. The temporal bones slip external to the parietals, and the zygomae slip inferior to the temporal part of the zygomatic arches. At full term the sphenobasilar joint behaves like an intervertebral disc: it is dynamically capable of universal joint movement, as well as lateral and vertical strain patterns.

At birth the cranium consists of a partly ossified vault (the calvarium), formed out of paper-thin membrane, and a partly ossified cranial base, formed out of cartilage. The cartilage begins to ossify as early as the seventh week after conception, the membrane a week later.

The triple-layer architecture of most cranial bones (smooth dense cortical bone on the outside, honeycomb or diploic bone in the middle, and another layer of cortical bone on the inside) does not become formed until the fourth year.

Cranial suture genesis begins with the genetically coded sutural shape, which is then personally tailored by posture and movement: motion (and impact trauma) determines the final architecture of the joints. Until his second year, an infant's individual cranial bones remain quite independent in terms of the possibilities for movement, which makes the countless falls of childhood relatively easy for the head to absorb and distribute – the

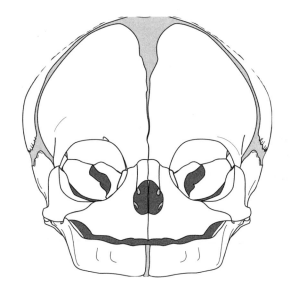

The symphisis mentis and metopic suture at birth

bones jar momentarily, held together and synchronized in their movement by the RTM system. Sutural interdigitation begins to appear by the end of the second year, and is completed in the fourth year. The full interlocking and formation of what Sutherland called the "articular gears" is in place by age six. The articular gears form in response to the path of motion of each individual suture or articulation.

The frontal (metopic) suture does not close until the fourth year. Both the occipital and sphenoidal cephalad portions do not ossify until the seventh to eighth year. If the sphenobasilar joint ossifies, it does so at the same time as the sacrum, between the twentieth and twenty-fifth year.

*Growth Tides* There are hormonal and bony growth tides throughout in-utero and postpartum life, upon which normal growth is dependent. At birth the brain is one-quarter of its adult size, then doubles in size in the next twelve months. Cranial bones grow and change shape to accommodate the growth rate of the brain, continuing to protect their ever-expanding charge. Bone growth is coordinated by genetic whispers, hormonal suffusions, neurological imperatives, and the pressure exerted by the brain. Under compression from the growing brain, the piezoelectric charge of bone becomes negative, thus attracting more osteoblasts.

Growth tides also take care of sutural interlocking. Failure of a suture to form when the appropriate tide arrives means that the bone cells have to wait for the next one. If there is none, the affected bone cannot develop normally. In hydrocephalus,

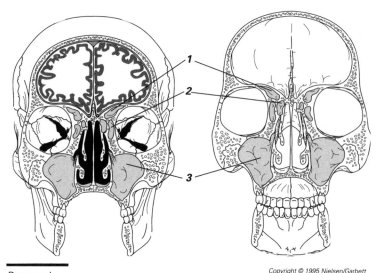

*Paranasal sinuses, anterior and posterior views*

*1* Frontal sinus
*2* Ethmoid sinus
*3* Maxillary sinus

the pressure of the artificially-enlarged hemispheres keeps the developing bones apart during the critical period from two to four years of age when the development of sutural interdigitation is usually at its height; after four there is no other growth tide to signal interdigitation.[49]

At puberty, the air sinuses of the sphenoid, maxillae, frontal, and ethmoid undergo explosive growth,[50] awash in the hormonal flux of sexual maturation.[51] If the maxillae have become immobile – through facial trauma, improperly fitted or monitored dental braces, or temporomandibular joint dysfunction – sinusitis or a torus palatinus[52,53] may result (occurring when the vomer cleaves inferior through the hard palate to produce a longitudinal, sausage-shaped protrusion down into the oral cavity).

*The Cranial Base* The cranial base provides support, protection, stability. It also provides apertures (foramina, fissures, orifices, alveoli) for the access and exit of the spinal cord, cranial nerves, arteries, veins, ears, auditory tubes, teeth and pharynx (the venous outflow is blocked every time we hold our breath, cough, or scream). It also houses our sense of smell, vision, sound production, and the beginning of our gastrointestinal tract. The brain needs entry and exit arrangements because it requires a profuse blood supply to provide for its needs for oxygen and glycogen. The cranial base also provides attachment for neck and thoracic muscles. Its sutures and many apertures and fissures permit further motility, which helps protect against fracture by allowing some absorption of shock through movement.

The function of the cranial base bones is to provide a strong and stable, yet fundamentally pliant, protective support for the cranial contents, able to

accommodate the rhythmic motility of the cranial wave. Stability and movement present a polarity, but these conflicting priorities are brought together by the flexibility of the base and vault bones and their sutures, and further accommodated to by the flexibility of the neck.

Distortions at the sacrum will tend to distort the cranial base and distortions of the cranium (not just of its base bones) will tend to disturb the equanimity of the sacrum. Sutherland called this immediate reciprocity "the core link."[54] The attachment of the spinal dura at the second sacral segment forms the "south pole" of Sutherland's "mechanism."

*The Cranial Vault* The cranial vault comprises seven bones:

■ The frontal (1 bone; excluding the orbito-nasal portion)
■ The parietals (2 bones)
■ The interparietal portion of the occipital bone (1)
■ The squamous portions of the temporal bones (2)
■ The sphenoid, greater wing portions only (1)

The bones of the cranial vault, or "calvarium," are the part of the skull that Buddhist monks traditionally use for their begging bowls. They all ossify out of membrane, and can be regarded in craniosacral work as behaving as specialized "stiffened membranes."

Where the cranial base is specialized for support, stability, and mobility, the vault is specialized for protection and malleability. Vault protection is achieved by smoothness, roundedness, responsiveness, and the ability to deform in a controllable way in response to severe traumatic impact. The vault is charged with protecting the cortex and deep brain structures such as the corpus callosum, limbic system, and thalamus.

The ideal way to understand the motion of individual cranial bones, and the skull as a whole, is to study this chapter in conjunction with a disarticulated cranium, a model of the reciprocal tension membrane, and an intact skull. If you do not have all of these elements, use the illustrations in this book to the optimum.

The neurocranium is an enclosed structure that behaves like a water-filled balloon (that is, according to the laws of physics that apply to closed hydraulic systems). If the balloon is placed on a table and pulled out sideways so that it fattens laterally, it shortens in its anteroposterior dimension, with some loss of height in the superior-inferior plane as well. This combination of movements represents what happens to the cranial vault during cranial flexion.

### The Viscerocranium

The viscerocranium is considered distinct from the neurocranium, that part of the skull that encloses the brain. The viscerocranium encloses some of the sense organs – the eyes, nose, and mouth. It consists of fifteen bones:

- The ethmoid (1 bone)
- The frontal (1 bone)
- The maxillae (2 bones)
- The zygomae (2 bones)
- The concha (2 bones)
- The lacrimals (2 bones)
- The palatines (2 bones)
- The nasals (2 bones)
- The vomer (1 bone)

Both the ethmoid and the frontal are transitional bones, part neurocranium, part viscerocranium.

The bones of the face are considered to "hang" from the frontal bone.[55,56] The delicate ethmoid, vomer, and palatines are the most pliant bones in the skull, which permits improved shock absorption in trauma and allows the cranial wave to reduce in amplitude between the more motile neurocranial bones and the more stable upper viscerocranial bones. The maxillae are an admixture of diploic bone, pneumatic (air sinus) bone, and thin laminar plate bone. The mandible is both the strongest and the most mobile bone of the skull. Both the mandible and the maxillae channel powerful mechanical and psychological forces to the neurocranium, particularly to the sphenoid and to the temporals.

# 17

# The Reciprocal Tension Membrane

*As the written word is a limited medium when it comes to describing structures that need to be visualized, the reader will gain a better understanding of this chapter with the aid of a cardboard or latex model of the falx and tentorium which are joined at the straight sinus (see p. 181).*

William Sutherland and Harold Magoun[1,2] named the combination of the endosteal dura and the specializations of the meningeal dura – the falx, tentorium, and spinal dura – the reciprocal tension membrane (RTM). This system also encompasses the spinal dural attachment to the second segment of the sacrum. The reciprocal tension membrane is a supportive, integrative, and protective system of membranous sheaths that arise from the firm but motile periphery of the neurocranium. It interleaves the cerebral hemispheres to stiffen them where they are the most unsupported. Tying the motility patterns of quite different bones together, it helps to provide mechanical congruity. Its greatest usefulness occurs after birth, when its memory of optimum cranial shape helps the child's cranial bones to regroup, a phenomenon most noticeable in the three days after birth.

## Meningeal Anatomy

There are three meningeal layers – the dura, the arachnoid membrane, and the pia mater. The dura itself has two layers. It is important to be able to visualize the relative position of these four layers in craniosacral work.

## The Dura

The outermost of the two dural layers is the endosteal. Firmly attached to the bone of the inside of the cranium, it is, plainly speaking, periosteum. The second dural layer is the meningeal dura, which forms specialized, freestanding arcs and sickles that separate the cranial hemispheres both vertically (from each other) and almost horizontally (from the cerebellum). Nowhere in the body does periosteum do this, so the presence of the meningeal layer justifies dura receiving its own nomenclature. The meningeal layer also forms tunnels through which the peripheral venous sinus network returns blood back to the straight sinus and the jugular vein. The slight elasticity of dura, and the shape and attachment of the falx and tentorium, seem to be responsible for some of the phenomena we deal with in craniosacral work.

Dura is formed mainly out of collagenous fibers. It looks a bit like properly cut prosciutto – pinkish, slightly translucent, with dense but delicate striations of connective tissue threading through it in areas of higher stress. When removed from the cranium, it has the tonicity of a soft fingernail. The 5 percent elasticity dura does have permits a small degree of movement between the bones it attaches to. It is essentially impermeable to cerebrospinal fluid, although some leakage is reported to occasionally occur in the spinal cord area and through the cribriform plate of the ethmoid into the nasal orifice. The dura is pain-sensitive in the area of its transverse blood vessels. It has been shown that there are pain receptors in the sagittal suture of monkeys,[3] and it is likely that human beings have a similar anatomical arrangement. We may have pain-sensitive stretch-receptors in all of our cranial sutures.

In craniosacral work we tend to focus particularly on the spectacular architecture of the falx and tentorium, making it easy to forget that the meningeal dura is tightly adherent to the endosteal, which spans the inside of the cranial sutures. (Even in dissection of cadaver specimens of deceased adults that have been used as teaching aids for several years, the meningeal layer has to be forcibly torn free from the endosteal, evidence of its adhesive tenacity.) This means that the meningeal dura plays an important role in limiting cranial bone motion.

Dura, particularly the falx and tentorium, seems to be accessible to awareness.[4] The falx cerebri and cranial vault dura is fed by the opthalmic branch of trigeminus, the tentorium and falx cerebelli by the upper cervical nerves. After some months of meditative experimentation, it is possible to find the neurological "way in," particularly to the falx, and to learn how to move your own cranial bones in conjunction with the active cooperation of the external muscles of the eye and the muscles of the jaw and neck. The ability to visualize the internal and external structures involved greatly enhances success in this endeavor.

### The Arachnoid Membrane and Pia Mater

The arachnoid membrane layer has, beneath its surface (that is, closer to the actual brain tissue), an intricate and beautiful system of fibers that help to hold open the space between the arachnoid and the pia mater. This space is filled with cerebrospinal fluid. This is called the subarachnoid space. The pia mater attaches to the brain tissue itself, and follows the convolutions of the gyri (which neither the dura nor the arachnoid membrane do).

The blood supply for the cranial meninges is via the meningeal arteries, chiefly the middle one (the anterior and posterior meningeal arteries supply surprisingly small areas of the cortex), and from branches of the internal and external carotid arteries. Venous blood drains from the brain by way of six sinuses: (1) the superior sagittal sinus, (2) the inferior sagittal sinus, (3) the straight sinus, (4) two transverse sinuses, (5) two superior petrosal sinuses, and (6) the cavernous sinus.

### The Dural Tube

The dural tube consists of meningeal dura, arachnoid membrane, and pia mater, all of which envelop the spinal cord. It is attached very firmly to the foramen magnum, then filamentous insertions connect it to the second and third cervical vertebrae, from where it remains completely free of attachment until slip-like insertions to the lumbar posterior longitudinal ligament and firm attachments to the sacral periosteum at the level of the

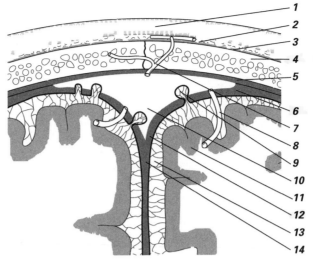
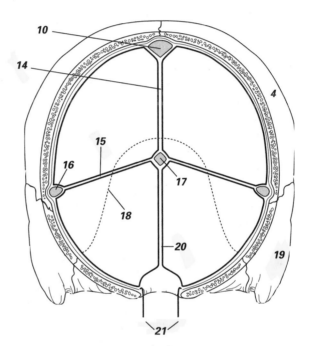

second sacral segment. From that point the dura merges with the periosteum that lines the sacral canal, which merges with the filum terminale, and the tendon of the pubococcygeus muscle.

## Three-Dimensional Architecture of the Reciprocal Tension Membrane

Brain tissue has the consistency of an over-ripe avocado; the meningeal dura neatly divides the hemispheres into compartments that help make up for the brain tissues' lack of tensility, and reduces the risk of concussion.

*Above:*
*A coronal section through the cranial vertex*

*Below:*
*A coronal section at the level of foramen magnum (schematic)*

*1 Skin and subcutaneous fat*
*2 Aponeurosis of occipitofrontalis muscle*
*3 Periosteum*
*4 Parietal bone*
*5 Endosteal dura*
*6 Meningeal dura*
*7 Emmisary vein*
*8 Superior cerebral vein*
*9 Arachnoid granulation*
*10 Superior sagittal sinus*
*11 Cerebral cortex*
*12 Arachnoid*
*13 Subarachnoid space*
*14 Falx cerebri*
*15 Tentorium cerebelli*
*16 Transverse sinus*
*17 Straight sinus (AKA "Sutherland's fulcrum")*
*18 Lambdoid suture*
*19 Temporal bone*
*20 Falx cerebelli*
*21 Spinal dura*

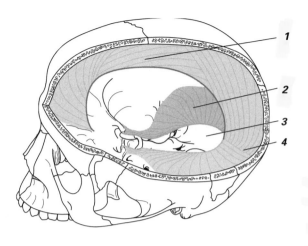

### The Falx

The falx cerebri is that part of the falx that separates the hemispheres of the brain. It is 1½ to 2 inches (4 to 5 centimeters) deep; viewed from the side, it is sickle-shaped, with the straight sinus acting as the handle, then the blade of the sickle curves around the superior aspect of the skull until the pointed end inserts at the crista galli of the ethmoid. Inferior to the straight sinus the falx is called the falx cerebelli. It is much smaller than the falx cerebri, and from the straight sinus continues inferiorly and anteriorly along the internal curvature of the occipital squama until it reaches the foramen magnum, where it bifurcates to attach to the perimeter of the foramen itself. The spinal cord is enveloped by a continuation of the meningeal dura, known as spinal dura mater.

In terms of the human field, the superior portions of the falx cerebri are part of the crown soul, and the Bindu ancillary soul center; the inferior part of the falx cerebri and all of the falx cerebelli seem to form part of the channel of the inner eye, which runs from the rear of the atlanto-occipital joint (at the acupuncture point Wind Palace, Governor Vessel 16) to glabella.[5]

### The Tentorium

Viewed from above, the paired structures of the tentorium cerebelli look like the compound-curvature, double-delta wings of the Concorde aircraft or the space shuttle. The tentorium is composed of a matched pair of these wings, which are at their widest in the middle one-third of their anteroposterior dimension. The posterior junction of these two dural folds is at the straight sinus, where their fibers are continuous with the falx. The tentorium is at its most superior point at the anterior end of the straight sinus. It is more inferior at its lateral and posterior margins. Looked at from the rear the tentorium has a downward slope known as a dihedral angle in aircraft design. The anterior attachment is to the clinoid processes of the sphenoid.

The tentorium is so effective in supporting the brain that it changes its apparent weight, as measured at the tentorium gap, from about 3 pounds (1.5 kilos) to just 2 ounces (50 grams). The specificity of force applied through the CV4 technique can have such profound and sometimes permanent effects precisely because of the connecting and interleaving functions of the reciprocal tension membrane. Energetically, the tentorium is part of the channel of the inner eye.

### The Tentorium and Falx Together

To describe the reciprocal tension membrane to clients, I use terms like "a membrane system inside the head," or "a system of partitions and reinforcing struts." For the healer, it is important to be able to visualize its architecture and distinguish its poles. A cardboard or latex model is a useful study aid. If you take a model of the reciprocal tension membrane up to eye level, and look at it from the posterior to anterior aspect, remembering to slope the wings of the tentorium at a downward dihedral angle, it looks something like a peace symbol.

Sutherland focused attention on the poles of the reciprocal tension membrane as places of particular mechanical importance. He regarded the membrane system as having six poles:

### The Six Poles of the Reciprocal Tension Membrane

- Anterior at the crista galli
- Posterior at the internal occipital protruberance
- Central at the clinoid processes
- Lateral at the petrous ridges of the temporals
- Inferior (1) at the foramen magnum

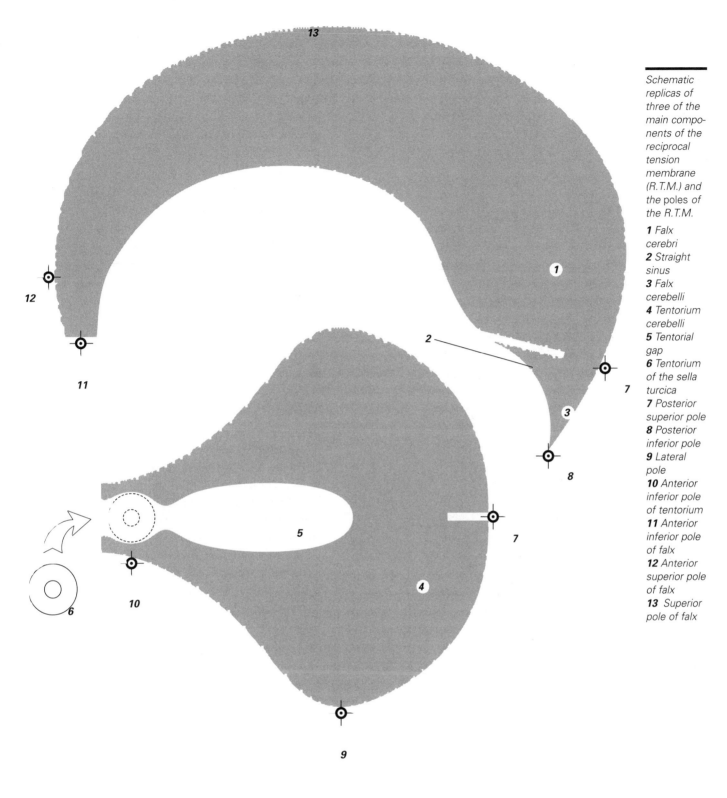

Schematic replicas of three of the main components of the reciprocal tension membrane (R.T.M.) and the poles of the R.T.M.

**1** Falx cerebri
**2** Straight sinus
**3** Falx cerebelli
**4** Tentorium cerebelli
**5** Tentorial gap
**6** Tentorium of the sella turcica
**7** Posterior superior pole
**8** Posterior inferior pole
**9** Lateral pole
**10** Anterior inferior pole of tentorium
**11** Anterior inferior pole of falx
**12** Anterior superior pole of falx
**13** Superior pole of falx

17·17

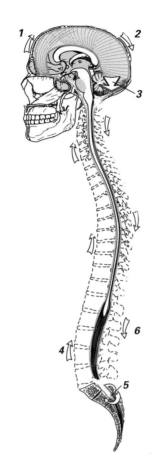

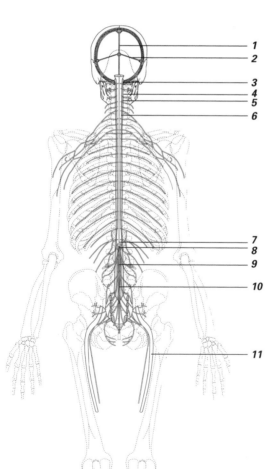

■ Inferior (2) at the level of the second sacral segment

### The Core Link

The connection made between the occiput and the sacrum by the largely (95 percent) inelastic tube of spinal dura – firmly attached to the perimeter of the foramen magnum and to the second sacral segment – forms the basis of what Sutherland called the "core link,"[6,7] which is part of the reciprocal tension membrane. It is important that the student realize that whereas the meningeal dura is tightly adhered to the inside of the cranium, it is free-floating in the spinal canal, separated from the surrounding bone structures by a boundary layer of fat. (The only exception to this free-floating is filamentous attachments that the spinal dura makes to the second and third cervical vertebrae.) The sacrum and the occiput can be likened to two clothesline poles and the spinal dura to the thin rope connecting them. The core link movement imitates the rhythmic expansile-contractile motility of a swimming tadpole.

The spinal dura acts on the sacrum somewhat like a sea anchor does on a ship: it stabilizes its movement by the smallest of amounts, modifies it, and sometimes even amplifies it if the "waves" (here the cerebrospinal fluid patterns in the brain and spinal cord) are right.

The spinal dura pulls upward during cranial flexion (which occurs during the in-breath during deep rest), causing the sacrum to make a circumductory movement identical to that of the occiput. That is, the sacrum moves as if paired to the occiput, so that both go in the same direction while the sphenoid is flexing ("similar motion"). Thus, as the occiput "flexes" (which is actually a backward-bending movement, and not true whole-body flexion), the sacrum enters into a movement exactly synchronous (in its case, true flexion) with the tip of the coccyx moving into the perineal space.

While the spinal dura is immediately affected by any kind of movement imparted to it, such as the spinal curvature you make while stretching the back in a full yawn, it does not necessarily transmit this to either extremity – occiput or sacrum – because there is enough slack in the spinal dura, and because the fat that encircles the spinal cord permits motion without necessarily moving the extremities.

## The Cerebrospinal Fluid

*The cerebrospinal fluid is the highest known element of the human body.*
– Andrew Taylor Still [8]

The cerebrospinal fluid provides buoyant support and shock absorption to the brain. It also forms a transport medium, mediating between the blood and the brain, which acts as an alternative and complementary suffusion and absorption mechanism to that performed by the blood-brain barrier.[9] That is, white blood cells, glucose, certain hormones, and neuropeptides enter the cortex from the cerebrospinal fluid which may not be able to do so from the arterial bloodstream.[10] Likewise, certain classes of drugs, such as some of those used in the treatment of AIDS, can reach the cortex through the cerebrospinal fluid, but not through the "tight junctions" of the blood-brain barrier.[11]

During early embryonic development, the eyes form by separating from the once-contiguous lateral ventricles. The eyes and the ventricles share similarities in internal fluids and basic structure.[12] The pressure in the eyeball rises above that of the ventricles, to become one-third greater – fifteen millimeters of mercury compared to ten in the ventricles. Touch the white of your eye under an eyelid and sense the pressure. The ventricles are at one third less pressure.

There are 125 to 150 cubic centimeters of cerebrospinal fluid within a normal cranial and spinal cord system,[13] with some 110 to 130 cubic centimeters of this is in the subarachnoid space and 15 to 20 in the four ventricles. Cerebrospinal fluid pressure is so low that it is often quoted in millimeters of water, where its range is 80 to 150.[14] The mercury pressure of 6 to 10 millimeters is approximately one-tenth of the diastolic (resting) blood pressure. However, cerebrospinal fluid is at almost twice the pressure of blood in the veins.

Cerebrospinal fluid production ranges from 0.3 to 0.6 cubic centimeter per minute,[15] giving total daily production of some 800 cubic centimeters,[16] meaning that there is complete renewal of the fluid approximately every six hours. Cerebrospinal fluid is produced by the choroid plexuses in all four ventricles, with the greatest production issuing from

the largest ventricles, the laterals. Under a light microscope, choroid plexuses look like tiny, densely branched fronds.

Anatomically, they are like miniature kidneys. (In traditional Chinese medicine, the brain is regarded as an outgrowth of the kidney, and its nature is regarded as being like the softest substance in the body, water. This "water" is said to be protected by the "hardest substance" in the body, bone, and the proximity of the hard and the soft concurs with the Chinese observation of body and energy organization through opposites.)

Cerebrospinal fluid is also produced in the ependyma and perineural spaces, with perhaps 35 percent of the total fluid coming from the ependyma, the tissue that forms the walls of the ventricles.[17]

In hydrocephalus an overproduction of cerebrospinal fluid, or a blockage in its circulatory sys-

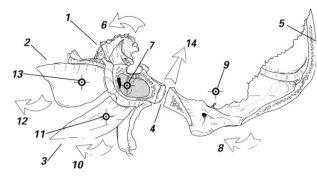

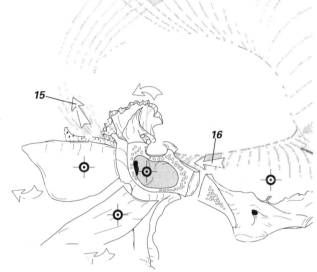

**Above:**
Flexion

**Below:**
Flexion detail, showing pull of the falx and tentorium

**1** Sphenoid
**2** Ethmoid
**3** Vomer
**4** Sphenobasilar joint
**5** Occiput
**6** Sphenoid flexion
**7** Sphenoid axis
**8** Occipital flexion
**9** ... around the axis of occiput
**10** Vomer flexion
**11** Vomer axis
**12** Ethmoid flexion
**13** Ethmoid axis
**14** Sphenobasilar flexion
**15** Superior pull of falx cerebri on crista galli of ethmoid
**16** Anterior pull of tentorium cerebelli by clinoid processes of sphenoid

*Circulation of
the cerebro-
spinal fluid*

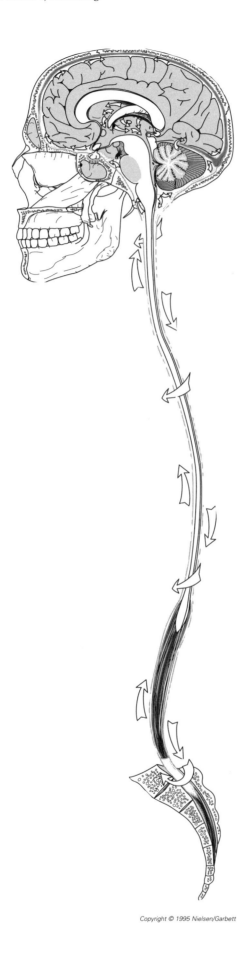

tem (commonly at the aqueduct of Sylvius), compresses then displaces brain tissue with the result that brain tissue starts to push on the cranial bones. The pressure exerted by the brain pushes the sutures apart. If the disease occurs suddenly, and before four years of age (the most critical time being between birth and age two), when sutural interdigitation is normally fully developed, the cranial bones separate easily from their neighbors. Lacking the normal stimulation of the presence of their neighbors, the bones' sutural edges form no interdigitations. They remain smooth. In contrast, hydrocephalus of gradual onset draws out the interdigitations of the suture lines, as they endeavor to keep doing their job even as the continents, so to speak, are drifting apart. Hydrocephalus is rare after the age of fifteen.

Cerebrospinal fluid has very limited compressibility[18] and, as far as the laws of physics are concerned, behaves like water. Indeed, it *is* 99 percent water.[19] Cerebrospinal fluid's specific gravity is 1.003–1.008, the same as seawater, from whence, in an evolutionary sense, it came. The body itself can be considered 90 percent seawater, and just as open to the tidal, fluid forces of sun, moon, and stars. Statistically speaking, the brain is about 95 percent water. The reciprocal tension membrane helps stabilize and "ground" this watery medium while giving it elasticity.

The cerebrospinal fluid buoys up the brain, effectively reducing brain weight at any one bony point of support thirty-fold.[20] Due to the suspensory and guidance capabilities of the reciprocal tension membrane and the cerebrospinal fluid in the subarachnoid space, the buoyed-up brain is able to move a few millimeters in anterior, posterior, lateral, and medial directions, as well as to rotate and circumduct. In short, the brain floats in a miniature, spherical ocean. Here is a way to approximate brain mobility: place a plum in a water-filled jar just big enough to contain it. Shake, rotate, or impact the jar on a hard surface, and note how the plum is remarkably immune to the transmission of sudden force. All that is missing in this simple model is a proxy for the subarachnoid fibers that span the space between the arachnoid membrane and pia mater, acting as springs to keep the central canvas of the brain in the middle of the trampoline frame of the cranium.

The fluid and its enclosure, the dura, are regarded as a semi-sealed hydraulic system[21] because the production and absorption rates of cerebrospinal fluid are so low as to not affect either the cranial wave or how the brain and spinal cord

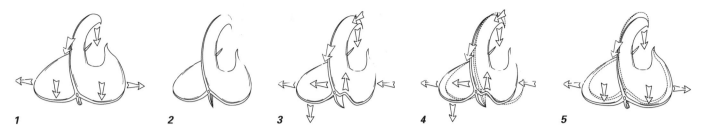

1      2      3      4      5

respond to trauma. In terms of the laws of physics, the fluid is usually regarded as a static medium within the closed hydraulic system, with movement described as of very low velocity and pressure. The combination of an infinitesimal production rate and a very low pressure is insufficient to propagate cerebrospinal fluid motion around the hemispheres in anything but the laziest of ways, much like hot water in a teacup describes slow convection currents.

The production of the fluid within the ventricles is, however, sufficient to maintain flow through them and out through the three foramina in the fourth ventricle, into the subarachnoid space that surrounds the brain and spinal cord. The dominant motion in cerebrospinal fluid is imparted to it through *being moved*, however, rather than moving itself. Movement is imparted to the fluid via the rhythmic tadpole-like contraction and expansion of the brain and spinal cord with each successive cranial wave, and by large body movements that change the spinal cord's position.

This closed hydraulic system does an admirable job of protecting the delicate brain. Since a sheer force cannot be transmitted through fluid, any impact pressure applied to "the mechanism" of the cranium is immediately widely distributed and dissipated through cranial bone deflection, sutural absorption, reciprocal tension membrane elasticity, and cerebrospinal fluid dissemination. The incoming arterial pulse has only a minimal effect on the fluid: as each successive systolic pressure wave (arterial pulsation) enters the cranium, brain tissues swell and displace venous blood in the superior sagittal and transverse sinuses, which also serves to promote cerebral circulation. Venous back-pressure and the volume of blood in the head do, however, affect cerebrospinal fluid dynamics.[22,23] For this reason, craniosacral practitioners may spend some time reducing venous pressure in the head before working on the head itself.

Another facet of cerebrospinal fluid protection and function in trauma can be demonstrated by placing a pitcher brimful of water on a table, then hitting the table sharply in a downward direction. The water in the pitcher mounts up in the center, which is the equivalent of what happens at the crown of the head when you land on your feet after a jump or fall. The pressure wave results in a superior and lateral displacement of the parietal bones at the sagittal suture. (The latest-model football helmets in the United States use packets of glycol – automobile antifreeze – to provide additional shock absorption for the brain. This is an intriguing duplication of our own system of cerebrospinal fluid, which is of a similar specific gravity.)

The way the brain is positioned is the result of the functioning of the reciprocal tension membrane and cerebrospinal fluid systems, and remains relatively constant in the earth's gravitational field. We therefore do not experience a sense of flotation, except on amusement park rides or while driving fast over a humpback bridge. Weightless conditions pose the problem of brain flotation, however, which is a major component in space sickness (which also results from unusual forces acting on the eighth cranial [vestibulocochlear] nerve and on the balance apparatus itself). Some 50 percent of astronauts suffer space sickness. In 1990, a Japanese newspaper paid the new Russian government some five million dollars to put one of its journalists into space in a Soyuz spacecraft. The luckless man spent five days in space inside Mir, the Russian space station, suffering from acute space-sickness. At one point a land-based commentator asked him how he felt, prompting a reply to the effect of "I feel miserable. How would you like it if you could feel your brain floating around inside your head all day long?"

## Diagnosis

The reciprocal tension membrane dissipates the force of moderate impact without passing shock on to damage the brain itself. In severe trauma, the forces brought to bear on the dura exceed its physical strength and tearing and hemorrhage may occur. Force can be transmitted from the point of impact directly across the cranium in a combination of osseous, fluid dynamic, and dural interactions. In some traumas the balance in the reciprocal tension membrane may be deviated. "Compression head" (a compression of the sphe-

*Similar and opposite motion of the tentorium*
*1 Similar motion: flexion*
*2 Neutral*
*3 Opposite motion: left side flexion, right side extension*
*4 Showing motion of drawing 3 from neutral*
*5 Showing motion of drawing 1 from neutral*

noid into its primary articulation with the occiput after a trauma) shows severely degraded cranial wave motion, or none at all.

Adhesions may form in the reciprocal tension membrane and core link system after severe trauma. The notable instance of this is in whiplash injury,[24] where you may see a delay of up to three years before a recurrence of the original neck and head pain symptoms felt after the accident. (Clients may also experience a clear connection between cranial and sacral pain.)[25]

Other than severe trauma, cranial movement and reciprocal tension membrane tensions vary in different individuals, and in the same individual according to his outlook on life at any given moment, and on his state of health. The dura can also be affected by emotional trauma, which may cause vascular changes and consequent tissue damage, or dental anesthesia, which may cause it to lose elasticity and take on a parchment-like feeling. After a severe case of influenza, an individual's reciprocal tension membrane feels wet and soggy, atonic. During violent vomiting, the diaphragm contracts so powerfully that pressure waves hitting the cranial base cause an energetic reciprocity with the similarly domed tentorium, causing the tentorium to feel as if it has been over-stretched (one client described this as being "like a concussion").

In multiple personality disorder, the membrane system takes on a different "feel" as the individual transits from one subpersonality to another.[26,27] You can sense this as it occurs from a change in bone fluctuation and energetic intensity – the texture suddenly alters. You can also tell by watching the "personality" expressed in the eyes – which change with each subpersonality. The subpersonalities have such different physiologies that some people with multiple personality disorder will keep a drawerful of glasses because the shifting of the personalities changes the focal length of their eyes markedly.[27] (How much of this change is mediated by lateral pterygoid, sphenoid, and palatine transformation?)

## Summary

■ The reciprocal tension membrane allows the cranial bones to regroup after birth. It maintains the shape of the skull in childhood.

■ The reciprocal tension membrane helps maintain the shape of the brain.

■ The reciprocal tension membrane checks, guides, and coordinates the brain's movement.

■ Both the reciprocal tension membrane and cerebrospinal fluid provide shock absorption for bones and brain, lessening the chances of bony fracture and allowing the brain to float supported by cerebrospinal fluid of nearly equal density.

■ The reciprocal tension membrane and cerebrospinal fluid affect hydraulic damping of the arterial pressure wave as it enters the cranium. First venous blood and then cerebrospinal fluid is displaced to make way for the swelling of the brain in systole.

■ The cerebrospinal fluid forms a transport medium, mediating between the blood and the brain, an alternative to the blood-brain barrier. Certain hormones, neuropeptides, white blood cells, and glucose enter the cortex from the fluid.

■ An immunological medium, the cerebrospinal fluid helps keep the brain free from viral and bacterial contamination. The cerebrospinal fluid performs many of the immunological functions that the lymphatic system does in the rest of the body.

# 18
# The Stomatognathic System

*As this discussion of the stomatognathic system focuses extensively upon the mandible and maxillae, it may be useful to first read the anatomy and physiology sections related to those two bones.*

The stomatognathic system consists of 27 bones:

- The occiput (1 bone)
- The temporals (2 bones)
- The sphenoid (1 bone)
- The maxillae (2 bones)
- The mandible (1 bone)
- The hyoid (1 bone)
- The clavicles (2 bones)
- The scapulae (2 bones)
- The sternum (1 bone)
- The upper two ribs on each side (4 bones)
- The 7 cervical and first 3 thoracic vertebrae (10 bones)

## Anatomy

The stomatognathic system consists of those parts of the head, neck, and upper thorax concerned with the muscular, osseous, ligamentous, fascial, and nervous system control of biting, chewing, and swallowing.

## Structure

The stomatognathic system is chiefly composed of the following:

- Tooth: constructed of enamel, cementum, and dentin
- Bone: in cortical, pneumatic, and diploic (cancellous) forms
- Joint: saddle synovial with meniscus at the temporomandibular joints; reniform synovial condylar at the atlanto-occipital joint; synovial at the sternoclavicular joint; cartilaginous at the intervertebral articulations; interdigitated, squamous, and harmonic sutural joints at the cranial sutures
- Muscle: fusiform, flat, bipennate, and multi-bellied types
- Fascia: superficial; cervical; prevertebral; infrahyoid; pretracheal; the fascias of temporalis, masseter, sternocleidomastoid, trapezius, and pectoralis major; galea aponeurotica

Every major component itemized above needs to be considered in working with the stomatognathic system. The energetic loading of the mouth, throat, and neck must also be taken into account.[1,2,3]

Within the anatomical realm the joints are the vital components, and the ones often afflicted with stiffness, crepitus, or pain. Of all the joints in the stomatognathic system, the temporomandibular joints are the most often afflicted,[4] followed by the atlanto-occipital joint. The temporomandibular joints act as the secondary joints of mastication; at a deeper level of understanding we see that the atlantoaxial joint[5] is the primary joint of mastication; this is known as "Guzay's Theorem." The temporomandibular joint and the atlantoaxial joint interact with each other continually to provide optimum stomatognathic system functioning.[6,7]

## Musculature

The muscles attaching to the mandible consist of the:

- Temporalis
- Lateral pterygoids
- Buccinator
- Orbicularis oris
- Hyoglossus
- Digastricus
- Geniohyoid
- Superior pharyngeal constrictor
- Masseter
- Medial pterygoids
- Depressor anguli oris
- Depressor labii inferioris
- Mylohyoideus
- Platysma
- Mentalis
- Genioglossus

The muscles attaching to the hyoid consist of the:

- Hyoglossus
- Geniohyoideus
- Digastricus
- Stylohyoideus
- Thyrohyoideus
- Genioglossus
- Mylohyoideus
- Omohyoideus (superior belly)
- Sternohyoideus
- Sternothyroideus

The suprahyoid and infrahyoid muscle groups – eleven muscles attaching to the hyoid – play an important role in the stomatognathic system. For craniosacral work, the chief muscles among these two groupings are:

- Lateral and medial pterygoid muscles
- Masseter
- Temporalis
- Omohyoid (superior and inferior bellies)

The lateral pteryoid muscle attaches to the medial aspect of the neck of the mandibular condyle, and the temporomandibular joint capsule itself. Note the importance of the retrodiscal ligament, which functions as the posterior attachment of the joint capsule, and therefore of the lateral pterygoid muscle, to the petrous portion of the temporal bone just anterior to the tympanic ring. This ligament plays a small but vital role in both temporomandibular joint and temporal bone dysfunction. It gets stretched anteriorly as the result of constant lateral pterygoid muscle tension, leading to the mis-seating of the meniscus with resultant clicking in the joint, and eventual deterioration in joint capsule shape and joint functioning.[8]

All of the muscles of mastication are part of the stomatognathic system, as are all the muscles that attach to the cranial base, the cervical spine, and the upper two ribs on each side. Since any of these may fault, they need to be considered in a complete evaluation of the stomatognathic system. Technically speaking, all are regarded as being in a closed kinematic chain. The effects of mandibular muscular status extend from the most superior point of the greater wings of the sphenoid[9] to the tips of the toes. The tongue, a strong, almost willful muscle, is an often overlooked component in work with the stomatognathic system (Feldenkrais work[10] expertly addresses it). All of the muscles that attach to the scapula also influence the stomatognathic system, although somewhat less directly.

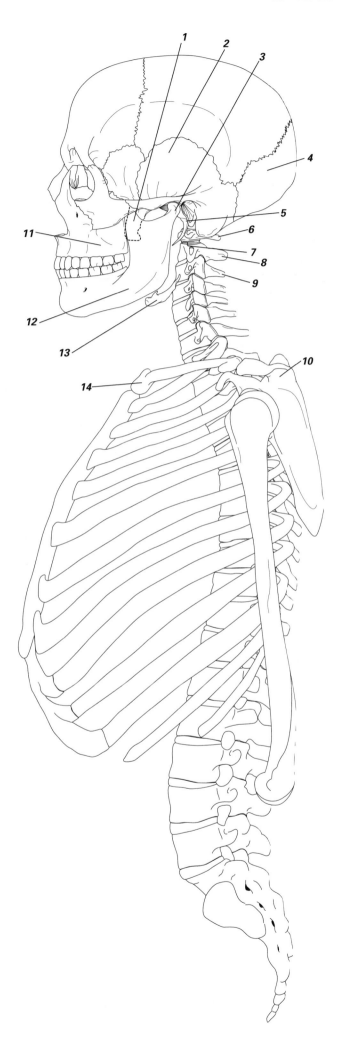

Principle components of the stomatognathic system

**1** Lateral Pterygoid plate (dotted line)
**2** Temporal bone
**3** Condyle of mandible
**4** Occipital bone
**5** Styloid process
**6** Atlas
**7** Base of dens
**8** Axis
**9** C 3
**10** Scapula
**11** Maxilla
**12** Mandible
**13** Hyoid
**14** Clavicle

## Evolution of the Stomatognathic System and Its Importance

For millions of years before the general adoption of cooking the hominids most likely to survive were those with the largest and strongest teeth, as large teeth lasted the longest and resisted breakage better. Mutations that increased tooth size gave the lucky owner a better chance of becoming the alpha male or female of the tribal group, and therefore of passing along large-toothed genes.

With the widespread adoption of cooking practices and the general use of tools for cutting, pounding, grinding, and making pastes,[11] teeth were no longer given the most challenging of tasks. Less used, they began to shrink,[12] as evolution (and fashion) dictated that massive teeth were no longer quite the drawing card they used to be. Individuals with big teeth began to look goofy. The trait started to disappear. (The importance of teeth to our pride in appearance is enormous. Witness the amount of money people spend capping their teeth and you'll understand their importance to the archetypes of the beauty and the hero. The villain, on the other hand, is often portrayed with bad or blackened teeth, or enormous ones like Count Dracula.)

Pottery and earthen ovens were first used ten thousand years ago. Pottery meant that food could be cooked into soups and stews, requiring even less chewing than a grilled meat. In the first areas where pottery was mastered, cemeteries suddenly appear full of skulls with no teeth: dental decay had begun.[13] The ancient Egyptians used crude dentures, some made of animal teeth. The Etruscans used improved dentures and also employed gold fillings. Two hundred years ago Robert Burns grieved in rhyme that there was no known pain worse than the toothache.[14]

### Physiology

The teeth play a central role in the functioning of the stomatognathic system. Attached to the alveolar ridges with gomphotic (peg and socket joint) articulations, each tooth is as independent as a cranial bone, and may be as much in need of unwinding as the sphenoid or the occiput.[15,16] Each has its own memories, its own history. The periodontal ligaments connect the teeth to their sockets and

are similar to the sutural ligaments within the cranial sutures. They are "wavy," and can become stretched under constant compression. If a tooth is removed and not replaced, its opposite partner will float upward (or downward) as a result of the loss of opposition. The ligaments straighten, releasing the tooth on a trajectory, so to speak, in much the same way that a stretched bowstring releases an arrow. If a tooth is replaced or crowned too high, it will stretch (compress) its opposite periodontal ligaments excessively.

We swallow, on average, 1,800 times per day;[17] twice a minute while awake, once a minute while sleeping. When anxious, stressed, feeling guilty, or trying to suppress feelings, we swallow more often and more awkwardly. Typically, each swallow means a compression of the teeth, and the possibility of reinforcing a muscular tension pattern that may already be hypertonic. Different dental schools idealize and theorize over the precise way that the teeth relate to each other, but unfortunately most of these theories are based on a model of an immotile cranium.

Competence in craniosacral work hinges on an understanding of the multitude of ramifications from the upper[18] and, particularly, the lower jaw. The place to begin this understanding is at the temporomandibular joint, and the place to deepen it is at the atlanto-occipital and atlantoaxial joints.

The occiput is host to the largest aperture in the cranium, the foramen magnum, a pear-shaped aperture whose narrower portion faces anterior. The pear-shape is caused by the reniform (kidney-shaped) occipital condyles, which crimp the foramen magnum and form the articulation with the first cervical vertebra. The shape of the foramen magnum is the result of a trade-off between the brain and spinal cord's evolved need for more space, and the first cervical vertebra's need to keep the condyles close together; the closer the condyles are, the more flexible a universal joint the atlanto-occipital joint becomes.

The meningeal dura has a firm dural attachment around the circumference of the foramen magnum[19] (forming what Sutherland called the "upper pole" of the core link). Once the meningeal dura parts company with the occiput it becomes known as the spinal dura, which envelops the spinal cord as it descends through the middle of the atlas, on its way to the second sacral segment, where it ends. The spinal dura has fine filaments of attachment to the second and third cervical vertebra,[19,20] but neither to the atlas, nor to any other vertebra. This is one reason that the area between the occiput and the third cervical vertebra is so prone to tension and displacement, which are both factors that affect the functioning of the temporomandibular joints.

The posterior aspect of the atlanto-occipital joint marks the location of an acupuncture point called Wind Palace (Governor Vessel 16), which denotes the beginning of the inner eye. The inner eye is a channel of energy running through the head, beginning at the atlanto-occipital joint, passing through the foramen magnum, and exiting at glabella. The atlanto-occipital joint is therefore deeply connected to the use of the inner eye. Head and neck positioning affect not only the stomatognathic system in general, and the temporomandibular joints in particular, but also inner-eye functioning.[21,22,23]

The temporomandibular joints are normally loose within their temporal fossae,[24] fluidly stabilized and contained by their joint capsule, menisci, ligaments, and spatially centralizing muscles. They have four ligament groups – the temporomandibular, stylomandibular, sphenomandibular, and retrodiscal – all allowing a great deal of freedom to the mandible. The first three ligament groups are not normally implicated in the kinds of stomatognathic system dysfunction treatable in craniosacral work, unless the mandible has been severely restricted in its motion long enough to permit ligamentous contraction. The retrodiscal ligament is frequently implicated (see below).

### Motion and the Neuromuscular Pattern (Engram)

The natural, relaxed neuromuscular pattern (engram) of the mandible allows the teeth to separate slightly with the slight impact of walking, as the lead foot hits the ground. The stomatognathic system engram keeps the teeth in their normal relationship to each other regardless of body position. This ability evolved to cope with such ancient sensual predilections as eating fresh figs while hanging upside down. It also enabled us to prepare for a fight by increasing the number of muscle fibrils in a contracted state at any one time. It encompassed our signaling apparatus of baring our teeth in fierce threat displays, and the ability to use our teeth as effective weapons when more than a threat display was needed. This engram can create problems when it is overloaded by the almost non-stop stress of modern times, leading to continual muscle fibril contraction, clamming up the stomatognathic system.

"Optimum psychological state" is a term sometimes used to define the condition in which the engram functions best. In this optimum state our nervous system functions within a fluid yet stable set of checks and balances that ensures a high level of health, and as a spin-off of this we have optimum stomatognathic system functioning.

The conventional dental model is a static one where the upper and lower teeth touch all day long. The cranial model suggests that the normal healthy relationship is one where the teeth have no need to touch except when chewing. In the liquid-electric model, the temporomandibular joints float freely at all times except when eating (when alternating compression and release patterns occur), but even then they float.

Optimum psychological state does not imply perfection, however. Over millions of years we have evolved multiple mechanisms to cope successfully with stress[25] and adversity of many kinds. What we have not evolved is the ability to cope with the kind of continual stress typified by life in big cities, a way of being which is appropriately described as "life in the fast lane."

The engram of the stomatognathic system is regulated from the highest level of the soul state; there is no tension in the system when we are at one with the world. The soul displays its status through the intermediary manifestations of the hormonal system, and its condition is interpreted and fine-tuned for its densest wavelength – the body – by the nervous system. The background role of the autonomic nervous system and the motor components of the central nervous system balance each other in health. The brain itself is often likened to a biological analog computer,[26] with the cerebral cortex operating (at its simplest level) on the basis of a binary system. Like a conventional computer, the brain fires signals and flips circuit switches according to a simple on-off pattern. In computer language, it creates either a one or a zero.

A "constant-on engram" occurs when a complex of cortical neurons become fixed in an "on," or firing, position because of either an imagined or real threat, or because of drug stimulation. This results in continual contraction of the muscles controlled by the neuron complex. If this occurs in the

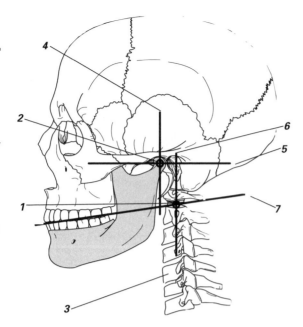

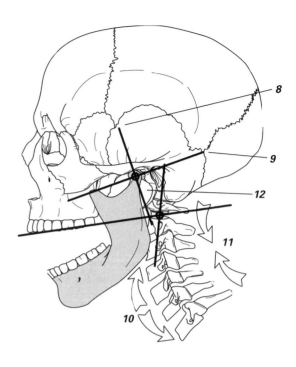

**Right:**
Guzay's theorum: *jaw closed*

**Far right:**
Guzay's theorum: *jaw fully open*

**1** *Primary axis of mandibular motion at base of dens*
**2** *Secondary axis of mandibular motion at temporo-mandibular joint (TMJ)*
**3** *Cervical spine tending to slight loss of curve when biting (schematic)*
**4** *Vertical line through TMJ*
**5** *Horizontal line through TMJ*
**6** *Verticle line through dens*
**7** *Horizontal line along occlusal surface of teeth*
**8** *Change of verticle line during translation*
**9** *Change of horizontal line during translation*
**10** *Elongation*
**11** *Contraction*
**12** *Alterations of forces along axes 4, 5, 6, 7*

nucleus of the motor branch of the trigeminus nerve, the mandibular musculature cause constant compression of the teeth and temporomandibular joints, leading to malaise, headache, fascial contraction, and eventual temporomandibular, atlanto-occipital, and atlantoaxial joint dysfunction, and cervical osteoarthritis.[27]

## Axis of Rotation

Although the temporomandibular joints seem to be the axis of rotation of the mandible – and are so in the immediate structural and physiological sense – a deeper look[28] shows that the atlantoaxial (first and second cervical vertebral) complex is the source joint for the mandible. In the liquid-electric model, the mandible's spherical axis of motion is at the atlanto-occipital joint, formed by an imaginary sphere 1 inch (2.5 centimeters) in diameter that rests at the base of the dens of the second cervical vertebra. Understanding the ramifications of this axis of movement allows you to radically improve temporomandibular and atlanto-occipital joint dysfunction.[29] To work with this model, you have to normalize the neck (especially the atlas and axis), occiput, temporals, and mandible – in other words, you have to treat holistically, attending to the whole stomatognathic system. Treating the whole system means treating the dreambody. Treatment that does not touch the soul will not rectify a dysfunctional component of the stomatognathic system, all it will do is achieve a rearrangement of symptoms.

## Interconnectedness

The teeth, temporomandibular joints, atlanto-occipital joint, and atlantoaxial joint collectively form one of the most interconnected areas of the body, in terms of postural and psychological reflexes. Only 5 percent of people in the Western world[30] have normal dental occlusion, temporomandibular joint function, and a mandibular axis of rotation at the atlanto-occipital joint. The great majority have multiple and imbalanced axes of rotation and moderate to severe alterations in intercuspation, with resultant uneven wear patterns and pressures on the teeth, temporomandibular joints, upper neck, and cranial sutures.

## Dentistry and Orthodontics

Many of the best dentists have studied craniosacral work, and test their clients' cranial motility patterns before and after all dental work. If such a dentist is not available to you, refer your clients to one who works with a craniosacral therapist in his office or refers his own clients for craniosacral work.

One dental school ideal begins with the static principle of centric occlusion (defined above, under Motion). As noted, most dental schools also accept as normal the upper and lower teeth being in constant contact throughout the day, while in the liquid-electric model of visionary craniosacral work we consider this entirely wrong, and instead posit fluidity and an absence of tooth contact at all times (except when eating) as the ideal.

Ideally, craniosacral clients should not have dentures fitted for size until their heads are functioning fluidly and normally, with their cranial waves balanced. The best dentures are built to fit in slight flexion, causing minimal impedance to cranial motility. The use of "soft layers" between dentures and gums creates an interesting effect throughout the craniosacral system: it seems to put energy into it and optimize the connective tissue environment, much like an air-soled sports shoe can improve lap times. (On the other hand, fixed bridges that span many teeth or the maxillary and palatine sutures do the opposite, and can create havoc.) If a soft layer is laid over a trigger point that was previously irritated by a hard denture contact, a whole body release can ensue, ending an old dysfunctional body pattern for good.

Dental splints allow muscles to relax, and are much easier to remodel than dentures or bridges – one of their big advantages. A dentist may not be able to get crowns accurate enough to eradicate muscle spindle irritation, but he can refine a splint to the point of no irritation. With the dental splint in, have the client clench, unclench, yawn, and triturate while you feel his sphenoid movement and energy patterns. Suggest that the dentist make the splint progressively thinner, and each time check the cranial wave until you sense interference coming in again; then have the dentist increase the thickness back to the last depth at which the cranial wave was unimpeded. The optimum splint erases the tense neuromuscular engram. (Splints typically are used for six to twenty-four months. Some Japanese dentists use a traditional enameled horsehair block, about one-quarter to one-half inch [one-half to one centimeter] deep in place of a splint. Enameled horsehair has just the right amount of "give" in it to allow the fluctuant motion of the cranial wave.)

Always check clients' bridges for an impediment in the cranial wave – especially those spanning an area from the front teeth to the molars, across the premolar area. Dental bridges can cause headaches, depression, and a cessation of the cranial wave similar to that found in compression head. If the orthodontic surgeon can use a hinged bridge, or simply cut the existing bridge in half at the median palatine suture, it may provide an immediate and enormous sense of relief.

Always consider the teeth when dealing with sphenoid distress. Dental disease and uneven wear patterns may be a reflection of sphenobasilar joint status, particularly a sphenoid torsion lesion.[31] Torsion, side-bending, and latero-flexion lesions also affect the atlantoaxial joint; thereby further stressing the teeth and temporomandibular joint.

The type of filling used to treat a dental cavity can have unexpected ramifications. Gold, now in fashion as a replacement for leaking amalgam fillings, has two disadvantages. The first is that it changes size with temperature alterations, which may cause problems with the bite. The second is that a change from amalgam (which contains mercury) to gold can create a galvanic current, affecting the electric field of the eyes or the optic nerves, or the piezoelectric motility patterns of the sphenoid, or all three, possibly leading to a distortion in vision. One way that gold fillings can have this effect is by altering the minute motility patterns that each eye habitually moves in. Ceramic inlays, now in their second generation, are a better – although more expensive – option.[32,33]

Another ramification of dental work extends into the dura: dental anesthesia can produce a slight short-term toxicity to the dura. The client experiences generalized fatigue and malaise at this time. Dental anesthesia may also give the cranial dura a parchment-like texture, making the cranial wave tight and dry in feeling. After some exposure to clients who have had recent dental anesthesia, you can begin to detect how long ago it was administered by the change of feel in the membrane system. Such changes are palpable up to six months later.

The extensive use of dental braces tends to imprison "the mechanism." That is, unless they are hinged at the median palatine suture, they inhibit or foreclose the cranial wave in the maxillae, and alter it in the mandible. This seems to result in temporomandibular joint dysfunction twenty years later, a connection that, while hard to prove scientifically, is noticed in clinical practice with regularity. (I mentioned this in a class in Germany recently. A woman's hand shot up. "Twenty years exactly," she said.)

The use of artificial joints to replace eroded temporomandibular joints had a brief period of popularity beginning in 1983. Some twenty-five thousand people had one brand of implant, the Vitek, fitted. It has subsequently been found to have a failure rate that may ultimately prove to be 100 percent. Those fitted with such failed prostheses are in far worse shape than people who never had the operation. The pain and disability they suffer makes some of them suicidal.[34]

## Diagnostic Considerations

### Energetics

Energetically, the stomatognathic system relates to vishuddha, the throat soul, expression. The neck represents flexibility in life, and the back of the neck fear of betrayal (encompassing the feeling of being stared at from behind, and worries about being stabbed from behind). The front of the throat is immediately concerned with survival: numerous reflexes cause us to shorten our neck whenever we are attacked, or fear attack (a glancing impact to the cricoid cartilage, such as taught in the martial arts, causes a terrifying loss of the ability to breathe; the dreambody knows this response and fears it.) We also swallow our truth when we fear the results of speaking it.

The shoulders are deeply invested with elements of aggression[35] (wanting to punch, but holding anger in) and responsibility (the world weighing too heavily on our shoulders). The shoulder muscles speak of pride in muscular power. The pectorals are the shields that protect the tender aspect of the heart.

The temporomandibular joints are the intimates of aggression, determination, and the tendency to withhold tender emotions from expression. We bite down on our teeth to get through a difficult event, compressing the temporomandibular joints. A German expression calls this "to bite on a sour apple." Sixty percent of those suffering from temporomandibular joint problems are women, who are often conditioned against self-expression in childhood. One student noted the relationship of this to the doctrine of "If you can't say anything nice, don't say anything at all," stating that her mother's variation of this was "Don't ask: if you were meant to know you would have been told."

The atlanto-occipital joint is extremely sensitive to the stress of everyday life, to posture, and to feelings of aggression, anger, and being weighed down with too many responsibilities. When "the world gets you down," the occiput is muscularly and energetically compressed on the atlas, and the head feels much heavier.

### Trauma and Dysfunction

When the mandible or maxillae are forced to change into a new position by any form of traumatic displacement, there may be a change in tooth intercuspation, usually with an increased wear rate and a negative effect on cranial motility.[36] The condylar relationship will alter, possibly predisposing to temporomandibular joint dysfunction, and the teeth will have an increased frequency of breakage.

The mandibular condyles constantly remodel according to patterns of use and psychological stress. The teeth support the condyles, which are, in turn, only an ancillary support to the teeth – rather like the outrigger on a Polynesian canoe supports it but does little of the buoyancy work. Normal chewing forces are taken by the teeth, the viscous and biconcave temporomandibular joint menisci, and the muscles of mastication. If a tooth or teeth are in a defective relationship in either the anteroposterior or a unilateral plane, muscle contraction may be overstimulated, resulting in the appearance of a constant-on engram.

The mandible is also influenced by remote factors such as foot pronation, pelvic imbalance, the status of the symphysis pubis, sacroiliac joints, linea alba, rectus abdominus, xiphoid process, sternum, and the upper three cervical vertebrae. The mandible, as a "bowled" structure, is also affected by the status (position, motion, and energetic loading) of the other bowled and domed structures[37] of the body, such as the domes of the respiratory diaphragm, the hard palate, the tentorium, and cranial vault, and the bowled structures of the soles of the feet, perineum, and cranial base.

It can take some months, occasionally years, for headache or backache to manifest after a poorly executed dental extraction, which may damage alveolar bone for some time. Always check the client's dental history – especially extractions, bridges, and crowns, but also of fillings. This is particularly true for clients with sphenoid-related cranial dysfunction.

Hyoid muscle imbalance reflects and reciprocates muscular imbalances within the postural spinal musculature. Since the position of the head dictates in large part the position and curvature of the neck (Sutherland's maxim "the head end tends to be the boss"), so the hyoid and cranial base, in particular, tend to reflect one another's relative status. The hyoid may float and be small in size, but it is capable of exerting a profound effect. Like the mandible, it is a pattern-setter. Experience has shown me that the hyoid is particularly connected to the frontal bone in an energetic sense. It can be very helpful to unwind both using a coupled straddle hold.

### *Faulting: Mandibular Displacement*

Mandibular displacement can be an indication of the following:

■ Malocclusion (This is a primary cause of mandibular dysfunction. Occlusion stimulates the periodontal proprioceptors and thus alters the engram of the muscles of mastication by sending "position" reports to the stomatognathic system, which adjusts the components of the bite to best ensure successful occlusion.)
■ Disturbed centric relation
■ Cranial lesion patterns, especially of the temporals and sphenoid
■ Muscular imbalance, particularly of the lateral pterygoid muscles
■ Eruption of a tooth due to iatrogenic causes

This might include an opposite and paired tooth being removed with no replacement installed. The erupted or prominent tooth can cause prematurity in contact[38] with its neighbors, thus causing the mandible to displace. In this case, corrective work will normalize the position of the errant tooth, and a new engram will evolve, hopefully erasing all trace of the maladaptive pattern. Ideally, this new engram will ensure complete intercuspation and normal contraversial (i.e., equal on opposite sides) temporomandibular joint positioning.

## Temporomandibular Joint Dysfunction

Craniosacral work is especially effective in dealing with temporomandibular joint conditions[39,40,41] because it honors motion. All strategies that assume immobility, or impose it, dishonor the sensitivity (not to mention the simple mechanical truths) of the stomatognathic system. Craniosacral work is one of the very best ways of working with temporomandibular joint conditions.

Poor finishing of fillings or poor-fitting crowns can create prematurities of contact (and therefore dysfunctional mandibular patterns[42]) or stress to the temporomandibular joints, or affect sphenoid motility patterns.

In chronic temporomandibular joint constant-on engrams, the periodontal ligaments are held in unending compression, locking the teeth down within their sockets, thus removing one important element in the chain of slightly flexible components[43] that constitute the stomatognathic system. In these cases the cranial wave may completely disappear in the mouth area. The whole muscular system, especially the masseters, temporalis[44,45] (notably its posterior bellies), and pterygoids will be in tender-to-touch hypertonicity. This puts the teeth in danger of losing a very important protection, their "bullet reflex." Bite down on an unexpected bullet in your grouse (it does happen), and the jaw springs open before the brain knows what has happened. This spares a fracturing of tooth enamel or, worse, a broken tooth. A hypertonic jaw is so locked down that the bullet reflex may be critically and disastrously slowed.

### *Treatment*

Mandibular and temporal balancing represent cornerstones of stomatognathic system therapy, but unwinding of the head upon the neck and the release of "archaic wounds" is the foundation. Balanced treatment begins with observation, listening, touching, and sensing; at the highest level the soul state needs to be sensed so that the vagaries and vicissitudes of the constant-on engram can be addressed at the causative level.

Consider spending as much time as needed, ten minutes or more, unwinding each tooth. (Unwinding pairs of teeth will give you left and right, then up and down, comparisons.) The canines – prominent, robust, and easy to get a hold of – are an excellent place to start. Use a slip of tissue between your gloves and the tooth enamel to prevent slippage. One dentist who works extensively with the cranial wave considers it a part of his treatment responsibility to unwind each tooth. He will not extract a tooth until he can pull it out using only his fingers – until this is possible, he believes that the tooth retains the inherent vitality to heal itself.

(While the subject is debated, it does seem that flossing is much more effective than brushing in keeping the teeth free of decay; performing both is of course ideal. Tell your clients seriously that it is not necessary to floss all of the teeth – just the ones they want to keep. The best advice for people who want to floss, but cannot bring themselves to do it, is to tell them to pull out twelve inches [30 centimeters] of floss each day and throw it away. After a few weeks of this, they usually drive themselves to stop the waste and actually use it. Toothpicks should be avoided, as they can destroy a healthy periodontal membrane. An alert and concerned dental association in Denmark banned the sale of dental picks in 1990.)

The normalization of muscle tonicity and suppleness is vital to optimal function within all aspects of the stomatognathic system. Muscle balancing can be achieved with a number of methods, such as biofeedback, acupuncture, Feldenkrais exercises, Rolfing, fascial release, reciprocal innervation techniques, trigger point therapy, Bio-energetics, unwinding, mandible and maxillae decompressions, and direct digital pressure techniques. Dentists use a multiplicity of techniques to achieve muscle balance – amongst which are correcting the height of fillings to within 3 microns, employing splints and other orthodontic appliances, and the use of braces.

Bio-energetic therapy can release stored tension patterns in the stomatognathic system, especially through cathartic oral expression and deep work with body armor patterns.[1,46] Sexual trauma to the mouth area is often the deep cause of temporomandibular joint problems, and a client who was not aware of the event would have even greater dysfunction – the "archaic wound" is very deeply buried.

Artists, hairdressers, violinists, and people who spend a lot of time on the telephone usually have occupational patterns that compress, sometimes forcibly, their temporomandibular joints. Ask a client who is a musician to bring in his instrument and watch very carefully as he plays. Let your eyes go soft, and move into a "glamour." Where is the compression? Where do the energy lines twist up? Where does it feel "all wrong"? Imitate the client's playing, and note how you feel. Ask him to watch your miming and point out what body usage could be improved as you mirror it back.

### Client Education and Practical Advice

Teach and then encourage clients with temporomandibular joint and stomatognathic system problems to do three things. The first is to notice when they swallow their truth, do not speak up, or otherwise stifle their self-expression.[47] Educate them to notice feelings of anger and aggression that they do not express and have no outlet for. Teach them that it is best to feel their feelings in the moment they experience them, and not to stuff them down, and lock them away, behind their teeth. In this way, even if they are unable to express them, they can *feel* them, which is infinitely better for body and soul than denial.

The second thing to teach these clients is to sit in a meditative posture for ten minutes immediately before sleeping, contemplating their day. One way to do this is to go back to the first memory of awakening, and continue a fast-forward through the day, reviewing especially the most pleasant and stressful events. This technique serves as a kind of refuse disposal, clearing the psyche of clutter. In this way nocturnal tension, with its resultant wear-and-tear on the temporomandibular joints and possible bruxism, may be greatly diminished. Sleep will be deeper, dreams more profound, and the stomatognathic system more relaxed throughout the night.

The third thing to teach clients, especially those with temporomandibular joint dysfunction who have not been given a splint by their dentist, is to use a pencil or quarter-inch (six-millimeter) wooden dowel as an adjunct in their practice of the first exercise. Having it set transversely between the sixth or seventh teeth while practicing the review of the day aids relaxation of the jaw muscles before sleep. The effect can be maintained by wrapping the pencil or dowel with one or more layers of waterproof tape each week or two, to gradually increase diameter until the optimum combination of comfort and effectiveness is achieved, one that diminishes temporomandibular joint tension. (Make sure the client is not being hard on himself by using too thick a dowel – driving oneself too hard for too long is part of the causative pattern in temporomandibular joint dysfunction in the first place, and precisely the pattern we are seeking to change.)

Encourage clients to learn to keep their teeth slightly separated all day long. Teach them to place the tip of the tongue softly just behind the upper front teeth, on the incisive bone, as a means to decrease temporomandibular joint tension and create a little spaciousness at the mandibular condyles. This alone may reduce temporomandibular joint distress.

Existing problems of the temporomandibular joint or neck can also be helped by some simple things: the client needs to discontinue chewing gum or tobacco, and eating such things as beef jerky, if at all possible. Stressful body postures – such as resting the chin on the heel of the hand for hours a day, or habitually carrying a shoulder bag on one shoulder – need to be discontinued (backpacks or fannypacks are superior to bags carried on one shoulder). Temporomandibular joint problems can be exacerbated by conventional diagonal seat belts, which impart a unilateral torsion pattern to the thorax, neck, and sternocleidomastoid of the compressed side. A racing harness is a viable, albeit flamboyant, option.

# 19

# *Quantum Cranial: the Liquid-Electric Model*

Heads behave in their own unique ways. I call the individual motion of each cranial bone its 'signature pattern,' because cranial movement patterns are as different from one person to another as signatures, fingerprints, or the convolutions of our brain. This chapter seeks to explain where they come from, what influences them, and the different patterns of cranial bone movement.

## Simplicity

Since the Middle Ages, healer-priests have used Latin in diagnosis and prescription, a language their often uneducated patients could not comprehend, and it has become customary to prove one's therapeutic knowledgeability by saying wondrous-sounding phrases that no ordinary mortal can understand the meaning of. This approach is outdated, and does a disservice to our clients. Bringing in simplicity, wherever appropriate, deepens the rapport between healer and client, and speeds healing.

During the federal inquiry into the 1986 space shuttle disaster, Richard Feynmann, the Nobel Prize-winning physicist on the panel of investigators said of the NASA scientists with whom he was conferring that: "They kept referring to the problem by some complicated name – 'a pressure-induced vorticity oscillatory wa-wa,' or something. I said, 'Oh, you mean it's a whistle!' 'Yes,' they said, 'it exhibits the characteristics of a whistle.'"[1]

If we really understand something, we can find a simple way to explain it. In the following discussion, after describing the origin and manifestations of the cranial wave, I am going to use the simplest words possible to describe the three principal phases, or patterns of cranial wave formation:

"similar motion," "opposite motion," and "liquid-electric motion."

Many teachers like to keep the cranial wave under technical wraps. I attended a cranial osteopathy seminar in England, hosted by an American osteopath from the Cranial Academy. In his sixties, the doctor was a model of professional integrity and reserve. He tutored expertly, a master of anatomical and physiological detail. During a tea break, an English osteopath asked him how cranial treatment actually worked. Our host gave an impressive-sounding left-brain answer, touching on correcting the lesion pattern and the resulting normalization of the membrane system. The student was unmoved. "That is all very well, but how does it *work?* How does the patient get better?" Taken aback by the intensity of the question, the American tried another left-brain tack, and talked about cortical optimum-seeking mechanisms and the hierarchy of somatic servo-loops. This was not accepted either. The man wanted the deeper truth. In a corner, our teacher looked around the small and interested group that had gathered around him. "Listen. This is energy work, it works because of intention and because of focus." He scanned the small group quickly, looking somewhat abashed by this admission, as if to say "But don't tell anyone!"

## Hyparxis

*Complete understanding of a client requires observation and action coming from the heart.*[2]

The ancient Greek philosophers used the term "hyparxis" to describe the ability to perceive the totality and interconnectedness of all things[3] – Mindell's "complete understanding." To use

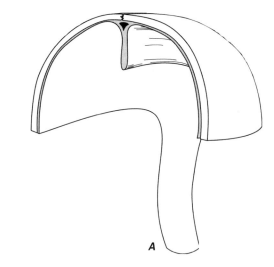

*Similar and opposite motion patterns of the parietal bones*

*A Spinal dura and falx cerebri: neutral*

*B Spinal dura and falx cerebri: similar motion – flexion*

*C Spinal dura and falx cerebri: similar motion – extension*

*D Spinal dura and falx cerebri: opposite motion*

*1 Parietal bone vertex moves inferior*

*2 Falx cerebri moves inferior*

*3 . . . and lengthens anteroposterior*

*4 . . . while parietal bones move lateral*

*5 . . . and spinal cord moves superior*

*6 Parietal vertex moves superior*

*7 Falx cerebri moves superior*

*8 . . . and shortens anteroposterior*

*9 Spinal dura moves cephalad*

*10 Parietal bones move medial*

*11 Left parietal moves superior*

*12 Falx cerebri moves left*

*13 Right parietal bone moves lateral*

*14 Left parietal bone moves medial*

*15 Squamous suture moves inferior*

*16 . . . while spinal dura rotates right*

*17 . . . while also moving inferior on left*

*18 . . . and superior on right*

hyparxis to understand the cranial wave, we must employ a minimum of three perspectives – one from each cerebral hemisphere and one from the intuitive heart. The left cerebral hemisphere interprets reality in a logical, linear way, the right in an intuitive, artistic fashion; the intuitive heart senses deep energetic and emotional truths. Only by using the bare minimum of all three can we begin to grasp both the totality and the nuances of what is. It is important not to get lost in minutiae, losing sight of this principle, while considering cranial motion patterns.

The interconnectedness of the body in craniosacral work, and the importance of intent in treatment, was first made clear to me during a craniosacral class, when the tutor asked me to put my hands on the model's sphenoid and close my eyes. I was instructed to let him know when I "had" the cranial wave. The moment I did so, the

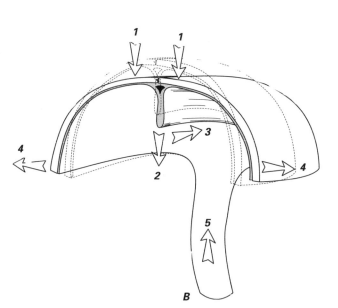

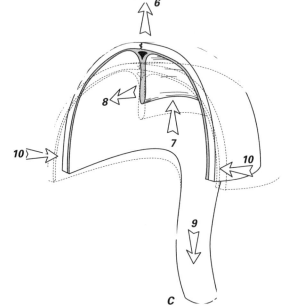

sphenoid moved very powerfully into a torsion pattern. It was amazing – I had never felt such a sudden change in a cranial movement pattern before. Then I was instructed to open my eyes. The tutor was at the model's feet, focusing his intent on them. He did it again – an almost imperceptible external rotation of the model's feet. Whatever further carefully calibrated and intent-full motion he made at the feet, wrist, or abdomen further torqued, side-bent, or sheared the sphenoid.

Years later, when a client unexpectedly lifted up her legs while I was palpating her temporal bones, I was amazed at the apparent amplitude of their displacement. Holding a man's temporal bones at the instant of death, Sutherland reported that they made two very large movements.[4] These experiences seem to demonstrate that the body is deeply

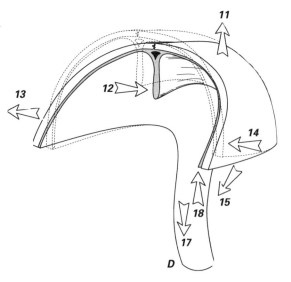

interconnected, and not just physically. What we feel in these moments is an admixture of bone movement, hydraulic change within the cranium, and the movement of the field.

The way bones feel and behave is also influenced by their "energetic loading." Thus the maxillae of a resentful housewife may feel loaded with anger, a long-suppressed desire to bite her way out. A Zen master's sphenoid feels loaded with the intense, almost blue-white energy of perception.

A bone's feel is also affected by its history. If it is home to a memory of physical or psychological trauma – an archaic wound – then both its field (and thus its "feel") and its movement will be affected. The presence of an archaic wound affects both piezoelectric charge and motion; the wound may have affected bone position and, in the case of a fracture wound, bone density and texture too. Archaic wounds are frequently found in the head, notably in the bones and joints that compose the oral cavity. A severe trauma may result in the complete absence of bone movement in the area of impact, or in a related area, such as occurs in "contre-coup" hemorrhage.[5] Such traumas may even have stopped movement in the whole head, a condition known as "compression head." When the traumatic memory is released to consciousness, processed and integrated, bone movement tends to resume.

## The Cranial Wave

The cranial wave is an involuntary motion that occurs in a watery medium.[6] A pulsation within a watery medium does not necessarily produce the kind of specific osseous rotations with precise axes beloved by the pioneering cranial chiropractors and osteopaths.[7,8,9] Rather, it produces wave movements, spirals, vortices, and motions reminiscent of the ripples resulting from the impact of a pebble on the surface of a pond. What is sometimes called the "cranial mechanism" is not a chronometer; it is a water-based weave of living tissue. The multi-layered genesis of the wave makes each person's cranial movement as unique as his fingerprints. As it passes through the head the cranial wave behaves in molding patterns that produce dilations and textures rich with interpretative nuance, allowing diagnostic interface with the spirit. The cranial wave is thus one way that both brain and spirit have of expressing their needs.

The cranial wave is variously described as the:

- Cranial Rhythmic Impulse (CRI)
- Cranial Respiratory Cycle (CRC)
- Sutherland Cycle[10,11]

- Cranial wave formation
- Third order, or Traube-Hering wave[10]
- Third force[12]
- Breath of life[13]

The 25-micron amplitude[14,15] of the cranial wave is such a minute motion (half the thickness of a sheet of writing paper) that we need to use different parameters to understand it than those used to explain gross body motion. The cranial wave is also affected in its amplitude and direction by the application of such discreet pressures that the everyday laws of physics do not seem to help us understand what is occurring. When the wave changes without any pressure exerted – only through the direction of the healer's intent – it is incumbent upon us to stop and think about what is really going on.

In visionary states, the healer can "see" the movement of the cranial wave; she can "see" still points. And if she becomes quiet and sensitive enough,[16,17] she can even hear the story of the bone she is focusing on, and see the light show of the structures.

### Wave Qualities

It may help to understand the cranial wave by considering it as having certain similarities to the breath. In physics a "phase change" is said to occur when water changes to ice upon freezing. Another phase change occurs when water changes to steam upon boiling. The cranial wave has phase changes, too, and like water, there are three principal phases, or patterns of movement, to cranial wave formations.

When we sleep, our breath is wholly autonomic, which is one phase, or quality, of our respiratory mechanism; when we sit and meditate we learn to gain complete conscious control of our breathing, and this phase of breathing is quite different than the first, that of sleep. When we get emotionally upset our breathing enters another, quite different, chaotic phase. There are, of course, overlaps between these and other phases of breathing.

A healthy individual's cranial wave frequency ranges from eight to fourteen cycles per minute.[18,19] The rhythm is hyperactive in fever, under the influence of amphetamines, and in certain kinds of drug overdose. When the metabolism is accelerated by caffeine, the cranial wave speeds up. In meditation, the cranial wave slows to its lower limits, where it synchronizes with the breath. It is reduced or may disappear altogether in the head after compressive head injuries.

A cranial wave that is faster below a certain spinal level indicates the possibility of spinal cord damage, a tumor, dural adhesions to vertebral bone, or a hematoma within the spinal canal.[20,21] The cranial portion of the wave increases after recovery from meningitis, but amplitude has often dropped because of dural and arachnoid adhesions, scar tissue, and the resultant loss of normal dural elasticity.

The cranial wave appears to be synonymous with what physiologists call "Traube-Hering Waves." These movements are also known as "third order waves," and are visible as fluctuant changes of arterial pressure spreading across the opened thoracic cavity of research animals. The frequency of the waves was recorded as slowing down during sleep. The waves seem to originate in rhythmic changes in the vasoconstrictor center. Further documentation occurred during the long-term observations of cerebrospinal fluid motion patterns in cats. In these experiments, cerebrospinal fluid was found to be displaced in the subarachnoid spaces by breath, beat, and the "third order" movement of Traube-Hering waves.[22]

When consciousness is operating at different levels, such as in a near-death experience or during a coma, the cranial wave may be markedly reduced, down to as little as two cycles per minute.[23] (This occurs because the electrical activity of the field is so minimal in coma that the cranial wave has little chi to fire and sustain itself with.) Thus, it is a common experience for nurses and family to sense that the essence of the comatose person is "gone" – that his soul is not present in the same field as the body, which seems lifeless, or "spiritless."[24]

Some of those who have had near-death experiences[25,26,27,28] report a sense of being afloat in a blissful sea of light, suspended near the operating theatre ceiling, up above their lifeless bodies. They describe a wave-like delicate rhythm, that seemed to move them back and forth in perfect, slow, ecstatic harmony. They recount never having experienced anything quite so perfect in their whole lives. But then a twitch is noticed in their "dead" body, and defibrillation and adrenaline were administered. The wave suddenly became chaotic and unendurably irritating. They recount a sudden, nauseating descent from ecstatic suspension, back into their damaged physical form. Electrical activity begins the moment the spirit merges with the body. (No defibrillator can make a dead body alive; only the return of the spirit can do that.) They felt as if they were now in a nightmare, where all rhythm and harmony had gone awry, a bad dream from which they had to wake up immediately. Thus ended their suspension in their own cranial wave, which was experienced in its purest, out-of-body form at the level where the spirit almost unifies with the soul.

It takes twenty to forty minutes after the termination of brainwave, breath and heartbeat at the moment of death for the cranial wave to cease;[28] this it does as the gyre slowly separates from the body. As the oldest pulse, it naturally ceases last. A Swiss friend found this uniquely verified when her dog had to be put to sleep. The formal, elderly vet administered the lethal injection, and quietly, within two minutes, the dog was dead. Then, ten minutes later, she said to the vet, "You know, he's still here, I feel him." The vet replied in his gruff voice, "It takes twenty minutes for the spirit to leave." My friend, herself involved in the esoteric, was touched that such an apparently conventional man understood this.

### Wave Formations and Breath

*Observations and recordings of the minute rhythmic motions of the live cranium have demonstrated that an expansile-contractile motion occurs synchronously with heartbeat and respiration, and also with a rhythmic periodicity similar to but slower than respiration.[29,30]*

Respiration may in fact be quite separate from the cranial wave. Emotions affect our breathing through complex pathways that alter diaphragmatic innervation, blood supply, tonus, and motion. Posture, mood, stress, and energy levels interact constantly to alter the status of heart and diaphragm, which in turn modifies the cranial wave formations that reach individual cranial bones.

The respiratory diaphragm is the most important central structure of the body. The physical heart sits on the central tendon of the diaphragm, to which its pericardial sac is firmly attached. The energy patterns of the spiritual heart imprint upon diaphragmatic action, and also affect cranial base functioning directly, through both the arteries that ascend to it, and through the connective tissue web of the mediastinum. This begins to explain a foundational axiom in visionary craniosacral work: that, energetically speaking, you cannot get the brain in the right place until you get the heart in the right place. Furthermore, the heart cannot be in the "right place" if the sacrum is not in the "right place:"

*Making his sacrum stiff: dangerous*
*The heart suffocates.[31]*

Diaphragmatic movement also affects the spinal cord by way of the rib articulations to the thoracic vertebrae and the diaphragm's attachments from the tenth thoracic vertebra to the fourth lumbar vertebra. Some of this motion is transmitted to the skull. When the breath synchronizes with the cranial wave, as it usually does within ten minutes of calm recumbency, the spinal cord moves superiorly in flexion as we breathe in.[32]

The strongest influence that the field exerts on the diaphragm comes from its local center of energy, which is Anahata, the spiritual heart. According to Indian yogis and South American native tradition, prana – the life force which is enhanced through appropriate use of the breath – is the most powerful component of our spiritual equipment.[33] Breath nurtures the spirit and is also an expression of it. We breathe "high, wide, and handsome" when we feel accordingly, while in states of depression we hardly breathe at all. The diaphragm is also influenced by Manipura, which encompasses both the solar plexus, and the movement center of the body, known as the hara, or lower dantian. It is further modified by Muladhara, the perineal center. (See Chapters 11 and 14 for more information.)

Sutherland noted that "the head end tends to be the boss." He was right and he was wrong. The head is the boss, but not the sovereign: the fluctuant field of the spirit plays that role. The spiritual heart is the "center of centers" of that field,[34] and, together with the hara, or lower dantian, is responsible for wave genesis, quality and frequency. Cranial wave formation is also modified by the status of the other five soul centers[35] (three of which are located in the head itself), particularly by the lower dantian. This is the production center of the physical body's chi: "The lower dantian is the furnace that produces life."[36] It is known as the "Sea of Chi" in acupuncture.

As a person moves into a meditative state his cranial wave begins to synchronize with his breath. When the breath meshes with the cranial wave, it is not simply an interesting physiological event – there are profound changes in the inner world of the dreambody. It is a time of deep harmony. The heart comes home.

A person living in tune with his cranial wave is at one with himself and his world, free of inner dissonance. He feels deeply nurtured, not by any external source, but by his Self. Reaching this state, he can begin to live in accordance with the ebb and flow of an ancient inner tide. Native

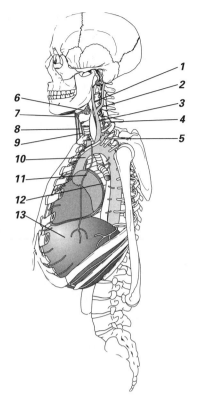

Domain of soft connective tissue web of the mediastinum
**1** External carotid artery
**2** Internal carotid artery
**3** Carotid artery
**4** Vertebral artery
**5** Subclavian artery
**6** Hyoid bone
**7** Superficial fascia
**8** Infrahyoid fascia
**9** Pretracheal fascia
**10** Ascending aorta
**11** Heart
**12** Pericardium
**13** Respiratory diaphragm

Americans call this living in "Indian Time." When one honors Indian Time, one does not turn up for a three o'clock appointment at precisely three, if to do so means rushing, and moving out of harmony with the Self. One arrives before, after, or even *at* three, as long as one stays in harmony with one's inner rhythms. Then one arrives in a whole, harmonious state. This is the right "time" to arrive. In another culture, a Zen nun described her enlightenment as the ability to eat when hungry, rest when tired, and sit when the time came to sit. Experiencing this level of harmony inside, the individual no longer searches for answers (or enemies) outside. She is home. Perhaps referring to this level of consciousness, the fifteenth-century poet Kabir wrote: "The God whom I love is inside."[37]

### The Long Wave

Hyparxis allows us to understand more about the cranial wave and some of its non-local characteristics, such as the long wave:

*She was sitting her final osteopathic examination. Three lecturers sat in front of an examination table on which lay a challenging patient that she had first to diagnose and then to treat. Towards the end of the treatment she decided to use a CV4, a cranial contact to the occiput. She knew that all three examiners were highly criti-*

*cal of the exactness with which students applied the CV4 – in fact it was popular wisdom in the School that it was better not to use a CV4 precisely because the three were so fond of finding fault in its application. If you wanted to pass your finals, you didn't use a CV4. But it was her evaluation that the patient needed it, and so she resolved to go ahead. She took great care to get it technically correct, and then settled into an expanded state of awareness, into a "glamour." Consciously she synchronized her breathing, then her own cranial wave, with that of her patient. By focusing her awareness she began to slow her perception of time down. The room changed. When she finished the CV4 she looked up, anticipating criticism. All three examiners had glazed eyes, and beatific looks upon their faces: they said nothing. She had inducted them into a glamour, too: their cranial waves had moved into an entrainment with that of the student and her patient.*

*She passed her examination.*

This cranial wave synchronization in groups and across distances is called "the long wave." The manifestation and the transference of the long wave has some things in common with the brain's "fifth wave."[38,39,40] The long wave is one of the factors responsible for the synchronization of bio-rhythms reported in study groups – for instance when large groups of young women are put into isolation together, such as for studies on circadian rhythms,[41] their menstrual cycles synchronize within two months. Not only that, but the cycles of other control groups totally isolated from them, but in close physical proximity, also move into synchronization.

Meditation, music, and dance seem to facilitate rapid long wave entrainment. Edward T. Hall has this to say:

*The power of rhythmic messages within the group is as strong as anything I know. It is . . . a hidden force, like gravity, that holds groups together.*

*. . . when people converse . . . their brain waves even lock into a single unified sequence. When we talk to each other our central nervous systems mesh like two gears of a transmission.*

*Rhythmic patterns may turn out to be one of the most basic personality traits that differentiate one individual from another.*[42]

## Ancient Origins: Breath and Beat

One of the most basic manifestations of life is rhythmic movement. To understand the origins of the cranial wave, and how it manifests in humans, it helps to study it in other creatures – this gives us both physiological and historical context.

Before breath and beat there existed an older rhythm, that of the cranial wave. It is the deepest and oldest movement pattern in the body, having its origins long before the evolution of lung and heart, in the fluctuant movement of single-celled amoebas 3.5 billion years ago. 600 million years ago, long before the advent of the cardiovascular system, the involuntary body movement of the first multicelled organisms circulated oxygen and nutrients (just as peristalsis does in our digestive tract today).

The human cranial wave is the remnant of this oldest of movements, which is seen in the common earthworm, which shortens itself in what we would call flexion, before elongating itself to move forward in a movement we call extension. Thus it propels itself through soil, and on the earth's surface. A banana slug curls in upon itself if it is alarmed, and then contracts and expands at a regular six cycles-per-minute until it senses the danger has passed.

The humble tadpole provides a good model of brain and spinal cord movement. The tadpole and our brain/cord complex have three things in common: their evolution, their shape, and their movement. The brain and spinal cord change shape in much the same way as the tadpole does while swimming, albeit much more discreetly. Both are fluid-breathing organisms: the tadpole lives in water, a formative aquatic stage transited on its way to becoming an adult amphibian; the human brain swims within a semisealed system of seawater-density cerebrospinal fluid. (The brain has managed the neat evolutionary trick of staying encapsulated within its own miniature ocean while its owner has made the transition to dry land.)

In more recent evolutionary time, the earliest aquatic cartilaginous fish and vertebrates swam their sleeping rhythm in harmony with the cranial wave, externalizing it. A shark sleeps while swimming at "idle," making lazy, rhythmic lateral sweeps of its tail. Sharks, in an evolutionary sense a primitive species, still depend upon movement through water to provide their oxygen needs – their gills cannot move enough water on their own to oxygenate the bloodstream, and a shark will suffocate if trapped in unmoving water. When the spinal cord of a shark is severed just below its medulla oblongata,[43] it continues to swim at its sleeping rhythm for several hours before dying – that is, its locomotor musculature has an inherent contractile pattern quite separate from that propagated by the motor centers in the shark brain.

The cranial wave ebbs and flows, echoing the distant tides of the oceans from whence we came. Many creatures externalize these slow rhythmic movement patterns. Elephants, for instance, sleep standing up, and "rack" – a rhythmic side-to-side swaying motion – as they do so, an externalization of their cranial wave. Dolphins sleep in two-minute pauses between surfacing to breathe, continuing to swim as their tails move in a ventral-dorsal plane.

Humans love to rock and be rocked. Rock a crying child and it is comforted. Nomad children rarely cry once they are on the moving camel's back. Rocking chairs allow us to bring outer body movements into a sympathetic frequency with our cranial wave. Latihan, Continuum, and tai chi allow us to express our cranial wave externally; these movements are a great joy and nurturance.

### The Source of the Cranial Wave

I suspect that it will turn out, once thorough hydraulic and electromechanical experiments are completed on live human subjects, whose cranial mechanics, piezoelectric balance and bioelectric field are not altered by the experimental apparatus, that the majority of what we feel as cranial bone motility is not bone motion at all, but rather the movement of the fluctuating field.

The ancient Chinese depicted the fluctuating field with the symbol of yin and yang energy dancing around a still center, the two perfectly overlapping. It expresses the higher truth that without the still point there can be no dance of opposites, and there is only the dance. The ancient Hindus depicted the same dance as two serpents ascending intertwined, the female "ida" energy forming a double helix with the male "pingala" energy. They called this dance "kundalini." In the western world this fluctuating field of energy is almost entirely unrecognized and undocumented, except within the chiropractic and osteopathic professions. Indeed, its very existence is often disparaged, dismissed out of hand, even made fun of. But absence of proof is not proof of absence.

Marion Woodman, a Jungian psychoanalyst,[44] posits the existence within the body of a "third force," which is neither physiological nor mechanical. The "third force" is the fluctuating field, which is composed of non-neurological energy, or "chi." T. F. Powys calls it "the oddity."[45]

This fluctuating field is measurable with appropriately calibrated electronic devices, such as those used to locate acupuncture points. Sensitive fingers readily feel this fluctuant field, just as they can detect the presence of an acupuncture point through exploratory touch. Very young children, psychics, and clairvoyants "see" it.

The fluctuating field *is* the spirit. It is a field of information and of intelligence,[46] "a single unified system of energy,"[47] whose fundamental texture is expressed in the quality of feeling we call "love."

The spirit is a quantum field of energy. The meridians and energy vessels of traditional Chinese medicine are maps of the more superficial aspects of this field. The chakra, or soul-center system, represents an understanding of a deeper layer of the fluctuating field. This layer exerts a stronger influence than the meridian field upon muscular status, and hence craniosacral bone motility, which is why it is important in visionary craniosacral work. (See Chapters 11 and 14 for further information.)

## Manifestation: Cranial Wave Interactions within the Cranium

The presence of this fluctuating field gives muscle fibrils the triggering impulse which enables them to contract and expand rhythmically, independent of the central nervous system. The rhythmic motion of the muscle fibrils in turn pulls and releases the muscle's nerve supply. The sum of these muscular and neurological motions feeds into the spinal cord via the spinal nerves, and is one causative component in the alternate cephalad and caudad movement of the spinal cord. The rhythmic motion of the cord is passed to the physiologically continuous brain, changing its shape minutely.

The cranium deforms massively during natural childbirth.[48] Part of the reason that cranial bones exist as separate entities, possess movement, and have an internal membrane system is to successfully navigate a large, fragile cranium through a narrow birth canal, and have it reconstitute itself postpartum. The architecture, motion, molding patterns, and elastic resiliency required for birth provide the blueprint for brain and cranial bone motion throughout life.

The presence of sutures in the adult cranium enables the brain to have a fluctuant motion that facilitates both its nurturance and its cooling.

Sutures also make the adult head more resilient to trauma: cranial bones are less likely to fracture if they have sutures that help absorb the shock of impact. The reciprocal tension membrane – a system of slightly elastic membranes, consisting of the falx and tentoria (two spatially distinct but physiologically continuous parts), which attach to the inner surfaces of all the bones that envelop the brain, coordinates the movement of the individual cranial bones. Forces delivered to the cranial cavity through the spinal dura are also transmitted to the cranium by the endosteal dura, or outermost layer of the dura. It is natural to focus on the spectacular architecture and fascinating motion of the falx cerebri and tentorium cerebelli when analyzing cranial wave motion; however, it behooves the student not to lose sight of the role that the very strong adhesion of the endosteal dura plays in limiting sutural motion.

Nerve tissue, being inelastic, transmits the muscular ebbing and flowing of the cranial wave up and down the spinal cord, to brain and sacrum, with little dissipation of the impulse. The cord's motion, occurring in the almost frictionless medium of cerebrospinal fluid, passes through the foramen magnum and alters the shape of the brain stem, cerebellum, and cerebral hemispheres. David K. Michael and Ernest W. Retzlaff describe downward displacement of the parietal bones resulting from the simulation of spinal column extension, and upward movement resulting from flexion.[49] (If a child has no observable cranial wave immediately after birth, the rhythm can be "jump-started" by circumducting both femoral heads several times. This provides valuable insight into the role that the energy field of the lower soul centers, joints and muscles play in helping produce and control the cranial wave.)

The fluctuant motion imparted to the brain is transmitted to the cranial bones through the interface medium of the cerebrospinal fluid. As the brain is moved by each cranial wave, cerebrospinal fluid in the ventricles, cysterns and subarachnoid space is displaced. This movement helps to nurture the brain through enhanced circulation of the glycogen-rich cerebrospinal fluid. The movement of the fluid also improves heat dissipation from the brain, assists the evacuation of used blood from the cranium, and enhances vascular circulation to the pituitary.

Spinal cord and brain motion are sometimes misunderstood as the genesis of cranial bone motility, rather than simply a unit in a chain of functioning whose original source is the field. The brain, lacking contractile fibers (except in a discrete area of the cerebellum) is almost a passive unit. As it changes shape, the pressure it exerts (through the interface of cerebrospinal fluid) on individual cranial bones changes. In the healthy head, all of the cranial bones displace to accommodate the expanding brain and its fluid buffer by rotating, tumbling, pulling closer together or pushing apart. Their sutures[50] stretch or compress, and the thinner cranial bones undergo plastic deformations. These activities produce changes in each bone's field: bone registers a negative piezoelectric charge when compressed, and a positive charge when pulled apart under tension.[51] Sensitive fingers feel this change of polarity, and know how to interpret it.

Muscles that attach directly to the vertebrae transmit cranial wave motion directly to the spine, and may modify the motion of the enclosed cord. Muscles that attach directly to the bones that compose the cranial base likewise transmit motion directly to the cranium. (Notable amongst these muscles are the sternocleidomastoid, the lateral and medial pterygoids, the masseter, and the trapezius.) The sphenoid is influenced by the muscles that move the eyeball, all but one of which attaches to it. As we have seen, the bones of the cranial base also admit the ascending arteries, which are tightly adhered to their cranial access foramina; thus, by way of these vessels and their supportive web of connective tissue, the mediastinum, the movement of the heart and breath subtly but powerfully influences the cranium.

The body's smooth, involuntary muscle moves under the control of the autonomic nervous system, and its peristalsis may be modified by the fluctuant field. When a healer moves a cranial bone in the needed direction with appropriate intent, the involuntary muscle of the abdominal cavity relaxes, and borborygmus results. This is one confirmation of the choice of cranial technique.

### Nomenclature: Flexion, Extension, and Still Points

The cranial wave is the spirit made manifest. The spirit loves movement, which we define in craniosacral work in terms of flexion and extension, and the spirit also loves stillness, which we call the still point.

During flexion the viscerocranium widens laterally, partly in response to the pull of the falx at the crista galli and the frontal. It is also affected by the tentorium, through the interface that the palatine bones make with the pterygoid processes of the sphenoid, and through the motility of vomer and zygomae. This combination of movements represents what happens to the cranial vault during "similar-motion" cranial flexion.

William Sutherland used the sphenoid's motion as the reference point for his model. He defined flexion as the movement of the sphenoid into forward-bending or "nose-diving" (see the similar-motion model, below). Extension he defined as the sphenoid's backward-bending. Whatever movement other cranial bones made at the time of sphenoid flexion Sutherland also defined as flexion. That is, when the sphenoid moves into flexion, the movement that all other cranial bones make at the same time is also called flexion (classical forward-bending) even if the movement is actually a classical extension. The midline cranial bones, he posited, flex and extend with the cranial wave as if they were meshed together by straight-cut gears.

Flexion and extension are good basic standards to describe the movement of midline bones. In the case of paired bones, flexion and extension make less sense, because in Sutherland's model the movements often occur around oblique axes (as, for instance, with the temporals and zygomae); this results in a complex molding pattern consisting of both forward-bending and lateral movements (in other words, the motion is actually a compound external rotation). It makes more sense, therefore, to describe flexion in the paired bones as "external rotation" and extension as "internal rotation." Sutherland called these motions "wobbling wheels," an apposite description from a man who grew up in the century of the covered wagon.

The correct technical way to describe how paired bones behave during similar-motion flexion is to say that "all paired bones rotate externally in flexion." It may help to use the mnemonic "fatten in flexion," as long as you remember that the cranial bones become wider – fatten – in the lateral plane, not in the anterior.

"Slackening" is a term used in the similar-motion model to describe what happens when the moving cranial bones "let go" of the reciprocal tension membrane. This possibility occurs, for example, when bones that form the perimeter of the attachment of the tentorium come closer together, as they do in similar-motion extension. But it is a misleading term: there is no actual slackening in the sense of the dural partition suddenly losing its tension and sagging. Rather, as soon as one part of the membrane system loses tension, other parts take it up, like a cat's cradle made of elastic bands.

Move one bone into apparent slackness, and the slack is taken up by the tension in the others, or by the falx. So there is (nominally) always balanced reciprocal tension in the membrane system. Exceptions occur in severe trauma to the head, neck, spine, or sacrum.

In terms of body energetics, flexion tends to be associated with feelings of expansiveness, amiability, and openness. Extension is associated with solitude, reclusiveness, and inner work.

### Still Points

A still point occurs when the cranial wave becomes quiescent, which happens every few minutes, as natural pauses in the rhythm, particularly when we are free of stress.[52] (When we are "stressed out," they are much less frequent, even absent.) Still points are to the cranial wave as sighs are to the breath – autonomic releases that "let off steam." They also allow a return to natural rhythm after a period of overload, or trauma. During a still point, the dreambody makes profound physiological recalibrations. These often manifest as deep relaxation, and the client often falls into a light sleep.

A still point has a duration of anywhere from two to fourteen normal cranial wave cycles, before motility creeps back in. The first movement is almost imperceptible, it is so delicate: a new being is being born, tenderly, and at first it hardly moves.

The still point is much more than a physiological pause. The Vedic scripture Yoga Veshishta[53] notes that "Bliss is the effortless suspension of breath." You crest a ridge while walking in the Himalayan foothills, and unexpectedly see the whole mighty mountain range extending a hundred miles into the distance: it "takes your breath away." Such experiences are natural still points. After orgasm, there may be a period of euphoria and still point that can last up to a minute.

*The still point is spaciousness.*
*It is timelessness.*
*The still point is close to death, and*
*deathlessness, both.*

When the still point occurs in the "yoga of daily life,"[54] this apparently spontaneous cessation of the cranial wave is a moment of satori, of spiritual at-oneness, even ecstasy.

## Craniosacral Motion Patterns

I acknowledge how important it is to focus, learn, and understand as much as possible, but I hesitate to codify this interactive dance into dogma, such as by saying "The sphenoid moves into flexion during the inhalation phase." (I itemize the liquid-electric patterns, as described below, only to help the student practitioner orient himself.) This cannot be more than the barest outline of what it really does, what its essence is like, what it needs, why it loves to dance, and how its force field can be affected by other people in close proximity to it. And it does not begin to explain why it dreams.

As someone who is cross-dominant (born left-handed but persuaded at school to become right-handed), I share with my cross-dominant peers a certain foreignness to the abstract and the theoretical. I never was good at math or geometry, I was good at artwork and essays. This is one reason that the elaborate descriptions of suture architecture and detailed mechanical theories of traditional cranial bone motion descriptions came hard to me.

There are other reasons. I don't know, experientially, that cranial bones move like the old textbooks say. Something about these mechanical theories has an imperfect ring to it. What I *do* know is that every person's head behaves in a different way, and the same head behaves differently on different days. I can sense and see the complexities of membrane, muscle, dura, cerebrospinal fluid, and brain, but I cannot convince myself that the motion patterns I feel are explained by a mechanical theory based upon these component parts, however complex. I am suspicious of unipolar truths, and attempts to provide mechanistic explanations for body functions. The body is an energy system suffused with consciousness. It does not, of course, behave or respond solely in mechanical fashion. What I know experientially is that cranial bones *seem* to move, and change their electrical polarities as they do so, and behave much more like electrically-charged fluids than the traditional concept of bones.

In laboratory tests at Michigan State University using a mechanically operated, computer-controlled parietal bone simulator, the test subject who reported the actual movement most accurately was a blind person who had no previous exposure to craniosacral work, but who had developed extraordinary palpatory skills. Several osteopathic authorities in the craniosacral field who were also tested on this apparatus reported findings at greater variance from actual movement than this "naive" subject.[55] Perhaps this was because the theories they base their work on are incomplete, and interfere with accurate perception, or because they are accustomed to interpreting much more than bone movement when they touch.

I have included the classical osteopathic axis of rotation and motion pattern in the description of bone motion in each bone chapter. These descriptions help us understand one way that an individual cranial bone may move under certain circumstances, or phases. There are three phases of motion, which I call similar motion, opposite motion and liquid-electric motion.

### I: Similar Motion

In this "similar motion" pattern model, all paired bones move into external rotation (flexion) or internal rotation (extension) at the same time, as if they shared a common hinge and diverged – or spread apart – with their movement pivoting at the hinge. Thus the parietals are said to hinge at the sagittal suture and diverge at their inferior borders (the squamous suture) during flexion. The squamous sutures then converge in extension.

As we have seen, Sutherland regarded the sphenoid as the single most important bone in his study of cranial and sacral movement patterns. He was sure the sphenoid was motor-driven by a contractile movement of the brain, transmitted to it through the pituitary stalk. According to his understanding, the sphenoid then passed its movement on to its bony neighbors through a system of sutural gears and bevels, whose movement was coordinated by the membrane system.

In this model the benchmark bone, the sphenoid, moves around a horizontal coronal axis, and each lateral extremity (each greater wing of the sphenoid) moves the same amount into flexion (forward-bending) as does its partner on the opposite side. Sutherland was the first to identify this phase of craniosacral motion. It represents the dominant, but not the only, paradigm in cranial osteopathy today.

### II: Opposite Motion

In the "opposite motion" pattern, all paired bones move in opposite directions, or alternately. That is, as the left parietal moves into flexion, the right moves into extension. They still move at the sagittal suture, but now the movement is more like a shear than a hinge. In this pattern the sphenoid also moves around a horizontal coronal axis, but the axis has an additional pivot point in the center of the sphenoid body. The greater wings alternate their flexion and extension movements around this

central pivot point, with one side moving into flexion while the parietal on that side also moves into
flexion. At the same time the other greater wing
and parietal bone are moving into extension. Major
Bertrand DeJarnette, the chiropractor who helped
develop craniology, was the first to thoroughly
explain this phase of craniosacral motion.[56]

### III: Liquid-Electric Motion

In the liquid-electric motion pattern, the cranial
bones are regarded as moving to get "out of the
way" of the brain, itself constantly changing shape
by minute amounts as the result of the rhythmic
pull transmitted to it by the spinal dura, and by
muscular and mediastinal attachments to the cranial base. The spinal dura, muscles and mediastinum all move as a result of changes in the fluctuating field, as described above.

In this model the cranial bones also move in
"opposite motion," or alternately, but are now
regarded as having a fully-floating source point
which is located in the center of the brain. The
movement of the brain is itself modified by the
other energy centers in the body, notably by anahata (spiritual heart), manipura (hara), and by
muladhara and svadisthana (perineum and sacrum).
In this model there are no axes, and no pivots.
Movement occurs in response to tissue changes
caused by a spiralling or curving motions of the
fluctuating field. The local cause of motion may be
a displacement around the moving sphere of the
brain.

Neurocranial bones float, as if they had neutral
buoyancy and were suspended in water, and are
pushed or pulled by tidal electrical, muscular, and
osseous forces. Viscerocranial bones, one step
removed from the influence of the brain, have
something closer to the classical chiropractic and
osteopathic axis of rotation, but one that is modified by the fluctuating field.

### Stress, Love, and other Modifying Factors

As noted above, the cranial wave can be altered by
many factors. The variance may originate in
aspects of consciousness (such as a burst of insight,
or a fearful attitude), or it may have its source in
emotional traumas, postural change and patterns of
habitual body movements. It may be altered by the
results of physical impact. Such changes may
remain in the tissue for thirty or forty years
through alterations in the field, the tone of fascia,
muscles, and membrane system, and the status of
sutures and joints, until they are finally addressed
and allowed to normalize.

Personality and posture also affect bone motion.
Individuals with open, wide-ranging, liberal consciousness and relaxed postures tend to have open,
mobile, cranial sutures. People with dogmatic,
restrictive life views and armored postures tend to
have heads (and bodies) that are restricted in freedom of motion. (There are always exceptions.)

Under extreme stress we revert to primitive
behavior patterns, such as fight or flight. These
responses are marked by dramatic changes in the
fluctuating field, which result in instantaneous
changes in muscular, respiratory, neurological and
hormonal system function. The respiratory
diaphragm, the main central structure of the trunk,
is hyperactive and its activity is mirrored by the
tentoria and the bones that make up the cranial
base. Athletes in world-class competition, for
instance, have heart rates that exceed 180 beats per
minute for several hours. At these times our cranial rhythm tends to be both tight and in a similar-
motion pattern.

During moderate stress, such as concentration
under deadline pressure while at white-collar work,
the diaphragm and tentoria are less active, and the
pattern tends to be more mobile and opposite
motion.

Specific cranial bones are home to specific psychological complexes, or spiritual energies. As
examples, the parietals are invested with the
energy of GV20, A Hundred Meeting Places, and of
the crown soul center; the mandible is plainly
associated with aggression; the sphenoid is the
home of our insight, the inner eye. Intensifications
in these energetic loadings may lead to changes in
the cranial wave formations.

### Repressing Perception

Let us say that a child of eleven senses a deeper
truth about her parents, that even though they do
their best to hide it from her, they no longer love
each other. The aspect of her sphenoid that is the
inner eye is at work. She perceives what is real, but
she does not *want* to see what she is perceiving –
the implications are too threatening and painful.
She represses the information, denies it. This
makes her sphenoid confused at the energetic
level,[57] and she contracts her lateral pterygoid and
temporalis muscles. Now under tension, her sphenoid no longer moves naturally, and this begins to
take its physiological and energetic toll. Her inner
experience is one of being "all twisted up."[58]

At best she wants to be the one who conserves
the marriage; at last resort, she wants to establish a
strong bond to at least one of her parents, so someone will take care of her if they do split up. Super-

ficially she seems fine. Inside, a storm of powerful and divisive emotions is building up. Her deepest emotion may be repressed anger. She may begin to grit her teeth in order to "bear it." She may begin to grind her teeth all night – bruxism – as the anger surface expresses itself unconsciously. Or her bruxism may be an instinctive effort to "chew through the problem" to its completion. She feels helpless. Thoughts occur to her such as: "Why does no one stop the breakup of my family? Why does no one reassure me? Why does no one take time to listen to *me?*"

Unable to process the pain on her own, she likely tightened her mandible and kept it all inside. Energetically a battleground, her sphenoid cannot function normally; scalp, neck, and jaw muscle tension begin to diminish its cranial wave motion. Her studies fall off, she finds she cannot focus so well. Her vision deteriorates, and she gets new glasses; her opthalmic specialist cannot understand why she needs them so soon. This denial builds up a subtle dissonance in the energy field of the sphenoid. Within six months she has a learning disorder.

In this case, the sphenoid (as inner eye) is seeing the real, but its insight is not permitted to surface, and be integrated into waking consciousness. It becomes repressed to the unconscious, surfacing as fantasies by day, dreams by night. The change in the status of the sphenoid will be apparent to trained fingers; they feel reduced movement, and energetic dissonance. The sphenoid does not feel "right."

If the healer stands back from the young girl, first with eyes closed, then open, her inner eye may "see" the tension in the sphenoid. The inner ear may hear what troubles it. The empathetic healer's heart may feel her sadness.

Discerning the deeper truth of a situation and simply sitting with her, the healer gives her a heightened chance of making a breakthrough in perception. (In shamanism this is called a "a rite of intensification.") This is especially true if the healer has a clear intention to facilitate honesty, clarity, and healing. Touching the sphenoid will help the process in almost all situations, just as touching the heart can soothe, and occasionally enlighten, the heartbroken. If the young girl can relax in the healer's presence, and begin to talk about what has really been troubling her, the sphenoid will tend to self-correct, all other things being equal. The energetic imbalance disappears once repressed perception is brought to the light of consciousness. The correction becomes permanent when she has the time, and the outside support, to integrate her perception.

### Inherent Tension

But all other things may not be equal. Something may have happened years earlier that also needs to be exorcised from the client's psyche, or is still going on. Alterations in muscular, fascial, or membrane system tonus, especially when they result in a reduction in cranial wave amplitude, are sometimes referred to as affecting "the level of inherent tension" within the head.

In inherent tension, a sphenoid may be held under tension from a postural stress such as scoliosis; it may be affected, via the mediastinum and the sternocleidomastoids, by an illness such as asthma. It may be held in a kind of "startle response" resulting from an emotional trauma that occurred years ago. Such postural, respiratory or emotional distress may have led to widespread contraction in her cranial musculature, compressing her sutures and her temporomandibular joints, and reducing the free movement of her sphenoid.[59]

This combination of contractions – some short term, some originating years earlier – results in a sphenoid that cannot move normally. Its sutures sit under compression or tension, perhaps both. The inherent tension will continue until the causative postural, respiratory, or emotional pain is exorcised. Touch the tense tissue in an evocative way, and its messages will burst into her consciousness. She may cry about what really troubles her for the first time. Lacking this contact, the inherent tension continues. Her mental and emotional clarity continues to suffer.

### Physical Trauma

The body can handle impacts much better when it is healthy and has recovered from all previous wounds. To continue with this example, if the young girl suffers a physical trauma to her already suffering sphenoid, it will be much harder hit: it has lost its normal resiliency. She is alone in the kitchen, and stands on tip-toe to take a heavy wooden breadboard down from a high shelf. Partly because she is feeling miserable deep inside, she is careless and the breadboard slips out of her hands and hits her hard on the forehead. Such a blow to the head, even if apparently quite innocuous, may easily jar the sphenoid out of its normal position, or wedge an interdigitated suture into immobility. She rubs her head, feels "kind of all right" for a few hours, but then develops a splitting headache. Her sphenoid is now dissonant, inherently tense, moving abnormally (if at all), and in a non-normal spatial relationship with its adjoining structures.

Real healing entails addressing one or all causative levels until they are resolved. She has to be listened to; she may need psychotherapeutic help; she could certainly benefit from craniosacral work; acupuncture may also help to normalize her field. The ability of the healer to sense what really troubles her is foundational to her healing. And unconditional love has to be present: it is the most powerful healing force known.[60,61]

## Treatment

In visionary craniosacral work, "the mechanism" of bones, brain, cerebrospinal fluid, and membrane system is regarded as part of a quantum mechanical field whose movement is affected not only by posture, stress and muscle attachment, but also by the presence of other energy fields in close proximity to it. Thus the clarity of consciousness of the client, and the intent of the healer – irrespective of whether the healer touches the client's body or not – affect both consciousness and the cranial wave formations.

There are two apparently contradictory approaches to excellence in craniosacral work. The first truth is that the only correct way to evaluate a client's cranial motility pattern is by sensing it in terms of whether they are the optimum patterns for this person. No outside reference can be used. Perfection is a personal, not a textbook, ideal. The healer uses hyparxis, and her tactile and intuitive perception, to sense whether the head is in its best possible state. (Does it look right; does it feel right; is it right?)

The second truth is that it is essential to have a data-base, or benchmark concept, of how a cranial bone *should* move according to the forces acting on it, thus deepening the healer's understanding of what is going on. It also helps to know what its motility pattern *should* be so that it can be compared to this benchmark standard to assess the normalcy, or otherwise, of its motion. The first truth is the higher one, the second may help students get started, and deepen their perception. However, this second truth may also get in the way (note the performance of the "naive subject" with the parietal bone simulator, as mentioned above). Properly used, one truth complements the other.

According to the second truth, parietal motion in this model tends to be alternating, with the left parietal moving into flexion, displacing inferiorly at the posterior margin of the sagittal suture, and moving more laterally at the anterior portion of the squamous suture. Simultaneously, its twin moves into extension. In this model the sphenoid moves into slight torsion and side-bending patterns as it moves into flexion on the left as the left parietal moves into flexion – because of the reciprocal motion of the paired parietals, and the effects of the reciprocal tension membrane, *it has to.*

In the liquid-electric model, the sphenoid is regarded as being propulsed by the spherical surface of the temporal lobes located inside the greater wings, and by the pressure exerted upon it from above by the frontal lobes of the brain. As mentioned above, its movement is modified by the activity of the fluctuating field, and by muscular and membrane system tension. The sphenoid moves three-dimensionally (and usually asymmetrically) in response to these and other inputs from distant bony or soft tissues. The motility of the sphenoid, and also its "feel," is also affected by its own piezoelectric charge, and that of adjacent bones.

It was sometimes suggested by practitioners of the similar-motion model that if one temporal bone moved into flexion while the other moved into extension, then something was amiss. The practitioner was then directed to assess which bone was moving in time with the sphenoid. That bone was taken as being in normal motion. The practitioner was then directed to shepherd the aberrant bone into moving in time with the "normal" side. But real-world cranial movement patterns are not composed of tidy mechanical symmetries, and it is a grave error in treatment to guide opposite-motion cranial bone motility into a similar-motion pattern upon a mechanical paradigm.

The high art is based upon discerning what the optimum pattern is for *this* head, the head you are working on, and not falling into a mechanistic trap of forcing a physiological pattern to conform to an abstract theoretical model.

Superlative cranial technique tends to use minimal pressure but great focus, that is, chi-kung, or direction of chi. Superlative techniques also tend to be asymmetric and three-dimensional, matching the movement of the spiralling and asymmetric field. This affects the field so deeply because this is precisely how the field itself operates in first creating, then coordinating bodily functions. Craniosacral work enables us to dance directly with the field, permitting us great effectiveness in healing, for the field *is* the hyphen in psycho-somatic.

When a healer touches a cranial bone with the intention to access its tissue memories, the smooth muscles of the abdominal cavity relax, and produce burbling sounds immediately. Long-repressed memories begin to surface to the awareness of both healer and client. The moment these memories are brought to consciousness, processed and released, the feel of the bone (that is, its field), its position and its movement all tend to change. Each cranial bone – or each tissue in the body – moves and communicates in its own unique ways. Movement *is* communication.

Once the healer enters an energetic entrainment – that is, links up her breathing, empathy, and intent – with the client, she deepens her access. She may then be able to direct her chi to influence a cranial bone without actually touching it. She may be able to induce an insightful still point in the client's cranial wave by entering a still point in her own being. (This phenomenon is acknowledged by most advanced adepts of craniosacral work.) Its modus operandi is explicable through one of the earliest insights of quantum physics, that the presence of the observer alters the behavior of subatomic particles.

It is treatment and healing that counts,[62] not theory. The healer needs to be present and responsive. She must not try to fit a body into a pattern. Rather, it seems to me that she needs to liberate the dreambody, free it from every restrictive pattern that it can function successfully without. (Most people have some need for deep defensive armoring; remove it all and the client is overexposed, and may quickly collapse, only to erect a new armor in order to get going again.) She needs to learn what "normal" is so that she can recognize, immediately, the abnormal. But sensing normal has very little to do with a pattern described in a book – this, or any other. Sensing normal is hyparxis, it is a finger-feel, a matter of the healer asking her spiritual heart and hara soul center if they *like* the textures of this motion, this energetic, the same way they like the feel of a cat's responsive body. The cat feels good to the fingers, which then want to play with it. Touch a faulted bone with that same quality of awareness and you immediately feel a little sharp pain of grief in your own heart.

## Bone Motion

These notes are collated here for your guidance, and to enable you to have an overview of how the whole head moves in the liquid-electric model. A more detailed rendition can be found in each "bone" chapter.

Since we transit many different levels of physiological and emotional stress each day, a particular head will tend to exhibit different patterns at different times of day. Optimum, liquid-electric motion patterns are likely to be as fluid as waves on the beach, and as reciprocal as walking. All heads show an admixture of nondominant components that modify the dominant pattern – typically, a head exhibits an admixture of all three patterns: similar motion, opposite motion, and liquid-electric motion. The dominance or weakness of individual components accounts for the wide cranial wave differences found between people, or in the same individual on different days.

What is presented here is best understood as reference material, not as "this is how this bone is supposed to move." It bears repeating that it is vital not to try to make a client's head fit the textbook pattern: this is poor practice, and almost always counterproductive.

### The Sacrum

In the liquid-electric model the dominant motion of the sacrum occurs around the circumference of an imaginary sphere whose lateral curvatures encompass the sacroiliac joints. This permits the sacrum the kind of emphatically fluid, ever-changing universal joint malleability that it needs to act as the meeting place of so many dynamic forces. Therefore, in this model, the dura is not seen as the motor for the cranial rhythm in the sacrum.

In the liquid-electric model the sacrum moves in a floating, universal joint motion reminiscent of its motion while walking. Thus each side of the sacrum in turn moves anteriorly during flexion. During flexion, one side of the body of the sacrum also elevates very slightly, with the base moving posteriorly and the apex anteriorly, into the true pelvis. The other side of the body elevates during the next cycle. The opposite occurs during extension. The apex of the coccyx thus describes a circular motion, and there is a torsional movement around the median axial plane as part of each flexion-extension cycle. This simple torsion pattern of movement is made into a compound motion when the slight displacement of the sacro-iliac joints is added. The tonicity of the lumbar, abdominal, perineal, and leg muscles – especially the hip rotator musculature – exerts a powerful influence on sacral position and motion.

The axial torsion movement of the sacrum is transmitted to the vertebral column. The lumbosacral facet joints assist in conducting this motion. The cranial rhythm of the vertebrae consists of fine rotational motions around the axial plane which pass through the vertebral bodies, which are modified by smaller torsional and side-bending components, such as occur in the lumbar spine when we walk. This movement is transmitted to, and echoed by, the occiput.

### The Occiput

Like every other neurocranial bone, the occiput responds to the movement of the brain, but it also receives strong inputs from the sphenoid, mandible, vertebral column, and the muscles that attach directly to it. It is affected by the action of the spinal dura, which is firmly attached around the perimeter of the foramen magnum. The movement and tensility of the whole RTM exerts a dominant influence on occipital motion. In particular, the occiput is affected by oscillatory motions transmitted to it from the temporal bones.

In the liquid-electric model, as the left tentorium flattens during left temporal flexion, the left side of the occipital squama moves anterior and slightly laterally. The opposite occurs during temporal extension. As each temporal flexes in turn, so does the occiput move to that side. This movement pulls the occiput marginally anterior and lateral, and circumducts the occipital squama inferiorly on that side. The basilar portion moves superiorly.

### The Sphenoid

The brain acts on the sphenoid like a gently pulsating, mobile sphere resting softly upon it, causing the sphenoid to move like a floating universal joint. It moves three-dimensionally in response to membrane system tensions, cerebrospinal fluid dynamics and sutural inputs from adjacent and distant bones. Its movement is also affected by its own piezoelectric charge, and that of adjacent bones.

The sphenoid receives input from the temporals and the occiput both through directly sutural articulations, and through the tentorium. The parietals and frontal also articulate with the sphenoid, and pass on some motion from the falx cerebri. Thus the liquid-electric motion of the sphenoid needs to be considered in relationship to its cardinal neighbors, the occiput, temporals, frontal and parietals.

The greater wings move in "opposite motion," or into flexion and extension alternately. As the left greater wing moves anteriorly during liquid body flexion, the left temporal bone also rotates externally into flexion. As the left temporal flexes it draws the tentorium both inferiorly and laterally, and the bone flares laterally at the squamous suture. During left temporal flexion, the left greater wing of the sphenoid moves into flexion and an inferior torsion.

Now let us consider occipital motion, and how it affects the sphenoid, before including the parietal bone component. As the occiput circumducts and moves to the left in flexion, the falx is pulled posteriorly, inferiorly, and slightly left laterally. The falx is thus moved towards the straight sinus, pulling on the parietal bones and deflecting their movement. The combination of these movements causes the parietals to move laterally at the squamous suture, inferiorly at the sagittal suture, and into very slight internal rotation. As the left side of the sphenoid nose-dives in flexion, it glides anteriorly off of the parietals, which are rotating in the opposite direction.

The pattern fluidly reverses in extension.

### The Temporals

The liquid-electric model differs from the traditional "similar motion" model in two important ways. First, it is a "opposite motion" model, where as the left temporal moves into flexion, the right moves into extension. Second, because of this opposite motion the RTM has a greater amplitude of motion, and more liquidity of motion (opposite motion means greater tentorium movement) thus increasing the mobility of both temporal bones.

As one temporal bone rolls out into external rotation (flexion) along the center-line of its petrous portion, the temporal squama moves anterior and laterally, and the mastoid processes move medially and posterior. As a temporal flexes it draws the tentoria inferiorly and laterally. It is able to do this because the opposite temporal is moving into extension, thus "paying out the slack" in the tentoria, and not relying on dural elasticity to permit motion, as per the traditional "similar motion" model. During left temporal flexion, the left greater wing of the sphenoid moves into flexion, and the spheno-basilar joint moves superiorly.

As one side of the tentorium flattens during the flexion of that side, the attachment of the tentorium at the superior petrous ridge allows the temporal bone to roll into external rotation. The squamous portions move laterally, into external rotation, and the tip of the mastoid process moves medially, inferiorly, and posteriorly.

### The Parietals

Parietal motion in this model is alternating, with the left parietal moving into flexion as the brain changes position inside it, displacing inferiorly at the posterior margin of the sagittal suture, and moving more laterally at the anterior portion of the squamous suture. Simultaneously, its twin moves into extension.

As the left greater wing of the sphenoid moves anteriorly during flexion, the left temporal bone rotates externally. As the temporal rotates, it flares laterally at the squamous suture. As the occiput circumducts and moves to the left, the falx is pulled posteriorly, inferiorly, and slightly left laterally. The falx is thus drawn inferiorly and slightly anteriorly, towards the straight sinus, pulling on both parietal bones and deflecting their movement in a caudal direction at the vertex and a lateral and medial direction at the squamous suture. The combination of RTM tension, brain motion, and sutural architecture causes the left parietal to move into internal rotation during its flexion phase. During parietal flexion the left parietal flares laterally at the squamous suture, and moves caudally at the sagittal under the influence of the falx. (Thus in flexion the temporal and the parietal bones are simultaneously flaring laterally at the squamous suture.) At the same time the right parietal is moving into extension.

### The Frontal

The frontal behaves like a large sphenoid, a bone with which it articulates through the sphenoid's lesser wing. As the left greater wing of the sphenoid moves anteriorly and inferiorly in flexion, so the left side of the frontal moves anteriorly and inferiorly. Simultaneously, the right side of the frontal widens laterally. When the left frontal is in flexion, the right is in extension. During left occipital flexion the frontal is drawn slightly posteriorly and left laterally by the falx at its attachment at the midsagittal line. (It moves posteriorly in flexion because the falx, moving posteriorly, inferiorly, and deviating slightly to the left during flexion, pulls on it.) The frontal moves laterally at each side during its opposite-motion flexion cycle in part because of this falx tension.

The frontal moves around an imaginary, fully floating sphere about the size of a pool ball, located just superior to the cribriform plate of the ethmoid.

### The Ethmoid

In this model the ethmoid does not move like the classical osteopathic cogwheel, but rather dilates, rotates, flares and contracts under the influence of its neighbors, which behave like robust fledglings in a small nest, dominating the waif-like ethmoid. It is only because of the ethmoid's delicacy that its neighbors can move so easily: the very thinness of its walls allows both easy deformation and ready reformation. Movements of the maxilla, frontal and sphenoid distort, or squeeze, the ethmoid. The ethmoid, deforming like a compressed sponge, absorbs the disparate motion of the frontal and moves into a midsagittal torsion pattern as a result, with minor flexion and extension components received from the oscillating sphenoid.

### The Vomer

The vomer moves in a complex 'wobbling wheel' fashion in the liquid electric model. The vomer is dominated by the sphenoid superiorly, the maxillae and palatines inferiorly, and the ethmoid anteriorly and superiorly. The vomer moves around the surface of an imaginary floating sphere about one centimeter in diameter (the size of a dime) which is located in the center of the vomer. The vomer moves small amounts in every plane, particularly the anteroposterior.

### The Zygomae

The zygomae move in a sequential, or "opposite motion" flexion and extension cycle which accommodates the liquid movements of the brain and sphenoid. The extensive but delicate harmonic-suture articulation with the sphenoid allows the transmission of fine motion; the massive interdigitated articulation with the frontal and maxillae transmit stronger motions. As the left greater wing nose-dives and moves inferiorly in torsion, the left zygoma dips inferiorly. The zygomae dance in perfect synchronization with the temporal bones of the same side.

### The Palatines

The palatines follow the maxillae. As the left greater wing moves into flexion with its component of slight inferior torsion, the left palatine also moves laterally and inferiorly. Simultaneously, as the right greater wing moves into extension and inferior torsion, the right palatine moves medially and superiorly.

### The Maxillae

In the liquid-electric model, maxillary motion echoes that of the sphenoid, and is uninfluenced by the mandibular teeth, which are taken as being separate from the maxillary teeth, except while chewing. Thus as the left greater wing moves into flexion and inferior torsion, the left maxilla moves laterally and inferiorly at its posterior margin. Simultaneously as the right greater wing moves into extension and inferior torsion, the right maxilla moves medially and superiorly.

*Mandible*

The mandible echoes the "opposite motion," alternating flexion and extension patterns of the temporal bones. It receives strong inputs from the sixteen muscle groups that attach to it. The left side of the mandible moves postero-inferiorly with left temporal flexion, while the right side of the mandible moves superolaterally with right temporal extension.

## The Speed Reducers

Because of their ability to absorb motion (and thus pass on little of it), Sutherland used the term "speed reducers"[63] to describe one function of the palatines, vomer, and zygomae. The motility of the frontal, temporals, and sphenoid is greater than that of the larger viscerocranial bones they articulate with. The speed reducers dissipate the difference in motion. But the name can be misleading – the frequency of the cranial wave is not reduced, only the amount of motion passed on. For instance, the frontal may move forty microns per cranial wave cycle, but the zygomae at their maxillary borders pass on noticeably less motion, perhaps five to ten microns,[64] to the maxillae.

The three traditional speed reducers behave as follows:

■ The vomer slips out of its V-shaped articulation with the underside of the sphenoid. This slippage successfully dissipates some unwanted sphenoid motion, ensuring that it is not transferred to the vomer. By its very thinness, the vomer allows further dissipation of motion by deforming slightly.

■ The zygomae have robust articulations to the frontal and maxillae, with an appreciable surface area that allows for a high degree of sutural plasticity, which thus aids in the dissipation of excess motion.

■ The palatines dissipate motion through their extensive sutural articulation with the sphenoid and maxillae, and also undergo plastic deformation.

The ethmoid acts a fourth speed reducer in the liquid-electric model. The deformation that the ethmoid undergoes with each cranial wave facilitates the movement of the whole cranium.

## Summary

The cranial wave is a manifestation of a fluctuant force field. In visionary craniosacral work, "the mechanism" of bones, brain, cerebrospinal fluid, and membrane system is regarded as part of a quantum mechanical field whose movement is affected not only by posture, stress, and muscle attachment, but also by the presence of other energy fields, particularly those in close proximity to it.

Since cranial wave formations are quanta phenomena, visualization, prayer, and the presence of unconditional love in the client's field have powerful effects. It explains the dramatic fluid-like movements that occur during cranial corrections, and helps explain why the involuntary muscles of the digestive tract respond so immediately to appropriate craniosacral contact.

The position, motility, and "feel" of cranial bones is affected by five principle factors:

■ The status of the fluctuating field is the primary determinant of the cranial wave. The local condensations of energy in the field known as the spiritual heart and the movement center, together with the status of the sacrum, exert formative influences on the quality and frequency of the cranial wave.

■ The cranial wave is a manifestation of a fluctuant force field that can be affected by the conscious intent of the healer. The status of the muscular, osseous, and energetic bodies determines the quality and quantity of brain, spinal cord, and cranial bone motion.

■ Bone motility is affected by the attachment of the membrane system within the head, and by muscles, ligaments, and fascia that attach outside.

■ Bone motility is also modified by changes in bone shape caused by the plastic deformations that result from internal pressure (such as tumors) and external forces (trauma), or by extremes of posture.

■ The motion exhibited by a bone is modified by its energetic loading. If it has an archaic wound, its field and its motility will both be affected.

# 20
# *The Central Nervous System*

The hemispheres of what was to evolve into the human brain began developing 250 million years ago.[1] One hundred million years ago they evolved lateral specialization, and very slowly began to grow in size. Sixty-five million years ago protohominid brain volume had reached 30 cubic centimeters, 20 million years ago, 200 cubic centimeters. Between 18 and 7 million years ago, the brain did not grow at all, and by 4 million years ago it had grown to 350 cubic centimeters. Then, after millions of years of no growth, or exceedingly slow growth, the human brain has quadrupled in size in the past four million years, to its present average of 1,360 cubic centimeters.[2]

At birth, the chimpanzee brain is half of its adult weight, the human brain only one-quarter.[3,4,5,6] The bulk of our fine neurological development occurs outside the womb, where the growing child's brain is exposed to a multitude of social and environmental stimuli.[7,8] The most decisive formative forces are usually social. The different ways children are brought up[9] – ranging from the idealized nuclear family model through single parenting to communal upbringing – account for some of the enormous variations in human outlook and behavior.[10] Less neurologically evolved species have far more uniform behavior, with brains essentially fully formed at birth, and with little left to the vagaries of conditioning. Learning about (and understanding the importance of) the formative forces that have shaped an individual is of course a vital component in healing, and one that forms the basis for most forms of psychotherapy and psychiatry.

## The Functional Anatomy of the Brain

The brain and spinal cord begin as the worm-like notochord, which proceeds to evaginate before bulging ever more at one end, like a pointy pale gray asparagus tip. The elongation of this tip, the brain, presents a problem: there is insufficient room in the womb to accommodate a long, pointy-headed fetus. Something much rounder is needed. Evolution has arrived at a compromise – the enlarging brain bud makes a gradual in-utero flexure at the level of the midbrain, until it is bent over anteriorly at about forty degrees from the centerline of the spinal cord.

The lack of "asparagus tip" space forces the hemispheres to become shaped like ram's horns[11] – the asparagus tip eventually folds in over itself. In the brain's gray matter we demonstrate our love of the spiral. The fornix and caudate nucleus are finally so curved as to make almost complete ovals.

The hemispheres of the brain are known as the cerebrum, or the forebrain. (Note the distinction between "forebrain," which refers to the entirety of both hemispheres, and "frontal lobe," which refers specifically to the anterior 20 percent of the forebrain.) The brain, weighing in at 3 pounds ($1\frac{1}{2}$ kilograms), represents less than 3 percent of typical body mass but consumes a minimum of 14 percent of the body's oxygen and takes 18 percent of the blood from each cardiac systole.[12,13,14]

The more a function is used, the more space it takes up in the brain. (Oliver Wendell Holmes notes that a mind that is stretched to a new idea never returns to its original dimension.) At birth, the hemispheres are identical in size and unspecialized in terms of dominance.[15] In the first few years of life,[16] the left hemisphere is increasingly called upon to specialize in "left brain thinking" –

## Functions of the Hemispheres

| Left hemisphere | Right hemisphere |
| --- | --- |
| Language | Gestalt thinking |
| Logic | Recognition of musical pitch |
| Verbal memory | Facial recognition |
| Happy and pleasant emotions | Negative emotions, anger, intuition [20,21] |
| Fine motor control | Large motor movement control |
| Spatial abilities | Mystical experience |

that is, linear and analytic thought.[17,18,19] The authority and "right to life" of the right hemisphere is gradually suppressed, until lateral specialization and the dominance of one hemisphere is in place. This dominance is then permanent. In 95 percent of human beings, the left hemisphere is larger than the right. This is not a new phenomenon: we can see it in hominid craniums going back hundreds of thousands of years.[17]

The pre-Socratic Greeks viewed the brain as a radiator of excess body heat. Socrates, feeling the deft softness of the cortex, reasoned that memory worked through a mechanism similar to the one whereby a signet ring leaves an impression on soft wax.[22,23] Brain is very soft: you can push a finger through an exposed cerebrum and hardly feel any resistance, or simply scoop it out with a spoon, like an over-ripe avocado. It is highly susceptible to vibration. As a result, the brain or spinal cord can be damaged by the shock wave from a high velocity rifle bullet hitting bone in a site distant to it, such as in a shoulder.

## Blood Supply

Blood is delivered to the brain via the paired internal and external carotid arteries, and the paired vertebral arteries. Brain tissue prefers to take up carbon monoxide and carbon dioxide before blood-borne oxygen, and is therefore very susceptible to poisoning by these gases. Carbon monoxide intoxication leads to feelings of irresponsible euphoria, which come on just before blackout. Drivers of high-performance racing cars learn to recognize this euphoria – there are no other signs of this colorless, odorless gas – and get out of their vehicles as soon as they can stop. This is an instance where the cerebral cortex (knowledge) overrides the hypothalamus (pleasure).

Venous blood is collected by the superior and inferior sagittal sinus and the lateral sinuses, and then merges at the straight sinus; 95 percent of the venous blood leaves the brain through the jugular veins.[24] The cranial wave motion of the brain and reciprocal tension membrane assist the evacuation of venous blood from the cranium. Vascular evacuation from the semi-sealed cavity in which the

pituitary rests inside the sphenoid's sella turcica is also facilitated by cranial wave movement. Lastly, systolic cardiovascular pressure wave also assists venous blood evacuation from the brain and cranial cavity.

## The Telencephalon or Cerebral Cortex

The hemispheres themselves began 250 million years ago. Their covering, the cerebral cortex, appeared about 200 million years ago. Anatomists cannot ascribe a location for consciousness, but they do know that intelligent knowledge of our own existence resides in the cortex. We have the one of the most enfolded cortices of all mammals, and one of the largest.[25]

Our cerebral cortex has six layers of nerve cells,[26] formed around a basic structural unit of a column, about ¼ inch (6 millimeters) thick. The surface area of the brain, measured with the cortex in place, is 6.6 square inches (600 square centimeters); the unfolded surface area of the cerebral cortices is 24 square inches (1,800 square centimeters).[27]

The cerebral convolutions (gyri) are generic – we all have them; their exact shape, however, is unique to each individual. The cerebral cortex has more nerve cells (a hundred billion) than the whole of the rest of the body, and a greater neuronal density than any other body structure. We have no less than 100,000 billion possible connections between our cortical neurons. Once the brain is formed, we do not grow new neurons and cannot replace damaged ones. Recently, however, scientists have been able to cultivate cerebral cortex cells in laboratory conditions for the first time,[28] opening up a whole new field of therapeutic possibilities.

We use the term "gray matter" in everyday speech to define our brain, but only the cortex and

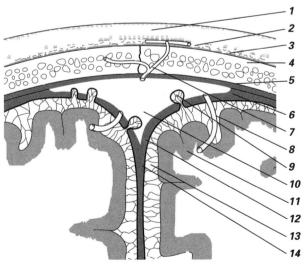

A coronal section through the cranial vertex

**1** Skin and subcutaneous fat
**2** Aponeurosis of occipitofrontalis muscle
**3** Periosteum
**4** Parietal bone
**5** Endosteal dura
**6** Meningeal dura
**7** Emmisary vein
**8** Superior cerebral vein
**9** Arachnoid granulation
**10** Superior sagittal sinus
**11** Cerebral cortex
**12** Arachnoid
**13** Subarachnoid space
**14** Falx cerebri

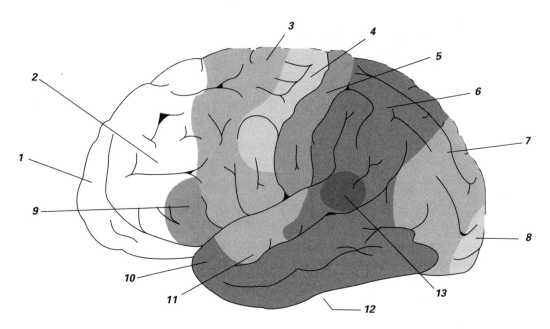

parts of the limbic system are gray, due to the absence of the myelin sheathing that makes the non-cortical brain tissue white in appearance. (The absence of the myelin sheathing allows for extremely high neuronal density and higher networking speed, in the region of two hundred feet per second. In the rest of the body, fast acting nerves have sheaths, and the slow acting nerves, where signals travel at three feet per second,[29] do not.)

Cutting-edge research on brain organization[30] indicates that the human brain may operate by sending a wave-like sweep of electrical energy throughout both hemispheres every 12.5 thousandths of a second.[31] More is now being learned in a single afternoon about how the brain works (using tagged glucose in Positron Emission Tomographs, or PET scans, and high-speed Magnetic Resonance Indicators, or MRIs) than in the previous twenty years of primate research.[32,33,34,35]

The cerebral cortex is the executive branch[36] of the brain. Its functions can be summarized as follows:

■ Organizing and accessing stored information to compare with new data
■ Remembering – handling most of the brain's memory storage
■ Social communication
■ Understanding and appreciating
■ Creating new possibilities, making decisions
■ Controlling precise motor skills

### Specific Areas of the Cerebral Cortex

***Wernicke's Area*** This is where the parietal, temporal, and occipital lobes of the cortex meet (it is level to the top of the auricle of the ear, and just posterior to it). Wernicke's Area is exceedingly important, as it integrates all sensory input, gauges its importance, and interprets its ultimate meaning. Thus, a stroke or traumatic wound to the area causes an extreme loss of thinking abilities. Wernicke's Area is usually well developed in one hemisphere only, usually the left. This unilateral development prevents confusion of thought occurring between the two hemispheres.

***Broca's Area*** Broca's Area[37] is located in the inferior to middle frontal lobe area, superior to the sylvian fissure, at the anterosuperior margin of the sphenoid's greater wings. It is the motor for speech,[38,39] controlling and coordinating the relevant movements of the mouth, tongue, and larynx. The evolution of speech is thought to have occurred at least three million years ago. (There is some debate as to whether Neanderthals, living as recently as thirty thousand years ago, could speak; if they lacked the ability, it may have been a vital component in their disappearance.[40])

### The Temporal Lobes

The temporal lobes are divided into a primary area, which interprets specific tones and acoustic volume, and a secondary area that deals with musical recognition and the interpretation of words. The area of the temporal lobes associated with the interpretation of hearing is about the size of a poker chip.

The temporal lobes are also concerned with memory. Memory is sometimes described as "information storage and retrieval." Our working memory is located in the most anterior portion of the temporal lobes, which is located close to the deeply scalloped posterior portions of the sphenoid's greater wings. The temporal lobes retain working memory (a few minutes to a few weeks) by electrochemical change in the molecules of their neurons.

Severe trauma to the left temporal lobe results in aphasia (loss of speech). Severe trauma to the right lobe results in impaired spatial ability – drawing, for instance, becomes almost impossible. The right temporal lobe seems to be the area of the brain most active in mystical and near-death experiences.[41]

## The Frontal Lobes

The frontal lobes are where we plan, make decisions, and pursue purposeful behavior, as well as where we carefully consider and evaluate threats, control fine muscle movement, and inhibit instinctive behavior – a human ability that has shaped much of our evolution. They also play an important role in regulating our emotions.[10]

## The Prefrontal Lobes

The prefrontal lobes take up the anterior 50 percent of the frontal lobe area. Their functions are less well defined than any other part of the brain. We know that this is where we carry out long periods of concentration restricted to specific subjects, and where we think through deep and complex problems. Part of our working memory is located in the prefrontal lobes. It is also where we elaborate thought and emotion, and where we plan our future.

The prefrontal lobotomy, an operation where fine surgical probes are introduced into the prefrontal cortex through the forehead or the eye sockets to sever neural connections, has entered folklore (as in the novel *One Flew Over the Cuckoo's Nest*). This procedure, initially popularized from the published findings of an Italian neurologist who based his report on the very limited basis of his work with just six patients, led to a popularizing of lobotomies that was only curtailed long after substantial evidence showed that the operation created many more problems than it solved. It made some psychotic or severely depressed patients more manageable, but it destroyed the sensitivity and intelligence of hundreds more.

## The Parietal Lobes

When you touch the parietal bones you are over the parietal lobes, home to both the motor and sensory cortices. They represent our control and awareness of our bodies. The motor area is divided into primary ("motor") and secondary ("premotor")

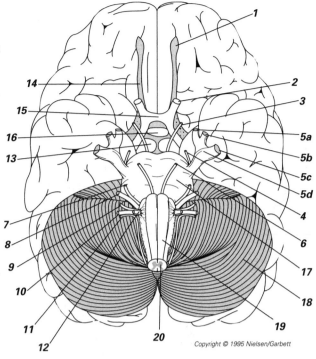

Copyright © 1995 Nielsen/Garbett

*Base of brain*
**1** *CN I: olfactory bulb*
**2** *CN II: optic*
**3** *CN III: oculomotor*
**4** *CN IV: trochlear*
**5** *CN V: trigeminus*
**5a** *CN V: opthalmic branch*
**5b** *CN V: maxillary branch*
**5c** *CN V: mandibular branch*
**5d** *CN V: motor branch*
**6** *CN VI: abducens*
**7** *CN VII: facial*
**8** *CN VIII: vestibulo-cochlear*
**9** *CN IX: glossopharyngeal*
**10** *CN X: vagus*
**11** *CN XI: spinal accessory*
**12** *CN XII: hypoglossal*
**13** *Mammilary body*
**14** *Olfactory stalk*
**15** *Optic chiasm*
**16** *Pituitary*
**17** *Pons*
**18** *Cerebellum*
**19** *Medulla oblongata*
**20** *Spinal cord*

areas. The motor cortex is about 1 inch (2.6 centimeters) wide.[42] It initiates movement, but can only produce crude movements on its own; it is the premotor cortex that refines the impulse into skilled movement.

The sensory, or somesthetic, area is where we interpret all our sensory input such as temperature, and the sensations of touch, pressure, and pain. There are primary and secondary somesthetic areas, posterior to the motor areas and extending almost to lambda, where the occiput reaches its most superior point. The primary area distinguishes between specific types of sensations, the secondary area interprets them much more finely and identifies objects through the sense of touch – such as a chair, a hat, a glass of cold water.

The parietal lobes are where we assemble our world: they are where letters come together as words, and words come together as thoughts. They are also where we link and synthesize ideas and information.

## The Occipital Lobes

The occipital lobes, also divided into primary and secondary areas, are devoted to the interpretation of vision. Visual information reaches the secondary occipital cortex via the optic nerves[43,44] (which pass through the lesser wings of the sphenoid), which cross over the optic chiasm (which lays on top of the jugum of the sphenoid), and have a relay station at the lateral geniculate bodies of the thalamus.[45]

The primary occipital areas[46] interpret light and dark spots and the presence of movement, which is of great and immediate survival importance to us. (The frontal lobes then evaluate whether danger is just implied, or actually manifested in the perceived movement.) The secondary areas refine and amplify vision, interpreting incoming visual information.[47] They also interpret the meaning of written words. The area of optimum focus on the retina is $\frac{1}{32}$ square inch (.8 square millimeter), but this is amplified and distributed to .9 square inches (6.4 square centimeters) of occipital cerebral cortex, a magnification of 600 times.

## The Corpus Callosum

The corpus callosum is a broad band of 200 million fibers[48] that forms the main connecting link between the hemispheres. Women have some 30 percent more nerve fibers in the posterior portion of the corpus callosum than men do,[49,50] which seems to give anatomical explanation[51] to women's greater skills in emotional and intuitive communication. Whether the female has the additional fibers because she has practiced communicating emotions intelligently much longer and more frequently than the male, or whether this increased number of fibers simply allows her to do this, is moot. The difference in the numbers of fibers is due to an estrogen "poisoning" of the male fetus' corpus callosum during the final stages of gestation[49] in what sounds like an arcane Greek myth, a kind of variation on the Oedipus myth – instead of the son killing the father, the mother kills off part of her son's sensitivity.

Cats have been domesticated for 20,000 years, and in this period of time have adopted a strategy of nighttime hunting. As a result, they, too, have a massive fetal kill-off of neuronal cells, but in the visual cortex.[52] As a fetus, a cat has 900,000 ganglion cells per eye; at birth, only 150,000. (Humans have 2.5 million ganglion cells in utero, 1.5 million during adulthood.) What domesticated cats have sacrificed is their color vision: as nocturnal hunters, they do not need it. The wildcats from which they have evolved hunt by day and have the full complement of cells. But since the neuronal cells are there in the cat embryo, they can be called upon again should human beings disappear, and domesticated cats survive to revert to daylight hunting. Thus, the cells are a kind of evolutionary bank account, ready to be drawn upon if there is a major change in the environment.

| **The Age of Brain Structures** | |
|---|---|
| *(in millions of years)* | |
| 500+ | *Brainstem, cerebellum, midbrain, and diencephalon* |
| 300 | *Limbic system* |
| 250 | *Cerebral hemispheres* |
| 200 | *Cerebral cortex* |
| 100 | *The lateral specialization of the hemispheres* |

From this, it is interesting to speculate that human males may have "decided" to rid themselves of a certain sensitivity, perhaps to become better hunters and warriors. Garibaldi was once described as having "the blind stupidity of a hero." Perhaps the male's callosum die-off permitted our warrior ancestors to face the woolly rhinoceros and not think about their own mortality, thus facilitating the success of the hunt. The female, on the other hand, had to be much more careful for reasons of childbearing and the vital importance of optimum male-female ratios to ensure the survival of the species. The full amount of cells available to the male in embryo form tells us that males can get their sensitivity back. We may even be in the midst of a reversal of this evolution right now, with more and more men joining men's groups, expressing their feelings, and coming out against wars of all kinds.

Occasionally a postmortem examination reveals that a person had no corpus callosum. But the adaptive capabilities of the brain meant that the abnormality went undetected throughout an apparently normal life.

## The Anterior Commissure

The anterior commissure is like a miniature version of the corpus callosum. It is located 1 inch (2.6 centimeters) inferior to the anterior third of the corpus callosum and contains about one million crossover fibers connecting the temporal lobes.

When the corpus callosum and anterior commissure are surgically cut (a process known as callectomy, sometimes used as a last-ditch treatment for chronic epilepsy[53,54]), the individual becomes a two-brained being, but usually adapts well. Upon careful testing in specially prepared laboratories,[55,56] callectomy patients display some deficits. One test sat the subject in front of a vertical partition two feet (two-thirds of a meter) deep, with a cutout for the face: this gave the subject two separate visual fields. A toothbrush was then placed in his left hand (which is connected to the right, or "artistic," brain, which is not good at categorizing and analyzing things). Using both eyes – and therefore both halves of the forebrain – the subject would be able to immediately identify the toothbrush, but the screen prevented this. Somewhere the subject knew he knew what the object was, but he could not make the connection – quite understandably, because the connection had been cut. Then the researcher left the room for a moment, and a video camera caught the subject moving the toothbrush deftly up to his left ear (connected directly to the left, or intellectual, hemisphere without the normal crossover that most brain inputs and outputs make either at the decussation of the pyramids or the optic chiasm). The moment he heard the sound made by brushing the bristles, he triumphantly identified the object.

## The Ventricles

The ventricles are spaces within the brain filled with cerebrospinal fluid. They perform at least three distinct functions.

The lateral ventricles are situated where they can act as oblique stabilizers and stiffeners in precisely the area of the brain that is the most unsupported – the central mass of the hemispheres, midway between the reinforcements of the falx and tentorium. They are the site for the majority of cerebrospinal fluid production, and the hydrostatic stiffness imparted by the fluid helps to brace the brain tissue. They also permit the conduction of heat out of deep core of the hemispheres, thus helping to cool them, as the cerebrospinal fluid leaves the core of the brain and proceeds to radiate its burden of heat by way of the subarachnoid space covering the external surfaces of the hemispheres.

In a study of fifteen identical twins[57,58] of which one was classified "normal" and the other as schizophrenic, fourteen of the schizophrenic twins had larger ventricles than their normal twin.

The third and fourth ventricles, while not placed strategically to provide stiffness, perform otherwise identical functions. They are midline structures, arranged like aircraft flying in air-to-air refueling formation (the third ventricle superior and anterior to the fourth). And, as in air-to-air refueling, they are connected by a fluid-filled tube, the aqueduct of Sylvius.

The third ventricle neatly splits the thalamus and hypothalamus in two. Viewed from the side, it looks like the head of a bird, beak poised to swallow the optic chiasm. The fourth ventricle is located anterior to the cerebellum, between it and the medulla oblongata. Sutherland called it "lozenge-shaped," a description that puzzled me until I arranged the "lozenge" vertically – like an upright, slightly elongated diamond.

Just above the optic chiasm lies the supraoptic nucleus. This, according to research on hapless hamsters,[59] is the location of the brain's central timekeeper.[60,61]

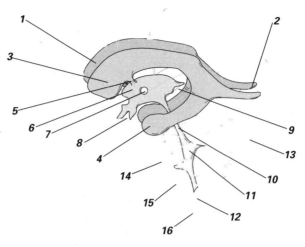

## The Diencephalon

Literally, diencephalon means "between the brain." It refers to all the structures that bound the third ventricle – the thalamus, hypothalamus, epithalamus, and subthalamus.

### The Thalamus

The thalamus, located in the center of the forebrain, is composed of multiple small (gray matter) nuclei. It rests on top of the mesencephalon (midbrain). The rest of the cerebrum, and especially the cortex, can be considered an extension of the thalamus' need for greater functioning capacity and memory storage. Before the hemispheres were, thalamus was. It is a crude analogy, but it might be helpful to think of the cortex as the thalamus' hard disk.

The thalamus initiates wakefulness and makes the preliminary classification of incoming information. It is the central switching station that directs information, both coming into the brain (afferent) and leaving the brain (efferent), working in very close coordination with the limbic system and basal ganglia. All somesthetic, visual,[23] auditory, and motor signals pass through it on their way to target destinations. All the incoming signals from the cord pass from the basal ganglia into the thalamus before being directed to appropriate areas of the cortex. Without the thalamus, the cortex is useless – the thalamus drives the cortex into activity.

### The Hypothalamus

The hypothalamus (meaning "below the thalamus") seems to be the place in the brain where our sense of identity resides. It could be considered "the brain of the brain." In directed energy cranio-

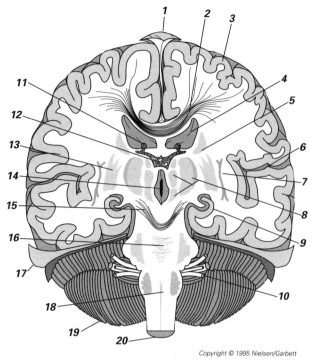

Coronal section of brain and cord

**1** *Falx cerebri*
**2** *Corpus callosum*
**3** *Cerebral cortex*
**4** *Left lateral ventricle*
**5** *Caudate nucleus*
**6** *Sylvian fissure*
**7** *Basal ganglia*
**8** *Thalamus*
**9** *Hippo-campus*
**10** *Cranial nerves*
**11** *Choroid plexus*
**12** *Foramen of Monroe*
**13** *Putamen*
**14** *Third ventricle*
**15** *Substantia nigra*
**16** *Pons*
**17** *Tentorium cerebelli*
**18** *Medulla oblongata*
**19** *Cerebellum*
**20** *Spinal cord*

sacral work, one sometimes points straight at the hypothalamus through the acupuncture point Middle of Man (Governor Vessel 26) – and the client feels that one is pointing straight at his secret core. The hypothalamus lies anterior and inferior to the thalamus, and also anterior to the red nucleus, and the mammillary bodies. It is located just superior and slightly posterior to the body of the sphenoid. The pituitary stalk runs superior and slightly posterior from the sella turcica to the hypothalamus.

The hypothalamus controls internal bodily functions and stimulates the autonomic nervous system. It is light- and pressure-sensitive. Medical students have a mnemonic for remembering hypothalamus functions as the "four Fs": fighting, fleeing, feasting, and sexual reproduction.

The hypothalamus is a central regulator for the following functions:

- Temperature
- Blood pressure
- Heart rate
- Blood sugar level
- Sexual arousal
- Fat metabolism
- Hunger/satiety
- Drinking/water balance
- Sleeping
- Balance in the autonomic nervous system
- Sense of well-being
- Carbohydrate metabolism
- Protein metabolism
- Emotional reactions essential for survival

### The Epithalamus

The epithalamus includes the pineal gland, which is situated posterior and inferior to the thalamus, at the posterior-most margin of the third ventricle. It forms the little lump of brain matter just superior to the superior colliculus.

The pineal gland is sensitive to light,[62] especially to seasonal changes in light, as well as to electromagnetic fields. It is sometimes called "the body's light meter." It also seems to exert homeostatic effects that are largely unknown, but may turn out to be mediated by melatonin, which some endocrinologists describe as our most powerful hormone. Melatonin is released in the late afternoon, and sets the hormonal foundation for sleep[63] some hours later. Thus, to avoid jet lag, air travelers are encouraged to expose themselves to afternoon sun upon arrival, to hasten the recalibration of their biological clocks. The pineal also acts to inhibit the onset of sexual maturity.

Jacob Liberman[64] has done extensive work on the use of light in healing. One facet of his work is the use of light to access unresolved emotional trauma. Yogic texts[65,66] ascribe aspects of higher consciousness to the pineal, including a role in the functioning of the inner eye.

### The Subthalamus

The subthalamus acts in concert with the basal ganglia to help regulate subconscious muscular activity.

## The Limbic System

The limbic system is known as "the mammalian brain" due to its specializations and commonality to all mammals. "Limbic" means "out on a limb" – that is, it is not part of the main "trunk" of the brainstem and thalamus. The limbic system is a border structure within the cerebrum – it borders, or surrounds, the thalamus and hypothalamus, with which it is closely associated. The limbic system is composed of the amygdala, claustrum, hippocampus, mammillary bodies, septum pellucidum, and basal ganglia.

The limbic system allows us to modify our behavior for different social occasions, control our temper, affect our own autonomic nervous system, and helps determine our mood and state of wakefulness. In other words, the limbic system gives us some degree of conscious control over behavior. It is where we interpret pain, in concert with the somesthetic part of the parietal cortex. Below a certain threshold of pain there is little limbic system involvement, such as when physical pain is described as "clean" or "just stretch pain." This is the "good pain" felt in deep tissue work such as Rolfing. When more severe, with sensations like nausea and deeper feelings such as terror creeping in, pain is described as "sickening" and "too much to bear." This level of pain means that the limbic system, which combines intellect and awareness of the body with our emotions, is involved. The limbic system has the ability to modify the hypothalamic functions, the "four Fs." It is one of the places where we can "rise above" our pain.

### The Amygdala

The amygdala (derived from the Latin for "almond"), located at the tip of the tail of the caudate nucleus, functions as part of the limbic system, sensing[67] and modifying social behavior to make it appropriate. More than any other area, it may be the place in the brain where emotions and intelligence are combined.[68,69] The amygdala also associates olfactory stimuli with stimuli from other parts of the brain.

The amygdala is called "the window through which the limbic system sees the world." It is intimately associated with tonic movements (such as raising the head, moving the body, circling) and occasionally with clonic (alternate or rhythmic contracting and relaxing of muscle tissue) movement.

### The Hippocampus

The hippocampus (Latin for "seahorse") interprets the importance of sensory information for the brain, and decides what is important enough (and interesting, fun, or euphoric enough) for long-term storage in the cortex. It places eligible new information into storage as memories,[70] and helps organize retrieval systems for the information by cross-associating and "contextualizing" the information with flags such as scents, emotions, and images.[71]

If the hippocampus is surgically removed,[72,73] or destroyed by a tumor, a person may still learn a new skill, such as hanggliding. But if you sit down for tea with him after he has become an expert hangglider pilot and ask him who taught him, and where he learned, and in what year, he will have no conscious memory of any of those facts. The hippocampus seems to play an important part in the loss of short-term memory that sometimes occurs with old age.

### The Mammillary Bodies

The mammillary bodies are two aggranulations of gray matter the size and shape of a pea, located immediately posterior to the hypothalamus, and anterior to the red nucleus and the exit of the occulomotor nerve from the mesencephalon. The mammillary bodies help regulate our wakefulness, and our sense of well-being. They are the target structure in directed energy work through the acupuncture point Ear Gate (Triple Warmer 21).

### Septum Pellucidum

Together with other discrete areas of the limbic system, this structure controls rage and mediates between conscious and unconscious levels of bodily activity. When we lose our temper, the septum pellucidum has lost its control over our social behavior and we have reverted to hypothalamic or cerebellar "fighting" functioning.

### The Basal Ganglia

The lateral parts of the basal ganglia are lateral to the internal capsule, which is itself lateral to the thalamus. The basal ganglia in particular need to be located so close to the limbic system because of their mutual and immediate coordination with, and connection to, the cerebral cortex.

Messages from lower brain centers, such as the pons and cerebellum, and the spinal cord pass directly to the basal ganglia, and from there go to the thalamus for directing to the appropriate areas of the cerebral cortex. The basal ganglia work in very close association with the subthalamus, substantia negra, and red nucleus.

They are particularly concerned in initiating movement, and in movement control in general, performing the background (gross body) movement control. Acting upon this robust foundation, the motor and premotor cortex fire signals that allow us to perform fine, dexterous movements (without this finessing from the cerebral cortex, we can only make crude, stiff-legged movements).

## The Internal Capsule

The internal capsule is the principle pathway of nerve fibers from the cerebral cortex to the lower regions of the brain and spinal cord. Many of its fibers originate in the premotor and motor cortex, from which they send information to be processed in the basal ganglia before being sent down the spinal cord to the body. The internal capsule is located between the basal ganglia and the cerebral cortex.

## The Midbrain (Mesencephalon)

The mesencephalon is a minute portion of the brain that connects many brain stem nuclei with each other and with the diencephalon. It coordinates movements, including control of most of the muscles concerned with eye movement, serves as a relay system, and analyzes the body's reaction to pain. The reticular activating system, extending upward from the spinal cord to the diencephalon,

Brain, cord and filum terminale

1 Superior sagittal sinus
2 Subarachnoid space
3 Corpus callosum
4 Pineal gland
5 Straight sinus
6 Cerebellum
7 Right lateral ventricle (part of)
8 Interthalamic adhesion
9 Third ventricle
10 Suprachiasmic nucleus
11 Optic chiasm
12 Pituitary
13 Mamillary body
14 Pons
15 Medulla oblongata
16 Spinal cord
17 Central canal of spinal cord
18 Spinal subarachnoid space
19 Lumbar enlargement
20 Conus medullaris
21 Cauda equina
22 Termination of spinal dura at second sacral segment
23 Filum terminale

passing through the medulla, pons, and mesencephalon on the way, controls many stereotyped movements; it helps determine the brain's basic activity level by filtering out, or letting through, incoming sensations. It actually excludes almost all incoming information – filtering down to a level that permits only one in a billion units of information through to higher brain levels. Many widely used substances, such as caffeine and nicotine, act on the reticular activating system to allow more information through; we feel more alert, but we also begin to become hyperactive, for which we pay a price in lost equanimity.

The midbrain contains the corticospinal and corticopontine fibers, which conduct motor signals from the cerebral cortex to the pon and spinal cord. The substantia negra ("darkly pigmented substance," the tissue that is destroyed in Parkinson's disease) controls subconscious fine muscular activity in the body.

Serotonin is the "Mr. Big" of the neurotransmitters. It helps regulate cognition, mood, and appetite (Prozac is a serotonin enhancer). It also balances the volume of information flow through the reticular activating system. Eighty percent of our serotonin is produced in the median and dorsal raphe, which are located at the junction of the spinal cord and brain, in the mesencephalon.

## The Brain Stem

The brain stem evolved more than 500 million years ago. It contains the mesencephalon, the pons, the medulla oblongata, the fourth ventricle, the olivary bodies, the decussation of the pyramids, and the pyramidal tracts. The brain stem is another structure that helps determine our level of awareness, warning us of vital incoming messages from our sensory apparatus as it passes through the reticular activating system. It is concerned with the management of basic bodily functions, especially the absolute essentials of respiration, arterial pressure and the sleep-waking cycle.[74,75]

## The Pons

The pons is located immediately inferior to the midbrain, between the cerebellum and the sphenobasilar joint, on the superior surface of which it rests. The pronounced convexity on the anterior surface of the pons causes the scalloped "bobsled run" curvature on the dorsum sellae (the posterior portion of the sella turcica) of the sphenoid and the superior part of basilar portion of the occiput. The reticular activating system runs through the pons, passing very close to the nucleus of the fifth cranial nerve, the trigeminus, a fact that explains aspects of both muscle contraction headache and temporomandibular joint dysfunction.[76]

Containing the nuclei for the fifth, sixth, seventh, and eighth cranial nerves, the pons performs a central role in eye and facial movements, hearing, and balance. The pons also affects arterial pressure and respiration rate.

## The Medulla Oblongata

The medulla oblongata controls vasodilation and vasocontraction, and also contains the same nerve cells that affect arterial pressure, heart activity, and respiration as does the pons – facts that explain why a CV4, which can change the level of electrical activity of these brain structures, can quickly relieve muscle contraction or migraine headache, and may work with cluster headache. It contains the nuclei for the ninth, tenth, eleventh, and twelfth cranial nerves, as well as the decussation of the pyramids (where the nerve fibers from the left hemisphere cross over to the right side of the spinal cord, and vice versa).

The medulla helps cause the scalloped contour on the superior aspect of the basilar portion of the occiput. It extends into the mouth of the foramen magnum, which helps explain why trauma to the atlanto-occipital area can so easily be fatal – the area encloses not simply spinal cord, but vital brain tissue. This is why hanging, as capital punishment, is so immediately effective.

The pyramids, which help control muscle contractions and tone throughout the body, are also contained in the medulla. We are targeting the pyramids when we vector energy to the brainstem with a CV4 with the intention of obtaining a "rolling wave" whole-body relaxation response. (This delicious phenomenon occurs when the pyramids recalibrate, and release a heightened muscle tonus throughout the body. The client experiences a wave of relaxation spreading down the body, as if his body were a Persian carpet being flicked in the air for dusting.) The olivary bodies,[77] another specialized part of the medulla, act as a relay station, sending incoming messages to and from the basal ganglia, cerebral cortex, and cerebellum.

## The Cerebellum

The cerebellum has tripled in size in the past million years. It has its own cortex, ¼-inch (6 millimeters) thick, and has some 30 billion nerve cells, compared to the 100 billion nerve cells of the cerebral cortex. Its vermis, a midline structure ¾-inch (1.9 centimeters) wide, coordinates stereotyped and subconscious movements. The cerebellar hemispheres coordinate voluntary movements with the cortex, in particular slowing outgoing motor impulses for a short fraction of a second, thus per-

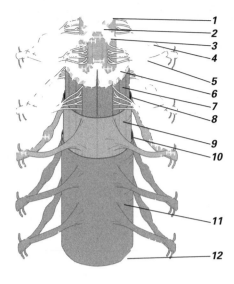

*Spinal cord, spinal nerves and meninges*

**1** *Dorsal horn*
**2** *Gray matter of cord*
**3** *Ventral horn*
**4** *Dorsal spinal nerve root*
**5** *Ventral spinal nerve root*
**6** *White matter of cord*
**7** *Pia mater*
**8** *Subarachnoid space*
**9** *Arachnoid*
**10** *Subdural space*
**11** *Dura*
**12** *Epidural space*

mitting us graceful motion.[78] If the cerebellum is destroyed, sequential and graceful motion becomes impossible.

Tentorium cerebelli means "little brain tent," and the cerebellum lies immediately inferior to its cover. The shape of the superior surface of the cerebellum, like a very shallow, scalloped roof, is the shape of the inferior surface of the tentorium, which separates the cerebellum from the cerebral hemispheres.

The cerebellum shapes the occipital squama, and the squama shapes the cerebellum. The partition of the falx cerebelli runs inferiorly from the straight sinus to the foramen magnum, helping cause the slight midline "waisting" of the cerebellum. The bulbous, miniature apple-shape of the cerebellum pushes into the occipital squama and causes it to become translucently thin in the areas lateral to the denser bone of the falx attachment and inferior to the tentorial attachments.

## The Spinal Cord

The spinal cord begins immediately inferior to the foramen magnum and ends at the level of the second lumbar vertebra. It ends there because it has ceased to keep pace with the lengthening of the rest of the body in utero, a development that has been accentuated by our doubling of adult body size in the past 3 million years.

The spatial relationship of gray and white matter is reversed from the hemispheres; in other words, unlike the brain where gray matter is on the outside, in the cord the gray matter lies at the center. So in the cord the delicate gray matter is enveloped by the more protected and robust myelin-sheathed nerves that make up white matter.

## A Summary of Brain and Spinal Cord Function

| Main level of neuronal function | Specific area | Neuronal function |
|---|---|---|
| **The cortex and higher brain levels** | Thalamus | Receives and relays all sensory input (except olfactory) and processes primary levels of sensations of pain, crude touch, and temperature |
| **The brainstem and midbrain** | Limbic system and thalamus | Subconscious body maintenance |
| | Reticular activating substance of medulla and pons | Arterial pressure |
| | Cerebral cortex, cerebellum and reticular activating substance, medulla, pons, and midbrain | Equilibrium, balance, and voluntary motor coordination |
| | The reticular activating system, basal ganglia, thalamus, hypothalamus | Wakefulness |
| | The limbic system, central segmental pathway and peri-aqueductal gray matter, opiate receptors in the spinal cord, endomorphins from diffuse areas of the brain | Pain control |
| | Hypothalamus | Rage, excitement, pain, pleasure, and homeostatic control |
| | Basal ganglia, cerebellum | Coordination of subconscious motor responses |
| | Thalamus | Basic perception of sensations, and the activation of the cerebral cortex |
| **The spinal cord** | | Relays ascending and descending impulses and handles the local reflex arcs, and damps pain messages via opiate receptors |
| **Components of movement control within the central nervous system** | | Cerebral cortex (telencephalon) |
| | | Basal ganglia (part of cerebrum) |
| | | Thalamus and subthalamus (diencephalon) |
| | | Red nucleus and substantia negra (mesencephalon) |
| | | Cerebellum (rhombencephalon) |
| | | Spinal cord |

Spinal cord white matter is composed of fiber tracts and glial cells ("astrocytes," meaning "little stars"[54,79]). Spinal cord gray matter is made up of nerve cell bodies and their axons, and synapses that relay signals between periphery and brain. The neurons are embedded in a matrix of glial cells. As looked at from above, the gray matter forms a shape reminiscent of four horns connected by a central, ovoid body, which is called the gray commissure. The anterior horn, or commissure, contains the motor fibers, the posterior the sensory. The spinal cord has a large number of opiate receptors, which act by reducing the release of pain emitter substances. Damage[80] to the opiate receptors in illness often leads to permanent and untreatable pain.

The spinal cord also contains vital reflex arcs that allow us to move our hands away from a hot dinner plate long before the brain knows what the arms are doing.

The spinal cord contains a central canal less than 1/24-inch (1 millimeter) in diameter. It contains upward-facing villi that waft cerebrospinal fluid cephalad. The villi are reported to degenerate between puberty and middle age.

# THE BONES

# 21
# Introduction to the Techniques

## Presentation of the Techniques

Each of the following chapters on an individual bone is laid out in a specific sequence designed to facilitate information flow and cross-referencing. Only the sacrum chapter has prone and side-lying techniques, and within it they appear in that order before the supine techniques. Within all the bone chapters (in the sacrum chapter, in each section – prone, side-lying, and supine), muscle techniques appear before bone (osseous) techniques. An index of all the techniques appears at the end of the book for ready referencing.

The discussion below provides an overview on session preparations and protocol, including important guidelines for oral work.

## Preparations

### Medical History

Begin by asking about related medical history, and whether the client has ever suffered a concussion, been knocked out, or been in a coma. Ascertain if he has broken any bones in his pelvis, spine, or head, or had brain surgery of any description. Cover the possibility of him being at high risk of stroke by gauging his general level of health, and noting his tissue tone. How is his blood pressure? Cover the possibility that he may have a brain tumor by asking if he has had any loss of nervous or hormonal system function, such as a loss of the sense of smell, balance, or any loss of sensitivity on his face or head. Persistent headaches, especially when they occur at night or upon awakening, are also indicative of possible tumor formation.[1]

Do not use a CV4, or any other compressive technique with clients at risk of stroke, with very elevated blood pressure, or who have a brain tumor.

Ask the client, "Is there anything else I need to know about?" – which allows him to tell you things you have not directly asked. For example, he may be diabetic, or suffer from epileptic seizures. These are not reasons to decline to treat the client; rather, they are conditions you need to be aware of in case symptoms or complications manifest during the session.

### Clothing and Jewelry

Jewelry, belts, denim or tight clothing, and contact lenses are best removed, if the client is comfortable doing so. There is no need to remove any other clothing except turtlenecks, which get in the way of occipital and temporal techniques. Make sure the client is, and will continue to be, warm enough.

### Supplies

See that you have massage lotion, examination gloves (see below), children's books (for parents to read to restless children), an audio system (to mask irritating extraneous noise that you can do nothing else about), a notebook for nagging thoughts, a case-history sheet, and a glass of water for yourself. Turn off the telephone, and put a "Do Not Disturb" sign on the door.

## Types of Techniques

Individual techniques may be unilateral, such as the Wrist and Elbow Corrections of the Spheno-basilar Joint, which you perform on one side of the body only. Others are one-side-at-a-time techniques, such as the Temporal Cross-Check, in which case the technique is usually described only from the left side and it is up to the practitioner to discern whether it is necessary to repeat it on the other side. Most of the techniques are bilateral, in which case you stay with the contact until it is effective or you recognize that it is not going to be. These differences are usually apparent from the description. What matters is feel – that the technique feels right to you and the client both, and that it feels effective. It is also important that the technique gives you sufficient sensitivity to track nuances in cranial wave formation as you begin to engage the cranial mechanism.

## Choosing Techniques and Client Empowerments

If a client has no symptoms, is clear mentally, and has a good energy level, there is no need for any interventionist craniosacral work. Instead, use directed energy, decompressions, and gentle balancing techniques. Should the client have symptoms, or be complaining of mental confusion or a low energy level, a deeper level of craniosacral work is warranted.

It is wise before touching the client to make sure he understands his role in the session. Consider giving three empowerments by saying:

■ "Please let me know if anything I do creates sharp pain." (Explain that there may be some feelings of stretch pain, but this should not be in any way alarming and should feel like "good" pain.)

■ "Please let me know if you have a strong emotion welling up that you do not feel comfortable staying with during this session."

■ "Please let me know if you have an alarming mental image, especially one that is persistent, such as the picture of a bone breaking, or you laying sick in a hospital bed."

## Client Position on the Table

All craniosacral techniques presented here are with the client laying supine on the table, except the sacrum techniques in sections labeled prone and side-lying techniques.

We gain better access to the client's head if it is further down the table than in other forms of bodywork. The optimum is established by laying your complete forearms, elbows included, on the table surface and then positioning your client so that the place where his occiput touches the table (as he lies supine) is level with your palms. This usually

results in the crown of his head being 8 to 12 inches (20 to 30 centimeters) from the top of the table.

When the client is prone, it helps to place a pillow under his ankles; when supine, under his knees. Consider having a chair with pillows on either side of the table so that you can bring the client's arms out to his sides – a valuable alternative arm position during a long session, one that helps open the channel of the spiritual heart all the way down to the fingertips.

## Posture and Body Use

To perform a technique correctly requires appropriate body use; this means ease and comfort for the healer and support and stability that makes the technique comfortable for the client. I have indicated with each technique where to stand or sit in relationship to the client on the table – these are guidelines based upon what I have found most useful. They may not work for you. Getting comfortable and having your body adequately supported may mean kneeling rather than sitting, or for a standing posture it may mean placing one knee or foot up on the table.

In taking up a contact, remember that the nondominant hand tends to be the more sensitive, the dominant the better for action.

Once I have taken up a contact, I find myself relaxing my hands in stages. When I first assume a position, my hand and forearm tend to have tension from the effort to establish a satisfactory hold. So once I have a good contact, I get myself comfortable, then relax my hand. Then, a minute or two later, I relax it even further. I find that a third conscious decision to relax gives total relaxation. A tense hand blocks information flow and becomes insensitive quickly. Use these relaxation commands for all techniques.

## Technique Pressure and Duration

I have not assigned a specific pressure value for touch in most of the techniques. This is because I have found, in teaching, that it is of little positive value to do so – tell someone to apply ⅕ ounce (5.6 grams) of pressure and, with the exception of physicists and gourmet cooks, most people have no idea how much pressure that means. Further, it may create trouble by placing a given textbook value before your own sensitivity to the client.

It is extremely important that you stay sensitive to how much pressure you are using when working on the head. In general, it can be said that craniosacral techniques involve much lighter touch, held for much longer, than beginners expect. When working with those who have had severe impact injury to the head, such as dashboard impacts in automobile collisions, stronger decompressive traction may be needed. But even in these cases, maintain sensitivity to the cranial wave formations.

Check with the client how your touch feels, and keep checking until you have gained enough experience that you can recognize when something is amiss, not responding normally to your touch.

Contact is taken up slowly and carefully, and also ended extremely slowly. (No single thing makes touch feel quite so reverential as the slowness with which you end it.) If in doubt, use a lighter touch. It is amazing how much how little will do. While reducing pressure is very often the secret to craniosacral work, there is another key element: the clarity of the healer's intention is every bit as important as the appropriateness of her pressure.

## Oral Work

It is important to explain to the client at the start of the session why you want to work in his mouth, and then ask his permission to do so as this is a private and energetically loaded area often carrying archaic wounds. Children often experience dentists as people to be frightened of, so any therapy that approaches their mouths has understandable negative associations. Oral work in adult clients may bring back the memory of dental trauma. There is also the possibility that the client experienced oral sexual abuse to consider – one present-day American study suggests that childhood sexual abuse happens to some 33 percent of young women.[2]

Contesting this figure as too high, other authorities say the actual incidence is lower.[3,4]

### *Examination Gloves*

The use of latex examination gloves is mandatory for all oral techniques (vinyl gloves are not adequate). The skin of your hands is regarded as always being broken, even if you have no visible abrasion (under a microscope, cuts become visible). Gloves are also expected in today's concerned climate.

Practice with gloves on to the point that you can overcome the inevitable loss of palpatory sensitivity that their use engenders. Wear the largest size glove you are comfortable with. If you cannot get large enough gloves, it sometimes helps your sensitivity to cut open the back of the gloves to about the level of the knuckles, so that they exert less pressure on your hands. As this does not expose areas where you will make contact, it does not affect the gloves' function as barrier agents, and may greatly enhance your effectiveness.

Mint-flavored gloves are slightly more agreeable to many clients than plain latex, and are worth locating. (The client tends to salivate more with mint gloves than with the unflavored variety, a problem in some dental procedures, but not in craniosacral work.) Washing off powder residues also improves the taste of latex.

### *Protocol*

If you have a choice, it is usually best to use your dominant hand inside the mouth. There are various ways to facilitate graceful technique. For example, ask the client to lick his lips before introducing your fingers, and enter the mouth by gliding along the biting surface of the teeth before moving medially or laterally. If more than one finger has oral placement, introduce your fingers one at a time.

### *Dentures*

Ideally, the client should remove his dentures before oral craniosacral work. Be discreet and tactful in asking, and if removing them would be an embarrassment to the client, you may find it better to allow him to keep them in until such a time that he feels comfortable removing them. (You cannot help a client who becomes so embarrassed that he never comes back.) The same applies to partial dentures, and removable orthodontic appliances – if possible, have the client remove them for the session. It is usually pointless to work on the maxillae or mandible with dentures in place.

## A Review: Coning-in and Assessment Immediately Before Touching

### *Coning-in*

- Wipe the slate clean before each session.
- Begin by standing at least 6½ feet (2 meters) away from your client.
- Take your space.
- Move to your expanded state: stand back, take a deep breath, open.
- Wait. Wait for your dust to settle. Wait for the client's mandala to come in.
- While breathing, circulate the light and deepen your stillness.

### *Assessment*

When you have the mandala, begin to look at its aspects, such as the client's posture and energy, with soft-focus, wide-angle vision. See the dorsal, ventral, and lateral aspects of his form – whatever you need to see the whole picture. Notice what changes occur in your consciousness while you begin to engage him so. Sense the space he takes up, his "energetic weight," his presence. Pay special attention to the head/neck/jaw/back lines in terms of what they tell you about his cranium's "aspiration content." Assess the client's chief characteristic, then begin an assessment of his energy and motility patterns. Finally, match the technique to the client or, better still, allow the information you have gathered about the client to create an entirely new technique.

## During the Session

During the session, move the client's hand and arm position every ten or fifteen minutes to avoid ulnar nerve numbness, which can be alarming to clients who do not understand that it can be brought on simply by the pressure of an elbow held at a right angle on the table surface. You will feel more cranial wave movement with the client's hands placed somewhere on his body, rather than on the table surface. (Solid surfaces tend to damp the wave, motile ones to amplify it.)

## Referrals

At the end of each bone chapter I present an itemization of other techniques. Besides craniosacral techniques, it provides a listing of other professional skills that I have found to be efficacious (it is by no means an exhaustive itemization of every possible alternative). Having a list of other professionals to refer one's clients to is an essential adjunct to practice. I keep a list of both male and female practitioners in every specialty, because matching another practitioner to your client may mean considering whether the client would work better with a man or a woman.

In deciding who to refer a client to, I tune in to the quality of the individual practitioner, which is much more important to me than whatever particular modality he may specialize in. Then I match the client to the practitioner, sensing their rightness for each other. In his introduction to The Secret of the Golden Flower, C.G. Jung[5] notes that when the "right man" makes use of the "wrong method," he finds a way to make it work, and work well; when the "wrong man" makes use of the "right method," nothing good comes of it at all. Thus, it is my experience that all professional skills are "right methods," no matter how disparate – whether surgery, astrology, or homeopathy – but that one has to search out the "right" practitioners.

# 22
# The Sacrum

**1** Dorsal surface

**2** Pelvic, ventral or anterior surface

**3** Sacral base, contact surface with L5-S1 intervertebral disc

**4** Superior articular process

**5** Lateral part, evolved from rudiments of transverse processes and ribs

**6** Articular surface, (L. facies auricularis, or ear-like facets) for articulation with iliac portion of coxal bone, together composing the sacroiliac joint

**7** Pelvic sacral foramina, points of exit for ventral nerve branches that are part of the sciatic nerve (L4-S3)

**8** Transverse lines, marking anterior fusion lines of five sacral segments

**9** Dorsal sacral foramina, for dorsal division of sensory and motor sacral nerves, and sensory middle clunial nerves (S1-3)

**10** Median sacral crest, a series of rudimentary spinous processes

**11** Lateral sacral crest, a series of rudimentary transverse processes

**12** Cornu, or little horn of sacrum, rudimentary articular facet for discontinued human tail

**13** Sacral canal with spinal dura attachment at second segment

**14** Sacral hiatus, aperture of the sacral canal which usually begins at level of third or fourth sacral segment

**15** Apex of sacrum

**16** Coccyx, usually composed of four vestigial vertebrae

**17** Cornu of coccyx, rudimentary articular process

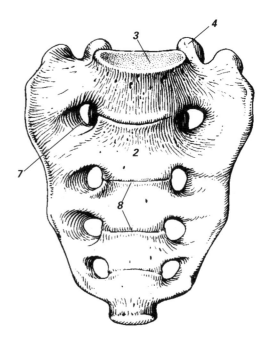

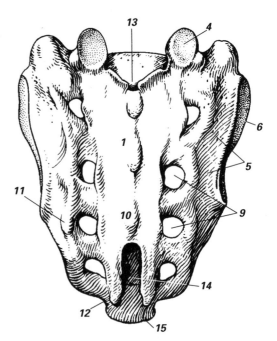

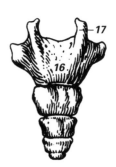

The sacrum is one of the best places to start a study of the cranial mechanism. It is, after all, the foundation. The sacrum plays a crucial role in many aspects of anatomy, physiology, body language energetics, and spirituality.

## Embryology and Osteology

The sacrum is composed of five fused vertebrae, each having seven centers of ossification, to give a total of thirty-five centers of ossification. Eight weeks after conception, ossification of the central part of the bodies of the upper three sacral vertebrae commences, followed shortly by the remaining two. The sacral vertebral segments normally fuse on their external surfaces between the twentieth and twenty-fifth year, when growth finally terminates. The segmental fusion lines are clearly visible on the anterior surface of the adult sacrum, where they are called the transverse ridges.

The symphysis pubis, one of the pelvic joint structures that profoundly affects and modifies the sacrum's motion, changes in texture and shape as a person gets older. It is usually fused by the age of seventy.

## Anatomy

The sacrum is a hand-sized biconcave bone, triangular in shape and complex in nature. It is located at the base of the spine, where it lies wedged between the ilia. The coccyx is located at the apex of the sacrum, and the fifth lumbar vertebra articulates at the sacral base. The sacroiliac joints form the articulations between the lateral aspects of the first, second, and upper portions of the third sacral segments and the ilia.

### Structure

The coccyx is typically composed of four rudimentary vertebrae and represents the vestigial human tail. The coccyx functions best when it articulates with the sacrum at a modest angle,[2] which does not impinge into the urogenital space and leaves adequate room for the rectum. This ensures easy anterior and posterior motion, and limited flexibility in all planes of motion.

In rare cases the tail that is visible during the fourth to sixth weeks of embryonic growth is not reabsorbed. It continues to grow, keeping pace with its cousins the vertebrae, and is still intact at birth. English midwife friends of mine were taught to snip it off immediately and slip it out of sight,

before the mother saw the child. (In medieval times, the presence of the tail was taken as a sign of the devil, and the mother and child sometimes put to death because of it.) The cutting off of the tail may take with it several coccygeal segments – sometimes only the first coccygeal segment remains. One client remembered her frustrated mother saying, while she was pranking around at eight years of age, "I always knew you were a little monkey, because when you were born you had a tail!" She always thought her mother had been joking, but the scar and the vestige of the coccyx proved it to be the truth.

The sacrum, composed of five fused vertebrae, is one of the strongest bones in the body. Cortical and cancellous bone makes up the vestigial vertebral bodies, which have thin remnants of intervertebral discs between them, often throughout life. You can introduce a probe in sagittally-sectioned cadaver sacrums and discover that the disc space is $\frac{1}{16}$-inch (1.5 millimeters) in thickness, even in the elderly. The "discs" lend extra flexibility – and therefore strength – to the sacrum and increase the shock-absorbing capabilities of the spinal column.

## Location

The sacrum is located at the base of the spine, between the ilia, the superior part of the coxal bones. It lies anterior and inferior to the posterosuperior iliac spines and sits wedged between the ilia like an arrowhead lodged point-down into a tree stump. The coccyx extends inferiorly to within $\frac{1}{2}$-inch (1.3 centimeter) of the anus.

### Landmarks

The cardinal visual and palpable landmarks of the sacrum are as follows:

- Sacral dimples at the level of the first sacral segment
- The prominences of the posteroinferior spines, which landmark the lateral borders of the sacrum
- The median crest, visible in those with minimal subcutaneous fat
- The gluteal crease, which hides the location of the coccyx, just superior to the anus
- The cornu, or "little horns," which look somewhat like the clinoid processes of the sphenoid

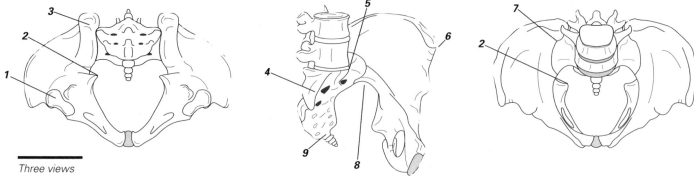

## Sutures and Articulations

The sacrum has two amphiarthrotic (slightly moving) joints with the ilia until age 40 in men and 50 in women, when it is regarded as having virtually ankylosed,[3,4] or fused,[5] with the ilia.[6] At the sacral base it has an intervertebral disc articulation with the fifth lumbar vertebra, and at its fifth segment a cartilaginous articulation with the coccyx.

The sacrum articulates with four bones:

- Both ilia
- The fifth lumbar vertebra
- The coccyx

## Weight

A medically prepared and disarticulated male sacrum weighs 3 ounces (85 grams) and a female sacrum 2½ ounces (68 grams). The male sacrum typically weighs more because it is denser and the male body larger; however, the female sacrum is broader.[7]

## Detailed Anatomy and Musculature

What were heretofore described as the innominates are now referred to as the coxal bones. The coxals are divided into three parts: the wings of the ilia, the bodies of the ischia, and the pubic bones.

The sacrum presents a foundation, or base, for the fifth lumbar disc to sit upon, known as "the base plane." Its angle is crucial in the complete analysis of low-back pain or dysfunction; an anteroposterior slope not exceeding 30 percent is desirable. Note how far posterior the final sacral segment protrudes. Get a sense of the typical position of the coccyx itself; it is usually located farther anterior than you would expect, making an acute angle with the fifth sacral segment. This acute angle, usually first caused by a fall, then exacerbated by perineal muscular hypertonicity, is a common finding in a musculoskeletal condition known as coccydynia, pain and dysfunction in the coccyx.

### *Musculature*

The muscles attaching to the sacrum consist of three specific groups.

On its anterior surface:

- Levator ani group
- Piriformis
- Coccygeus

On its lateral surface:

- Gluteus maximus

On its posterior surface:

- Iliocostalis
- Longissimus
- Multifidus
- Erector spinae
- Latissimus dorsi
- Longus and brevis rotatores

## Physiology

The sacrum is wedged between the ilia by the considerable dynamic forces of the bipedal[8] or "orthograde" posture. This is where the arrowhead is lodged in the wood. The more overweight the person, the more forcible the wedging.

## Axis of Rotation

The classical axis of rotation is across the transverse axis of the second sacral segment,[9,10,11] which is also the attachment of the dura. This is the "south pole" of the spinal portion of the reciprocal tension membrane.

## Motion

The sacrum acts as a differential to accommodate the differences in motion of the surrounding structures. That is, it gives and takes substantially, particularly before the age of 50, or longer in the healthy subject. As with any oscillating structure, in the classical model it is said to move around an axis, or in the sacrum's case, a faint vertical axis; however, in the liquid-electric model the sacrum's dominant motion is around a large, imaginary fully-floating sphere. Where these axes intersect lies a theoretical spot called the "point of resolution" of sacral motion. Optimum movement around this point of resolution is the healer's objective in the classical model: the balanced sacrum.

Both mobile (the whole sacrum moving in relationship to the coxal bones) and motile (the sacrum changing its shape in response to changes in outside forces and the cranial wave), the sacrum is moved externally by almost any leg, low-back, or hip movement, which is known as its "mechanical activity." It also moves within the pelvic girdle, and in upon itself, under the influence of the "core link" (see below). Not only does the sacrum move around compound transverse and vertical axes in the classical model, and changes its internal density with core-link oscillations, it is also capable of moving around the strong ligaments along its L-shaped auricular (Latin: ear-shaped) sacroiliac surfaces.[12,13]

### Osteopathic Model

In the osteopathic model (similar-motion model), the action of the spinal dura, which pulls superiorly on the anterior lip of the sacral canal during flexion, causes the sacrum to swing about its horizontal axis. This moves the sacral apex into the true pelvis (in women, the location of the birth canal) in flexion. Both sides of the sacrum move synchronously. The movement of the sacrum, according to Sutherland's classical model (see The Core Link, below), transmits motion to the occiput and vice versa. The movement of the sacrum imitates that of the occiput. There is a degree of slack within the spinal dura, but it is "potential slack"; that is, the dura may respond to spinal movement, but it does not necessarily transmit this to another pole – a bone or a suture may take up the slack. ("Pole" refers to the specific boundaries of the reciprocal tension membrane – for example, the anterior pole of attachment of the falx is at the frontal bone.)

### Liquid-Electric Model

In the liquid-electric model, the sacrum is not regarded as having any specific axis of rotation. Its predominant motion occurs around the circumference of an imaginary floating sphere, which envelops the sacrum and whose lateral curvatures encompass the sacroiliac joints. This permits the sacrum the kind of emphatically fluid, universal-joint malleability it needs to act as the meeting place of so many dynamic forces. The musculature of the whole body, its movement triggered by fluctuations in the field, is taken as the source of the cranial wave, which is imparted to the spinal dura.

Thus, the dura is not seen as the motor to the cranial wave in the sacrum, except in dysfunction.

In the liquid-electric model the sacrum's floating, universal-joint motion is reminiscent of its motion while walking. Each side of the sacrum moves anteriorly in turn during flexion, which is where the vertical axis motion occurs. During flexion, one side of the body of the sacrum also elevates (moves superiorly) very slightly, with the base moving posteriorly and the apex anteriorly into the true pelvis. The other side elevates during the next cycle, and the opposite occurs during

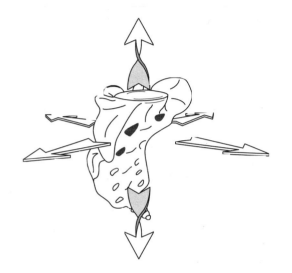

*Sacral micro-movement possibilities*

extension. The apex of the coccyx thus describes a circular motion. There is sacral torsion around the axial (vertical) plane as part of each flexion-extension cycle. This simple torsional pattern of movement is rendered into a compound motion when the slight displacement of the sacroiliac joints is added. The spinal dural attachment at the second sacral segment further modifies sacral motion, as does the respective tonicity and emotional status of the lumbar, abdominal, perineal, and leg muscles – especially the hip rotator musculature.

The axial torsion movement of the sacrum is transmitted to the vertebral column, assisted by the lumbosacral facet joints. The cranial wave of the vertebrae consists of fine rotational motions around a vertical axis passing through the vertebral bodies, which are modified by smaller torsional anteroposterior, and side-bending components. This is echoed at the occiput.

Intraosseous pliancy adds a final ingredient to sacral motion. This pliancy is permitted through the sacrum's inner cancellous composition (the bony connective tissue matrix that permits minute amounts of motion in every direction), its vestigial intervertebral discs, the fifth lumbar disc itself, and the sacrum's amphiarthrodial joints with the coxal bones.

## The Core Link

The connection made between the occiput and the sacrum by the spinal dura – firmly attached to the perimeter of the foramen magnum and the second sacral segment – forms the basis of what Sutherland called the core link.[14] This is a 95 percent inelastic tube of spinal dura that surrounds the delicate spinal cord like a loose-fitting hose pipe and connects the foramen magnum to the second sacral segment.

## Diagnostic Considerations

The sacrum cannot be overestimated in any assessment of the role it plays in determining cranial dynamics and pelvic balance.

### Energetics

The coccyx and the perineum (excluding the genitals) comprise the root soul center. The root soul acts as the accumulator of earth energy, which rises upward through the legs. It extends downward from the symphysis pubis and perineum all the way to the soles of the feet. A healthy root soul is capable of saying: "This is where I stand, this is what I stand for!" The root soul is concerned with security, stability, safety, and finding a good home. Stability is the need for grounding, and sometimes the root soul has an intense need for home, stability, and support. Safety may turn upon the struggle for survival. The root soul is also the source of energy for the ascent upward toward the light at the crown.

The sacrum is the sacred bone. A highly energized bony structure, it is the location of the second (sacral) soul center – the sexual band, which encompasses the location of the ovarian and sperm palaces and of sensory pleasure. The sacrum is the collection point and "launching pad" of the spiritual energy, which has its source at the root soul. This spiritual energy represents the creative exuberance of the energy field. In Taoism,[15] the sacrum is known as "the immortal bone."

We often treat the sacrum with directed energy techniques, known in the East as *chi kung* or *kime. Ki* in Japanese and *chi* in Chinese refer to the vital force of the body, its field.[16] *Kime* and *chi kung* direct or transmit energy across space or into the client's body.[17]

In working with the energetic components of the sacral area, I often combine the root and the sacral souls, with four equally important aspects that I identify by the mnemonic "the four Ss": stability, support, sexuality, and spirituality. ("Support" refers to the way the sacrum and low-back register whether we feel supported by those who love us. Low-back pain is almost always associated with feelings of a lack of support – in body language, "No one is behind me backing me up.") The psoas muscle[18] is a bridge between the *hara* (an ancillary soul center) and the sacral and root souls, spanning all three. It represents our deep sensitivity and reacts to the fear of being judged by contracting.

As Alexander Lowen noted, if because of religious belief or social circumstance pelvic movement is not allowed to be naturally and simply sexual, then the pelvis tends to stiffen. The body needs to move, and this need for movement, not permitted in the pelvis, tends to be transferred to the mouth area, where it shows up as talking – which is a movement of the mandible rather than the pelvis – about sex, usually (such is the human condition) about other people's sexuality. A person who can neither move his pelvis sexually[19] nor his mouth in gossip, begins to harden his belly, disassociating from all feelings[20] – the beginning of psychosis. The alternative is to understand the following relationships:

■ Movement is natural; movement is essential; movement is expression.[21]
■ If movement cannot be expressed sexually, it becomes oral.
■ Allow the belly to feel so that the mouth can express.
■ Allow the mouth to express so that the belly can feel.
■ Allow the mouth to express so that the pelvis can move.

Here is a summary of diagnostic questions to ask yourself for the root and sacral souls.[22]

■ How does this person meet his sensual and sexual needs? (Is the sacrum fluidly able to move in the anteroposterior plane?)
■ Is he too hard on himself (rigid sacrum)?
■ Is he too soft (a collapsed fifth lumbar disc, a dissolute life)?
■ Does he not give himself any fun, any pleasure? (Can the sacrum sway sideways?)
■ Does his sacrum want to support the life he is leading?

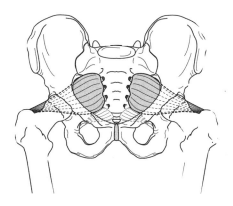 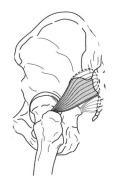 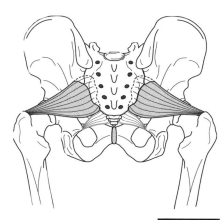

*Left to right:*
*Anterior,
lateral, and
posterior
views of
piriformis
(shaded) and
coccygeus*

- Is he open to doing new things in his life, expanding?
- Do his attitudes permit a pleasing flexibility of approach?
- Does he know where he stands on important issues?
- Is he ready and able to take a stand?

### Trauma and Dysfunction

The piriformis muscle originates from the anterior aspect of the first to fourth sacral segments, the greater sciatic foramen, and the anterior surface of the sacrotuberous ligament and inserts into the superior border of the greater trochanter, just posterior to the obturator internus and the gemelli. It is innervated by the fifth lumbar and first and second sacral nerves. The piriformis is an abductor of the thigh, an external rotator, and a minimal extensor to the femur. As far as the low-back and sacrum are concerned, it is a major source of trouble.

A hypertonic piriformis can cause malaise, mild personality change, and sacral deviation. (Of course, sacral deviation will be mirrored in the occiput.) By itself, this one muscle can extend sciatica down to the popliteal space at the knee. It is wise not to overlook it in any client examination. There are many approaches to the piriformis – long lever facilitative techniques to the legs, direct digital pressure as in Rolfing and shiatsu, and deep massage across the fibers as in "muscle springing."[23] The piriformis is also amenable to unwinding and reciprocal innervation (discussed in the techniques section below).

Energetic conflict in the sacral area will affect the legs and feet. Symptoms in the legs can be survival issues, the need to move on (with movement sometimes being frustrated by someone who won't let go[24]), support issues, or conflicts in sexual relationships. As the children of countless generations of nomads, we are genetically programmed with the urge to travel, to walk off our troubles by going on a "walkabout," or to walk forward to a new

relationship after four years in order to locate a new gene pool. In the Middle Ages, the church instituted the pilgrimage on foot to the Holy Land as a way for pilgrims to walk off homicidal spleen. If we feel imprisoned when we experience these powerful drives, and do not bring them to the light of consciousness where they can be felt and understood, they can lead to hip arthritis and low-back dysfunction, among other things.

The sacrum exerts a strong influence on the bones of the head, especially those that make up the cranial base, namely the occiput, sphenoid, ethmoid, temporals, and frontal. I have seen remarkable effects on the cranium from balancing the sacrum, such as sinusitis of several weeks' duration clearing up in an hour, and headaches either appearing or disappearing from five minutes of work. The ethmoid is particularly sensitive to sacral unwinding and decompression, a phenomenon that is explicable through core-link physiology.

The acute angle between the sacrum and coccyx that some clients have is usually first caused by a sudden fall, then exacerbated by perineal muscular hypertonicity. Sacrum Coupled with Symphysis Pubis, and Unilateral Piriformis and Coccygeus Release (techniques discussed below) help to normalize the sacrum and coccyx. A small but surprising number of cases of sciatica and low-back pain are entirely resolved by unwinding the coccyx, likely through the release of the piriformis and coccygeus muscles, which allow the sacrum – and therefore the fifth lumbar vertebra – to return to normal position, energy, and movement.

The sacral techniques described below may be applicable for sciatica, back pain, and pelvic stiffness accompanying pregnancy, low-back pain, and stress-related illnesses. The chapter Bad Backs includes a description of disc injury in lumbar and sacral conditions.

*The Heart of Listening*

**Above:**
The male pelvic diaphragm

**Below:**
The female uterus, vagina, and supporting structures

**1** Sacrum
**2** Coccygeus
**3** Piriformis
**4** Sacro-iliac joint
**5** Ischial spine
**6** Iliococcygeus
**7** Ala or wing of coxal bone
**8** Anterior superior iliac spine
**9** Anterior inferior iliac spine
**10** Pubic ramus
**11** Urethra
**12** Symphisis pubis
**13** Anus
**14** Pubococcygeus
**15** Uterus
**16** Cervix
**17** Vagina
**18** Obterator internus
**19** Urogenital diaphragm

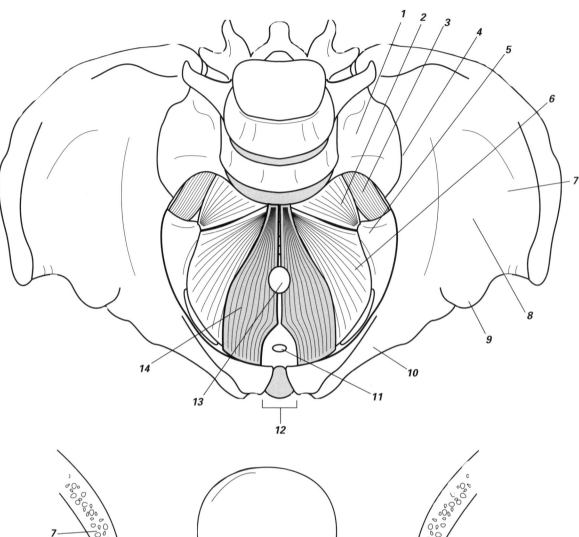

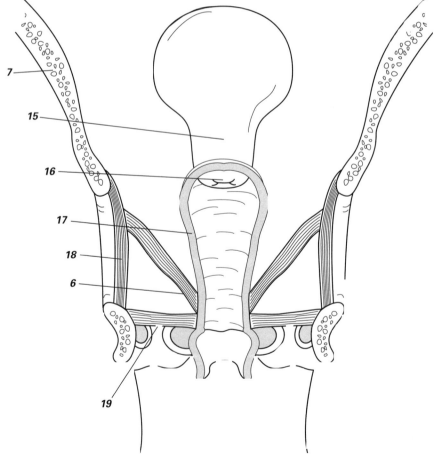

72

## Interconnectedness

The sacrum is one of the most interconnected bones in the body. The core link explains one polarity of the sacrum – a vertical pole extending upward; the ilia make up the other – a lateral and inferior polarity encompassing both legs. The sacrum moves in a compound multipolar way as we walk,[25] and is affected by the reciprocity between the anterior and posterior lumbar muscles and the abdominal muscles. It moves with the cranial wave and with every breath.

## Visualization

The basic challenge in visualization is to be able to create a complete picture of your target structure, in this case the sacrum and pelvis. This image needs to eventually encompass an alive, malleable sacrum, motile within itself, acted upon by muscles and discrete fascial and electrical forces emanating from trunk and limb, and limited by ligaments. In addition to changing shape from the forces of the cranial wave, it also moves in space with each breath. Another layer of the picture is the textures, colors, and considerable energetic weight of the root and sacral soul centers.

## Overview: Sacral Holds

All four bony polarities of the sacrum – the two lateral auricular surfaces, the base and the apex – need to be brought into balance. The relationship of the sacrum with the ilia and the hip joints laterally, and the thigh and abdominal musculature anteriorly, needs to be taken into account.

When the client is prone, place a pillow under his ankles; when he is supine, place a pillow under his knees to free any residual hamstring tension from pulling on the pelvis.

These sacral holds can be seen mechanically, as applications of corrective pressure, or as a dance with the dreambody. When we touch the sacrum, we are touching the source of sacredness, a place where, in the Eastern tradition, two serpents meet. In the Western Arthurian legend, two dragons meet there. In this myth, the King is intent upon building his palace upon a certain rock, but it keeps falling down. In a vision, Merlin sees two dragons fighting chaotically in a cave underneath the rock. The cave is located, and the dragon's power subsumed to the King's function as protector of the realm. The myth tells us that we cannot build our palace (our spirituality) upon its foundation (our sacrum) unless we first harness our dragons (our primal power).

## PRONE MUSCULOSKELETAL TECHNIQUES

### Gluteus Medius Release

Our adoption of the upright posture more than four million years ago has placed enormous stress on the gluteus medius and piriformis, two of the muscles most intimately associated with standing.[26,27] When the piriformis is hypertonic, the gluteus medius likely is as well. Use sensitive, deep tissue probing to locate hypertonic elements of the gluteus medius. Work either along the muscle fibers to induce release, or across them to facilitate their return to normal.

### *Jitsu* on the Inferior Gluteal Fold

This technique comes from the deep form of shiatsu, known as *jitsu* shiatsu, or potent shiatsu. It uses forearm pressure applied to one gluteal fold at a time from the opposite side. To work with the left leg, come around to the right side of the client and define his inferior gluteal fold. Place your left forearm in the fold, with your ninety-degree flexed elbow nestled in the space between the client's thighs. Introduce and sustain pressure at an angle directed through your left humerus at the client's left femoral shaft. It helps to vector your force mainly laterally, but with slight anterior and supe-

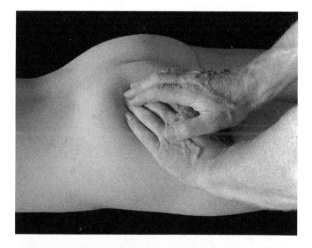

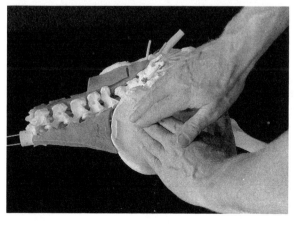

*Gluteus Medius Release, two views*

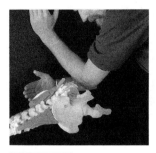
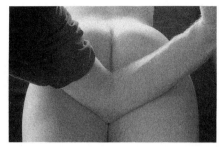

*Jitsu on the Inferior Gluteal Fold, two views*

rior components. Move your right hand to support the lateral aspect of the client's left leg from just above the knee to the hip joint area. Maintain your pressure with the aid of your body weight – place both feet well behind you, so that all of your body weight passes through your left humerus. After three to five minutes, your forearm contact will be able to palpate the posteromedial femoral margin, emerging as the hamstring muscles tonus subsides under the application of uninterrupted pressure.

This technique is very helpful in softening the "street armor" of more rigid people. Although you are getting very close to the sciatic trunk, this technique can help in selected cases of sciatica. It certainly helps free the hip and sacroiliac joints and induce deep states of relaxation.

### Unilateral Flexed-Knee Perineal Work

Stand to your prone client's left side, adjacent to his hip joint, and place your left hand under his knee (between the knee and table) and your right hand on the sole of his left foot. Now smoothly walk toward his head, collecting his knee and

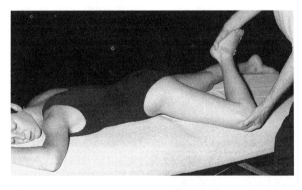

*Unilateral Flexed-Knee Perineal Work, smooth uptake of the position, with one possible contact shown below*

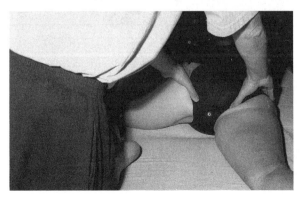

bringing it laterally into full flexion up to the level of his chest, so that it can rest on the table surface close to his rib wall. You help drive this movement with your contact on the left foot.

This position opens up the perineum for delicate work around the bony borders of the true pelvis (in women, the birth canal perimeter). The position is reminiscent of childhood naps, and promotes deeply relaxing and consciousness-changing work. Hunt the "feel" of the tissues until you find contraction or hypertonicity. Work to return normal space and tonus to the levator ani muscles, going slowly and meditatively. You can easily spend thirty minutes per side, to make a one-hour perineal session, ending with supine sacral balancing, possibly a CV4, Temporal Palming, and Frontal Anterior Decompression to harmonize the four primary poles of the cranial membrane system.

Use this technique with coccydynia, sciatica, and low-back pain that is not aggravated by the knee position.

## PRONE OSSEOUS TECHNIQUES

There are three basic sacral holds in cranial work – one prone and two supine. The prone technique is best for a client whose body size exceeds your own, or whose sacrum is exceedingly bony. The supine outside-leg approach is the technique of choice for most palpation of the sacrum as it allows for the most sensitive palpation of its fine motility patterns. The inside-leg approach affords more of a direct line at the sacrum, but necessitates more bodily contortion on the healer's behalf, which increases proprioceptive noise, and thus reduces her sensitivity.

In the context of a sixty- to ninety-minute treatment, it is usually better to begin with prone techniques for the sacral area, so these are listed first. Side-lying appears before the supine techniques. Application of the techniques in the order listed below gives the most effective response. Techniques for working with the musculature appear first. Prone contact is best with a client whose body weight exceeds your own, as a supine contact would quickly render your palpating hand insensitive; its drawback is that you have to have the client turn over in order to work on his head. Prone contact has the added advantage of enhancing the client's contact with his own hara, and with Mother Earth. It also gives clients a feeling of being less vulnerable.

## Basic Split-Finger Hand Configuration

With your dominant hand, locate the tip of the coccyx with your middle finger for landmarking, and leave it there for the moment. Now arrange the fingers of your non-dominant hand by splitting them two and two between the middle and fourth fingers. Place the heel of this hand on the fingertip that has located the coccyx; removing that finger, guide the coccygeal tip into the shallow depression between the thenar and hypothenar eminences. Place your hand in such a way that two fingers contact the sacral surface on either side of the median crest. Depending on the relative size of your hand to the client's sacrum, you will find that your fingertips are approximately at the level of the fifth lumbar spinous process. This is the basic configuration used in most sacral contacts.

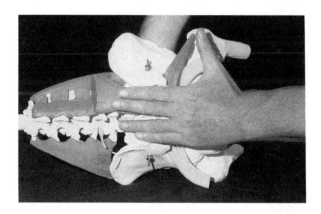

## Still's Technique

This is a traditional osteopathic maneuver involving circumduction, traction, compression, and knee flexion with the femur, combined with counter-strain pressure on the gluteal, piriformis, and coccygeus muscles of the same side. Your primary contact is with an ankle "trap," your secondary contact is with the heel of the hand over the sacroiliac joint, or buttock musculature. This is a mobilization technique, and also tends to gap the sacroiliac joints. Use it prior to supine normalization of the sacrum, psoas release work, or core-link work with the spine.

Stand at your client's feet. Grasp one foot, arch and calcaneus, with both hands. This part of the technique can be used as a method of lumbosacral decompression, gently alternating tension and compression at the feet to gap and facilitate the sacroiliac joints. Alternatively, you can proceed to gentle tractions and rotations to the ankle, gradually increasing the arc of movement and the pressures involved until it becomes a facilitative technique of the hip and sacroiliac joints. Add the final

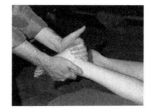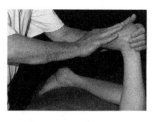

*Still's Technique, tension and compression with calcaneal contact*

component by introducing one hand as pressure/counter-pressure over the lateral aspects of the posterosuperior iliac spines.

## Sacrum Prone Technique

From the client's side, use your non-dominant hand to take up the basic split-finger sacral contact, then place your dominant hand transversely over the non-dominant hand to give you enough contact pressure to sense the cranial wave. After two to three minutes the cranial wave of the sacrum will begin to come out to you. You can use both hands, working together, to begin shepherding and molding the sacrum back into its optimum movement, position, and energetic state.

*Far left: Basic Split-Finger Configuration, showing contact with bony structures*

## Sacrum Prone Still-Point Induction

Still points are cessations of the cranial wave and occur spontaneously during craniosacral work. You can also induce a still point with either technical or sensory means, or a combination of both. The technical approach depends upon "chasing the dragon" – in this case, following the sacrum the way it prefers to move (i.e., moves with the greatest ease) until it has used up all of its movement and enters an "I quit!" mode.

To "chase the dragon," assume the sacral contact described above (or one of the supine techniques described below) and wait until you can feel the cranial wave, and differentiate between its flexion and extension phases. Begin to flesh out your

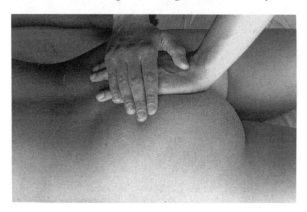

*Sacrum Prone Technique*

picture of sacral status, and differentiate the nuances of what you are feeling. For example:

- Does this sacrum prefer to move into flexion or extension?
- Is there a greater amplitude of movement on one side of the sacrum?
- Does the pivot of sacral motility appear through the second sacral segment or elsewhere, or is this sacrum behaving in such a natural fluid-electric way that there is no single axis of movement?

Lodge this information in your short-term memory; I find visual images the best way to do this, but find your own way. Then choose a moment to begin initiating the still point at a change in the cycle between flexion and extension. For example, say that flexion is the way that the sacrum moves more easily. Begin gently following the tip of the coccyx anteriorly as it swings into each flexion cycle. As it reaches the soft limit of the anterior swing, stay there – do not follow the sacrum back into extension, but rather wait, and resist the sacrum's return. This is a kind of passive resistance. Each time the sacrum resumes its flexion phase, which it will do according to its own rhythm, follow the swings anteriorly. Sometimes

you will feel the bone give a couple of little squirms, rather like a puppy getting comfortable in its basket, as you near the still point. Then there comes a moment when all flexion and extension has ceased and the sacrum no longer squirms, swings, or pulsates. This is the still point. Now wait again, patiently, until the dreambody makes the first move. Meanwhile, a great calm descends.

In contrast, the sensory approach to inducing a still point dispenses with any technical analysis. It focuses on asking the bone where it wants to go and helping it go there softly and supportively. Continue until it can move no more, and rests in its still point.

## Bilateral Ischial Tuberosities Pressure

Position yourself at the client's feet, and place the heels of your hands directly upon his ischial tuberosities. Modulate pressure and vector as becomes appropriate, using this as a diagnostic and directed-energy contact. (The pressure may end up being quite emphatic.) Take care in lumbar disc injury situations. This technique is good for separating the sacroiliac joints in a cephalad direction. Since the ischial tuberosities are energetically paired with the temporal bones' mastoid processes, pressure here may help you relieve temporal symptoms.

To use it as a decompression, after the initial cephalad intention gently reverse pressure until the bones begin to float free at the sacroiliac joints. This is wonderful.

## *Hara* Contact

This is a Bio-energetic technique[28] excellent for initiating energetic releases or whole-body "streaming." Sit to one side of the client, adjacent to his *hara,* which is the ancillary soul center related to movement. (It is located about 1 inch, or 2.5 centimeters, inferior to the navel.) Arrange your hands anterior and posterior, with both thumbs pointing inferiorly.

Clear your own field, find spinal center, then focus on your hands. It is almost as if you withdraw energy from your own hands – making them very passive contacts, almost soft vacuum cleaners – gently sucking in the client's energy so that a new confluence can begin to stream through his *hara.* This is very useful in working with people who are described as "rigid types" in Bio-energetic therapy.

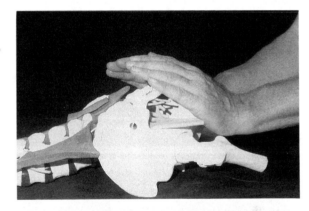

Pressure on the ischial tuberosities, bilaterally

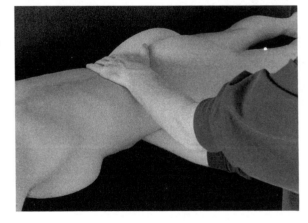

Hara Contact

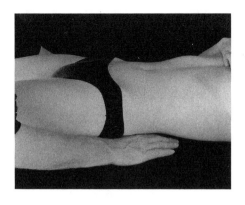 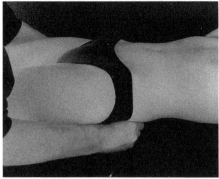 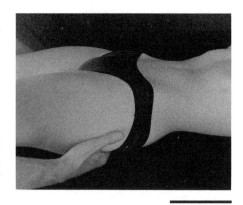

*Reposition-ing the pelvis*

## SIDE-LYING OSSEOUS TECHNIQUES

### Sacrum Work during Pregnancy

Make sure the client is lying comfortably on her side. Use a pillow for her head, and possibly another between her bent knees. Apart from the imbalance caused by lying on one coxal bone and not the other, this is a perfectly good way to work with the sacrum. Applying an anteriorly-directed pressure to the sacrum and a posteriorly-directed pressure to the anterosuperior iliac spines will relieve the low-back pain of pregnancy 90 percent of the time. Continue until you feel the cranial wave return to normal.

## SUPINE MUSCULOSKELETAL TECHNIQUES

### Sacrum: Reposition Pelvis

If you reposition the client's pelvis prior to beginning other supine sacral work, he will feel more comfortable, and you will have better results. The following is a simple, deft lifting and repositioning technique designed to place the pelvic girdle centrally on the table, with the lumbar spine slightly decompressed and the buttock muscles moved laterally and inferiorly. It is a good way to ensure that the pelvis is straight and level on the table before you begin interactive work with the legs or pelvic girdle.

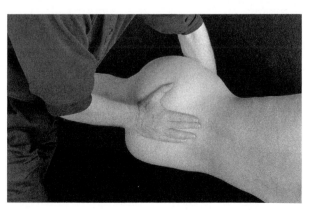

Stand at the client's feet, or bring a knee up on the table between his calves (if you cannot reach the sacrum from this position, stand to one side of the table adjacent to the client's thighs). Adopt a wide stance, and reach over to place both hands palms down on the table surface lateral to the iliac crests. Perform an external rotation of your forearms, bringing your hands under the client's buttocks, and move inferiorly and medially to the lateral sacral borders. Make a firm contact with the sacrum, wait until you can register the cranial wave, and then perform a cantilevered lift to the sacrum during the client's out-breath. Lift the sacrum clear off the table, and the moment you sense the point midway between the extremes of flexion and extension, replace the sacrum smoothly onto the table surface. This facilitates full cranial wave motion in the sacrum.

### Psoas Muscle Release

Come around to one side of the table, let us say the right. Bring the client's right knee into full flexion, and sit in the space thus vacated. Place the flexed knee in the crook of your right shoulder, just medial to your acromion process. You now can control movement of the right leg entirely by your shoulder contact, freeing both hands to locate and release the psoas muscle.

To locate the psoas, trisect the distance from the client's umbilicus to his left anterosuperior iliac spine. (With female clients, it is important to stay well clear of the ovaries, which are located 1 inch [2.5 centimeters] medial from the anterior spines.) Place the curled backs of your right-hand fingers at the middle trisection, reinforcing with your left hand. Increase your pressure slowly in a posterior

*Far left:*
*Sacrum work during pregnancy*

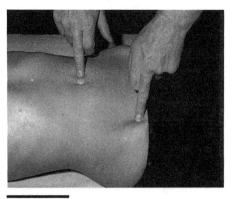
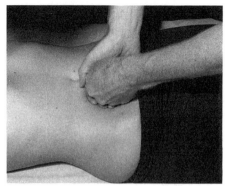
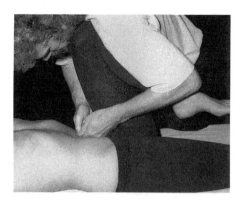

**Above:**
*Psoas Muscle Release, landmarking and basic contact*

**Below:**
*The psoas muscle (shaded)*

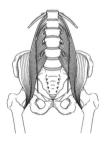

direction, making small rotatory movements with the backs of your fingers to "squidge" the small intestines clear of the psoas muscle belly. Once you can feel the 1 inch (3.9 centimeter) thick bulk of the psoas, begin to work transversely medial to lateral across its fibers to release hypertonicity. Your right hand stays soft, for sensitivity, your left hand provides the drive.

Begin to combine this direct work with the psoas with femoral rotation. Rotate your own trunk, and with it the client's left leg, by first moving toward his head, then medially, then inferiorly, then laterally, and finally toward his head again. While you are adducting the femur, traverse the psoas from medial to lateral. This combination of direct muscle work and rhythmic rotations of the femur works by returning rhythm and release to the hypertonic psoas. The final component is to instruct the client to breathe out as you bring their femur medially and inferiorly. This further relaxes the abdomen.

## Iliacus Release

Access the iliacus muscle with your fingertips and finger pads around the lip of the iliac crest. Trace the arc of the iliac brim as far posterior as you can, applying finger pressure and intention to release the iliacus. (You can also release the iliacus with a reciprocal innervation technique. For a reciprocal innervation technique, get the client to flex the thigh of the "good" side repeatedly against resistance.)

*Iliacus Release*

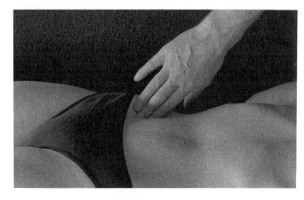

## Unilateral Piriformis and Coccygeus Release

The coccygeus is a short, squat, triangular muscle that is a strong stabilizer of the sacrum at the "south pole" of the core link. Its attachments are from the fifth sacral and first coccygeal segments to the ischial spine.

**Approach #1** Sit or kneel beside the table at a forty-five-degree angle from the client's legs, facing his heart. Slip both hands under his buttocks until you reach the lateral sacral border. Apply fingertip contact to the border and fingerpad contact to the belly of the piriformis and coccygeus muscles. Tune in to the motility pattern and energetics of the muscle tissue and wait for release and balancing to occur. This is especially useful in working with sciatica.

**Approach #2** Stand at the side of the client's thighs and bring what was your inferior hand in the last technique between the client's legs, and take up a coccygeal contact, working with inferior-directed decompression of the coccyx (thus moving across the long axis of the muscle fibers). The superior hand continues to carry out its lateral lengthening of the piriformis (moving with the long axis of the fibers) as in approach #1. This is the most powerful craniosacral technique for these two muscles.

## Bilateral Piriformis and Coccygeus Release

This uses the same outside-leg technique as above to work simultaneously with both lateral borders of the sacrum. It is excellent for working with unilateral sciatica, particularly those resulting from long automobile drives.

## Piriformis: Reciprocal Innervation on the Floor

To use a reciprocal innervation technique with a stubbornly hypertonic piriformis, lay the client down on the floor with his "good" side against a stout wall and that knee flexed. Place one hand on the hypertonic piriformis, and palpate it while instructing the client to (isometrically) push his "good" leg laterally against the wall. Have him push during a long out-breath, and relax during the in-breath. Repeat the pushing and piriformis contraction on the unaffected side until the client approaches exhaustion, ill humor, or both. Then allow him to drop his leg and rest deeply. The motor cortex will now fire signals for complete relaxation to *both* piriformis muscles. You may instruct the client to repeat this three to five times per day, for up to five minutes each time. This may work when nothing else will.

## SUPINE OSSEOUS TECHNIQUES

For these techniques, place a pillow under the client's knees to free any residual hamstring tension on the pelvis.

## Hip and Sacroiliac Facilitation

This is one of Andrew Still's "rhythm and movement" techniques;[29,30] Still understood instinctively the importance of moving the body in tune with the cranial wave. It consists of long, slow, almost lazy movements designed to free up hip and sacroiliac restrictions. Stand to one side of the table and collect the client's calcaneus with the palm of one hand. Place your other hand under his knee, flexing it, or on the patella itself. Move the knee in a circular or ovoid rotation, first toward the head; then medially, inferiorly, and laterally, before coming toward the head again. This helps the psoas to release by first contracting and then stretching. Allow t'ai chi-like "water nature" into your own knees: flow-back and forth, flow around, be fluid in your own body as an example and incentive to the client to be fluid in his.

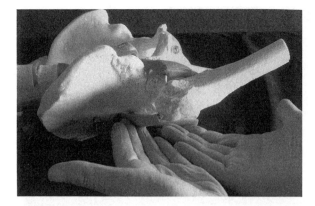

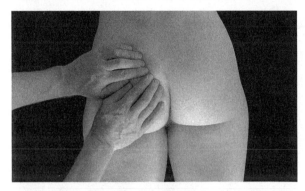

*Unilateral Piriformis and Coccygeus Release, approach number one. In the lower photo the technique is photographed prone, for clarity.*

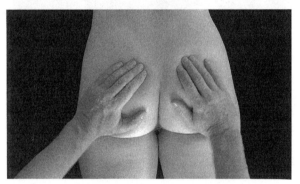

*Bilateral Piriformis and Coccygeus Release (shown prone for clarity)*

## Sacrum Cantilevered Lift

This technique allows elegant access to the sacrum, although mastering its timing takes some practice. It gives a primary sacrum contact with the non-dominant hand and leaves the dominant hand free to assess and treat other components in the pelvic or core link mechanisms.

Feed your dominant hand transversely under the sacrum, with your thumb posterior to the first sacral segment. Then, during the client's out-breath, isometrically stiffen your hand and wrist under the sacrum, and drop your body weight toward the floor (mean it!) while simultaneously stiffening your elbow so that it acts as a fulcrum to

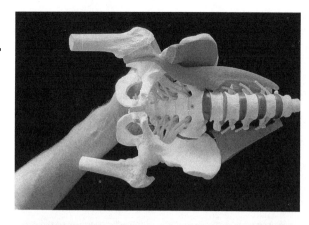

*Sacrum on hand, Outside-Leg Technique with hand position shown below*

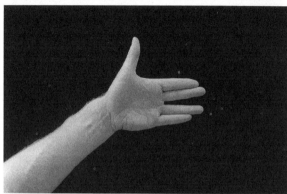

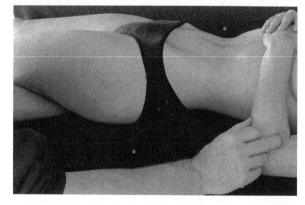

*Sacrum Outside-Leg Technique, with right middle finger on Large Intestine 10; hand positions shown below*

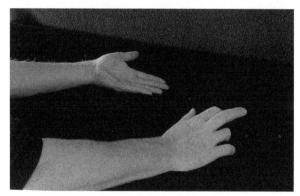

cantilever the client's pelvis up off the table surface. In the short moment that the sacrum is off the table, take up contact with your non-dominant hand configured in the basic split-finger hold, and then remove your other hand.

## Sacrum Outside-Leg Technique

From the side of the table, use the basic split-finger hand configuration to take up a sacral contact from outside (and under) the leg. Ask the client to lift his pelvis very slightly off the table for the greatest ease in taking up contact. Use your non-dominant hand to contact the sacrum. I like to make initial contact with my free hand to the acupuncture point Arm Three Miles (Large Intestine 10), which is located just distal to the elbow in a little depression on an extensor tendon.[31] (This is the place that becomes acutely tender in extensor tenosinovitis, or tennis elbow.) This contact completes a sensitive energy circuit with the sacral hand, and it allows you to access the pelvic and sphenoid areas energetically, which enhances the information available mechanically. Sense if some other technique or contact is more appropriate in each person you work with.

The sacrum outside-leg technique is especially useful because, after some practice, it can be maintained for long periods without losing sensitivity in the hand making contact with the sacrum. It is the foundation sacral hold in visionary craniosacral work; advanced techniques often stay with this primary contact, while using the free hand to assess and treat other components in the pelvic girdle or core link mechanisms. The outside-leg approach is the most sensitive technique, but some healers find it painful as it necessitates extreme adduction of the wrists. If this is true for you, prone sacral work or the sacrum inside-leg technique will give better results until your wrists gain more mobility and become free of discomfort.

## Sacrum Inside-Leg Technique

Here you stand to the side of the table and take up the standard split-finger contact with the sacrum by placing your forearm between the client's legs, which gives more direct access to the axial plane of the sacrum and is therefore better for lumbosacral decompression and unwinding, as well as the pubic bone compression techniques. The best way to initiate contact consists of a graceful move that requires no effort on the part of the client. Reach over the client's body with your dominant hand and take a firm contact at the anterosuperior iliac spine and hip joint area, then, bending your knees, roll the client toward you. As the sacrum is exposed, slip your non-dominant hand between his legs and take up sacral contact.

## Sacral Steering Wheel

With both hands placed transversely under the sacrum, this technique allows for full control of the bone's motility patterns. Take up contact so that your fingertips overlap the sacral border on the further side while the heels of your hands overlap the nearer border, which allows additional contact with some gluteal, piriformis, and coccygeal fibers. This is an excellent technique for an indurated, resistant sacrum. Having two hands under the bone allows for more physical capability in unwinding, lumbosacral decompression, working with lumbar disc injuries, and hip joint dysfunction.

## Lumbosacral Decompression and Unwinding

Place one hand between the legs, taking up the standard split-finger sacral contact, and the other transversely under the lumbar spine. Make sure that the fingertips of the sacral hand touch the palm of the lumbar hand. Differentiate the sacral spinous processes from the lumbar. Begin to sense the movement of the lumbar spine as a whole, and compare it with the movement of the sacrum. Then move to the direct palpation of each lumbar spinous process, perhaps localizing on them with a finger and thumb of your lumbar hand. Sense the relative motility of the sacrum compared with the fifth lumbar vertebra to gain insight into the stresses causing the vertebra's dysfunction. Move to listening to the other lumbar vertebrae, sequentially listening to, and then testing the movement of each.

Another possibility is to move into energetic work, focused on the spaces between the spinous processes. This is a shiatsu practice, excellent for clearing the spinal field for kundalini work. (It can be done with the client lying prone or supine, or kneeling.) Slight alterations in intention, pressure, and vector may exacerbate or completely ameliorate low-back pain.

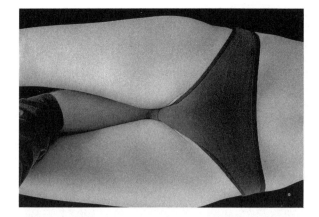

*Forearm alignment for Sacrum Inside-Leg Technique*

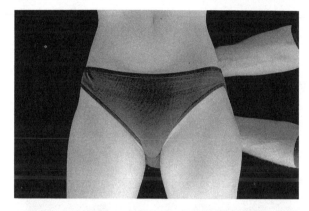

*Sacral Steering Wheel, with bony contact shown below*

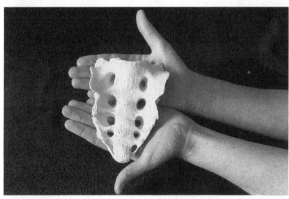

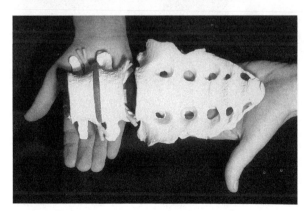

*Lumbosacral Decompression and Unwinding*

## Sacrum Coupled with Anterior Superior Iliac Spine

From the side of the table, assume an outside-leg sacral hold with your non-dominant hand, waiting until you have a relaxed hand and a distinct and clear picture of sacral motility. Then move your free hand to encompass the client's anterosuperior iliac spines, placing the base of the index and middle fingers of your hand on the distant spine (allowing your fingers to lie over the tensor fascia lata area), flexing your wrist sufficiently to clear the abdomen, and then allowing the fleshy part of your forearm's flexor muscle group to rest on the other anterior spine. You now have a three-point

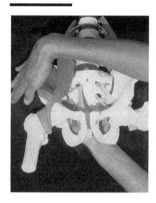
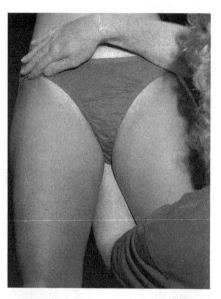

*Sacrum Coupled with Anterior Superior Iliac Spine, two views*

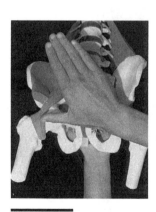
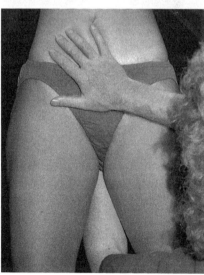

*Sacrum Coupled with Symphysis Pubis, two views*

pelvic hold: one hand underneath the sacrum, and one arm spanning the pelvic brim with two contacts.

Focus on the movement of the ilia, the "wings" of the coxal bones. The element of movement caused by respiration is very pronounced, and if the cranial wave is not in sync with the respiration, detecting it can be challenging. Note the effects of ilial respiratory excursion on the client's true pelvis. Are the bones moving synchronously? Is the pattern one of the coccyx and ischial tuberosities moving into the true pelvis at the same time (Sutherland's model)? Or is it the liquid-electric model, where one tuberosity moves into the true pelvis while the other moves out of it? Optimizing the client's pattern can be very important in preparing pregnant women for natural and healthy childbirth.

## Sacrum Coupled with Symphysis Pubis

This technique releases the perineum (the "pelvic diaphragm") by applying posteriorly-directed force at the symphysis pubis. This is a private area[32] – sexually loaded, sensual, and often traumatized – so consider explaining to your client beforehand why you want to use the technique and clear your own consciousness of any stray sexual or sensual thoughts before making contact.

First take up an inside-leg sacral contact with your non-dominant hand, standing at the side of the table. Next, place your free hand on the client's belly just below the navel, then work downward in gentle steps until you make a firm base-of-thumb contact with the symphysis pubis. Arrange your thenar eminence transversely on the most anterior portion of the pubic eminence.

Focus on the sacrum, waiting until you have a sense of sacral rhythm, position, and energetic status, then transfer your focus to the pubic eminence. Begin to first introduce, then fluidly increase, posteriorly-directed pressure on the pubic eminence until the sacrum responds. If it suddenly "kicks free," you have proof that the levator ani muscle groups have been in tension, inhibiting sacral movement. In this case, continue your pressure until you feel the intervening tissues unwind and relax; working pressures may plateau at ten to twelve pounds (four to five kilograms). There may be many different planes of motion as the sacrum unwinds.

As a powerful and capable straddle hold to the pelvic diaphragm, this technique is another important one in preparing women for childbirth. In your mind's eye, link your upper and lower hands and begin to visualize the anatomy and physiology of the true pelvis, in particular its bony margins and the perineal musculature. Analyze the forces acting upon both the units you are touching, and on the tissues that lie between them.

If you sense any kind of force – torsion, shear, or compression – faulting the pelvis, introduce corrective pressures using one of the ten options for interaction[9] or unwinding. Unwinding is usually the best.

In cases where direct work on the symphysis pubis would clearly be offensive to the client, take up the prone sacral contact and apply anterior pressure until the pubic bones make a firm and definite contact with the table surface. Mediate pressure to the levator ani group through this medium until you feel complete release.

## SUPINE COMPLETIONS

### Ventral Sacred Energy Vessel Hold

Move into respiratory entrainment. Perceive a contact area somewhere between symphysis pubis and the costoclavicular notch. Slowly establish contact with your forearm, going down with the client's breathing pattern, until you have established a firm but extremely sensitive contact. Wait. Wait until you can feel a continuity of movement patterns under the entire length of your contact. Begin interactive work to bring the sacred energy vessel into harmony. This is especially useful with clients who have been involved in severe trauma, whether physical, psychological, or psychic.

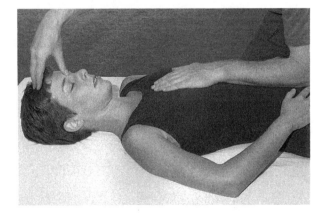

### Lumbar to Vertex Sweep

This can be a very good way to connect the energy of the sacrum with the head, by way of the spiritual heart.

Stand at the head of the table, employing a long, strong leg stance. Place both of your hands under the client's large paraspinal back muscles, as far down toward the sacrum as you can comfortably manage. Once you have a definite energetic contact with the back, select a movement to travel from your contact point to the crown – either a very slow movement like a massage stroke, or step-by-step movements in one-vertebra increments. Pay full attention to the variables of micro-movement timing, pressure, and poignancy as you ascend. Great abysses of emotional pain often lie behind the heart, as well as betrayal issues. As you sweep up the neck, lift the head free of the table so that you can elegantly and usefully traverse the suboccipital muscle attachments, freeing and unwinding as you go. Gently place the head back on the table, much as you placed the sacrum at the completion of the Sacrum: Reposition Pelvis technique.

### Other Techniques That Can Affect the Sacrum

- Leg, back, and arm unwinding
- Temporal techniques
- The CV4
- Mandible unwinding
- Lateral Pterygoid Release
- Rolfing
- Acupuncture
- Bio-energetic therapy
- Feldenkrais floor and table work
- Foot reflexology
- The perfect golf swing
- Reichian bodywork

*Far left:*
*Ventral Sacred Energy Vessel Hold, with second hand in an optional contact with the inner eye*

# 23
# *The Occiput*

**Etymology**

**Occiput** *from the Latin ob caput, meaning abutting the head*

**Cranium** *from the Greek for a helmet*

**Squama** *from the Latin for a fish scale*

**1** *Foramen magnum, or biggest hole, transmits medulla oblongata*

**2** *Basilar part, part of occiput that lies anterior to foramen magnum*

**3** *Lateral or condylar part, lies lateral to foramen magnum*

**4** *Squama, or squamous portion, part of occiput located posterior to foramen magnum*

**5** *Occipital portion of interdigitated mastoid suture, articulates with temporal bone*

**6** *Occipital portion of interdigitated lambdoid suture, articulates with parietal bone*

**7** *Occipital condyle, articulates with superior articular facet of atlas, composing atlanto-occipital joint*

**8** *Condylar canal, transmits condylar emissary vein from sigmoid sinus*

**9** *Hypoglossal canal, located anterior and lateral to foramen magnum, transmitting CN XII, hypoglossal nerve*

**10** *Jugular process, or spine, located lateral to jugular foramen, remnant of vertebral transverse process*

**11** *Intrajugular process, divides jugular foramen into lateral passage for jugular vein, and medial passage for CN IX, X and XI, glossopharyngeal, vagus and spinal accessory nerves*

**12** *External occipital protuberance, or inion*

**13** *Cruciform eminence, formed by attachment of falx and tentorium*

**14** *Internal occipital protuberance, located at center of cruciform eminence*

**15** *Groove for superior sagittal sinus*

**16** *Groove for transverse sinus*

**17** *Groove for sigmoid sinus (continuation of transverse sinus)*

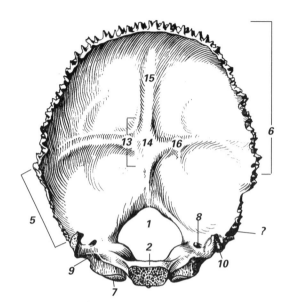

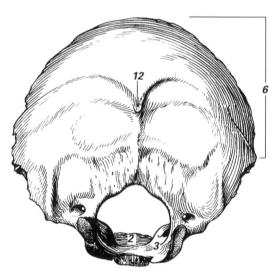

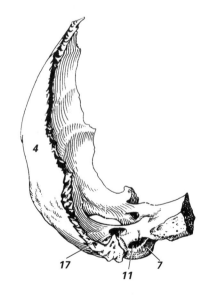

## Embryology and Osteology

All of the bones that comprise the cranial base begin as cartilage. The occiput begins to ossify in four distinct parts: one squamous, two condylar, and one basilar. The squamous part begins to ossify from cartilage in its inferior portion and from membrane in its superior half. It ossifies from as few as one or as many as eight nuclei, which appear eight weeks after conception, and usually unite soon afterward. When the cartilaginous and membranous centers fail to unite, the resultant tri-angular-shaped bone, wedged between the parietals just inferior to lambda, is called the interparietal bone. The two condylar and one basilar parts of the occiput each develop from a single ossification center.

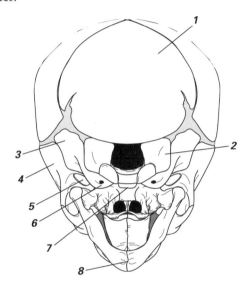

At birth the occipital bone consists of four parts: an expanded portion, the squama, which lies posterior and superior to the foramen magnum, two condylar parts, which form the sides, or lateral aspects, of the foramen, and a basilar part, which lies in front of the foramen.

The squama unites with the condylar parts by the time the cranial suture become defined at the end of the fourth year. By age six the basilar portion unites with the condylar, and the occiput unifies.

## Anatomy

The occiput is a robust, hand-sized, moderately complex, biconcave bone. It is similar in size to the sacrum. It has four aspects, the squama, two condyles, and a basilar portion where it articulates with the sphenoid.

### Structure

The structure of the occiput is entirely composed of robust cortical and diploic bone. Both the occiput and sacrum have apertures for, and attachments of, the spinal dura and enclosed cord, and both have a pronounced triangular, biconcave form. They are almost twins, separated by the spinal cord.

## Location

The occiput is located where the neck meets the head. Its most superior point, at lambda, is slightly higher than the apex of the eyebrow line. At its most inferior point – the occipital condyles – it articulates with the atlas (the first cervical vertebra). Its most anterior point is anterior to both the ear canal and the temporomandibular joints, where the basilar portion of the occiput articulates with the sphenoid (the sphenobasilar joint). Its lateral extremes lie posterior to the mastoids, at asterion. The lambdoid suture is 2 inches (5 centimeters) posterior from the mastoid tip.

### Landmarks

The inion, or posterior occipital protuberance, is external to the internal occipital protruberance (I.O.P.), the posterior attachment of the straight sinus. Both are located approximately dead center in the squamous portion, on a horizontal line drawn posteriorly from the pupils of the eyes. The I.O.P. is formed by the pull of the dura at the straight sinus, which is named "Sutherland's Fulcrum" within the cranial osteopathic world, in honor of Sutherland's contribution to our understanding of cranial mechanics.

The inion is more prominent in the Celtic peoples. Neanderthals had a bony bun at inion,[1] and the early European Neanderthals may have passed a remnant of this landmark on to Cro-Magnon man (our direct ancestors), especially in the Neanderthal heartland, the Yugoslavian region.

## Sutures and Articulations

The occiput has simple interdigitations with the parietals, robust and heavy intersection with the temporal mastoid area, free borders with the petrous portions of the temporals (i.e., the two bones come very close to each other, but do not form a suture). The occiput has either an intervertebral disk-like, cartilaginous articulation, or an ossified articulation with the clivus of the sphenoid. This depends upon age, history of trauma,

*Far Left:*
*Newborn cranial base*

*1 Occiput, squamous portion*
*2 Occiput, condylar portion*
*3 Temporal, petrous portion*
*4 Temporal, squamous portion*
*5 Temporal, tympanic ring*
*6 Carotid canal*
*7 Occiput, basilar portion*
*8 Symphisis mentis*

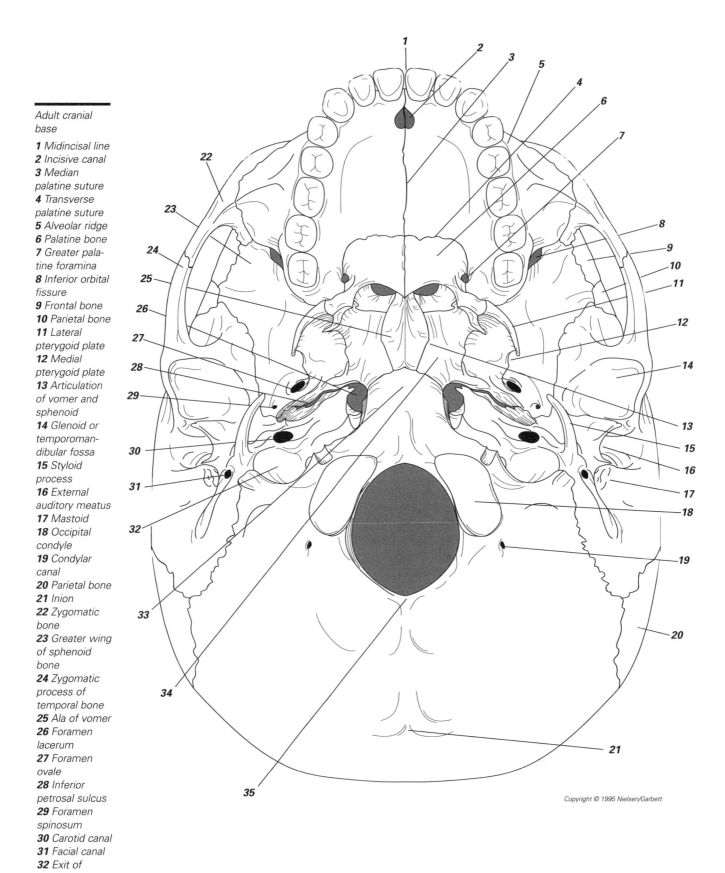

Adult cranial
base

**1** Midincisal line
**2** Incisive canal
**3** Median
palatine suture
**4** Transverse
palatine suture
**5** Alveolar ridge
**6** Palatine bone
**7** Greater pala-
tine foramina
**8** Inferior orbital
fissure
**9** Frontal bone
**10** Parietal bone
**11** Lateral
pterygoid plate
**12** Medial
pterygoid plate
**13** Articulation
of vomer and
sphenoid
**14** Glenoid or
temporoman-
dibular fossa
**15** Styloid
process
**16** External
auditory meatus
**17** Mastoid
**18** Occipital
condyle
**19** Condylar
canal
**20** Parietal bone
**21** Inion
**22** Zygomatic
bone
**23** Greater wing
of sphenoid
bone
**24** Zygomatic
process of
temporal bone
**25** Ala of vomer
**26** Foramen
lacerum
**27** Foramen
ovale
**28** Inferior
petrosal sulcus
**29** Foramen
spinosum
**30** Carotid canal
**31** Facial canal
**32** Exit of
jugular vein
**33** Basilar
portion of
occiput
**34** Body of
sphenoid
**35** Ipisthion

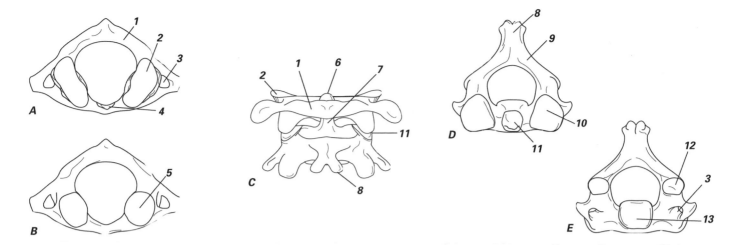

genetics, and the attitudinal openness of the individual.

The occiput articulates with six bones:

- The first cervical vertebra (atlas)
- Two temporals
- Two parietals
- The sphenoid

## Weight

A medically prepared, disarticulated occiput weighs 2 ounces (57 grams).

## Detailed Anatomy and Musculature

The occiput is largely composed of diploic bone of moderate complexity. It is marked by the largest aperture in the cranium, the foramen magnum – from the Latin, meaning "largest hole" – a pear-shaped aperture whose narrower portion faces anterior. The pear shape is caused by the reniform (kidney-shaped) occipital condyles, which crimp the foramen magnum and form the articulation with the first cervical vertebra. Thus, the shape of the foramen magnum is the result of a trade-off between the brain and spinal cord's evolved need for more space and the first cervical vertebra's need to keep the condyles close together (the closer the condyles are, the more flexible a universal joint the atlanto-occipital joint becomes). Since displacement or fracture at this level is almost always fatal, we have evolved this pear-shaped compromise.

Each condyle has two foramina. The eleventh cranial nerve, the hypoglossal, passes through the hypoglossal canal, which neatly tunnels through the condyles just superior to their articular surfaces. By any normal standard of nomenclature, these would be called the condylar foramina, since they pass directly through the base of the condyles, yet that name is actually given to foramina lateral to the condyles, barely passing through them at all, that allow passage to the meningeal branch of the ascending pharyngeal artery and an emissary (outgoing) vein.

The occiput is marked by distinct muscle attachment ridges on its external surface. The inion is the point of attachment for ligamentum nuchae, a vestige of a once-massive ligament that forms the mane ridge so prominent in grazing animals (it is at least sixty-five million years since our ancestors were muzzle-feeding grazers).[2] Now ligamentum nuchae helps us support our heads for less earthen activities, such as reading.

The occiput has pronounced ridges on its inner surface, caused by the pull of the falx and tentorium components of the reciprocal tension membrane. The occiput is remarkably thick and dense at these ridges. Note that:

- The falx cerebri (above I.O.P.) produces an indistinct double ridge of bone on the inside of the occiput. This is because the falx bifurcates before attaching to the bone to provide greater tensile stability. The superior sagittal sinus runs in the bifurcation, protected by it.

- The falx cerebelli (below I.O.P.) produces a much sharper and well-defined single ridge of bone.

- The tentorium produces well-defined double ridges of bone lateral to I.O.P., helping to form the cruciform eminence, at whose center lies the ipisthion. They are well-defined because the tentorium supports some 30 percent of the weight of the cerebral hemispheres. The transverse sinuses are located in the bifurcations that the tentorium makes just before attaching to the occiput.

The occiput is also robust at its anterior-most part – the thick strut of bone called the basilar portion, which articulates with the sphenoid at the sphenobasilar joint. The occiput is paper-thin, however, at relatively non-stressed parts of the squamous portion (if you hold up a disarticulated occiput to a window, even the light of an overcast day diffuses through the bone at these points). If

*Atlas, axis and atlanto-axial complex*

*A Atlas, superior*
*B Atlas, inferior*
*C Atlanto-axial complex, posterior*
*D Axis, superior*
*E Axis, inferior*

**1** *Posterior arch*
**2** *Superior articular facet*
**3** *Transverse foramen*
**4** *Articular facet for dens*
**5** *Inferior articular facet*
**6** *Tip of dens*
**7** *Base of dens*
**8** *Bifid spinous process*
**9** *Lamina*
**10** *Superior articular facet*
**11** *Dens*
**12** *Inferior articular facet*
**13** *Body*

you can examine either a disarticulated or intact skull, locate the transverse and sagittal crests on the internal surface of the occiput and note the location of the I.O.P. and inion. There are also exquisitely fine grooves on the internal surface of the occiput caused by the posterior meningeal artery. These are especially noticeable in proximity to the jugular foramina.

The jugular foramina, bracketed by both the temporal bones and the condylar portions of the occiput, allow passage for the following:

- The jugular veins
- The inferior petrosal sinus
- The ninth cranial nerve (the glossopharyngeal)
- The tenth cranial nerve (the vagus)
- The eleventh cranial nerve (the spinal accessory)
- The sigmoid sinus
- The posterior meningeal artery

The configuration of the occiput at the jugular foramina is interesting, particularly for its "jugular spine," a sharply pointed vertical spike of bone that stands guard over the posterolateral portion of the jugular foramina. This is the last vestige of the transverse process of the single vertebra the occiput has evolved from.[3]

### Musculature

The muscles attaching inferior and anterior to the foramen magnum consist of the:

- Rectus capitis lateralis
- Rectus capitis anterior
- Longus capitis

The muscles attaching posterior and lateral to the foramen magnum consist of the:

- Occipitofrontalis
- Trapezius
- Splenius capitis
- Semispinalis capitis
- Rectus capitis posterior minor and major
- Superior obliquus capitis

## Physiology

The occiput can be considered to be paired with the sacrum. They sit at either end of the spinal column, firmly connected to each other by the flexible but largely inelastic tube of the spinal dura mater.[4] Both admit the spinal cord, the occiput as the medulla oblongata, the sacrum as the corda equina. Both have firm dural attachments; the attachment around the circumference of the foramen magnum form the superior pole of the core link, the adherence of the spinal dura to the second sacral segment forms the lower pole of attachment. The dura, like the spinal cord itself, is inelastic. Movement is possible because the spinal cord and its enveloping dura have extra "slack" that they can pay out.

## Axis of Rotation

The axis of rotation of the occiput is classically described as lying in a horizontal and transverse, or coronal, plane. This is located ½ inch (1.3 centimeter) above the anterior third of the foramen magnum,[5] not passing through the occiput itself (the occiput is the only bone in the cranium whose axis of rotation lies external to the bone).

Occipital movement in the liquid-electric model consists of motion around the surface of an imaginary sphere 1 inch (2.5 centimeters) in diameter located just superior to the foramen magnum. There is no single axis. However, the occiput does behave as if moved by the surface of the brain, which can be regarded as the occiput's floating propulsive sphere. This sphere acts like a mobile universal joint, permitting occipital motion in every plane. Flexibility is the chief energetic characteristic of the occiput, and the mobile-sphere axis permits maximum occipital flexibility.

## Motion

Movement at the sphenobasilar joint is permitted either by a disk-like pad of cartilage, or a thin plate of connective tissue (a synchondrosis[6]) at the joint itself. If neither disk nor cartilage is present between the two bones, and they have fused,[7] then the intraosseous pliability of the cancellous bone of the clivus (the posterior part of the sphenoid body) and the presence of the sphenoid air sinus lend flexibility to the bones and permit the required small degrees of movement. The motion of the basilar portion of the occiput is a decisive factor in the behavior of the sphenoid, and thus of the whole head.

### Osteopathic Model

In the classical osteopathic model (similar-motion model), the occiput circumducts, or moves in an anterior and inferior direction, in flexion. This is not true flexion (forward-bending), yet it is called flexion as it is the motion made while the sphenoid – the standard of reference – moves into flexion. During flexion the basilar part of the occiput moves superiorly at its junction with the clivus.

### Liquid-Electric Model

In the liquid-electric model, as the left side of the tentorium flattens during left temporal flexion, the left side of the occipital squama moves anterior and slightly lateral. The opposite occurs during temporal extension. As each temporal flexes in turn, the occiput moves to that side. This movement pulls the occiput marginally anterior and lateral, and circumducts the occipital squama inferiorly on that side. The basilar portion moves superiorly, with a hint of internal rotation. During left temporal flexion, the left greater wing of the sphenoid also moves into flexion, and the sphenobasilar joint moves superiorly.

## Diagnostic Considerations

### Energetics

The head is "in charge," as seen in our titles "head of department" and "headmistress." When sailors navigate they set a "heading." We give a chafing horse "its head." We have "brainstorming" meetings, and members of Congress are sometimes described as having "skull" sessions to plot legislative strategy. We "lose our heads," "blow our tops." When we are behaving oddly, others may call us "numbskull."

Authority does not turn his head: the rigidity of the responsible, of authority figures, shows up strongly as upper neck and occipital rigidity. Releasing the occiput can allow joy and life to flow back into the being.

The occiput is the eighth vertebra of the cervical spine, and as it evolved out of a vertebra, its chief energetic delight is, like a vertebra, in movement, especially flexibility. The back of the neck is somatically connected to feelings of betrayal – being stabbed from behind. The occiput is also connected to memories of birth trauma,[8] particularly cases of the umbilical cord being twisted around the neck and occiput.[9] Since the occiput receives the spinal cord, and supports the cerebellum and hemispheres, it is sometimes involved in issues of allowing yourself to be supported in life. We love to sink our weary heads back in the feather pillows.

The occiput is also where "I don't know who I am" meets with "I am."

The neck is also power. When the German army swept through France in 1940, the French army and British expeditionary forces were overwhelmed. Winston Churchill sent a message to the French government that no matter what they did, Britain would fight on. The defeated French generals thought Britain would be demolished by the blitzkrieg tactics of the German storm troops. "In three weeks England will have her neck wrung like a chicken," the French generals forecast to their own Prime Minister. Learning of this comment soon afterward, British Prime Minister Winston Churchill stood before the Canadian Parliament on December 30, 1941 and, pointing dramatically to his own squat, bulging neck, pronounced defiantly: "Some chicken ... some neck!"[10]

The inner eye is a channel of energy running through the head. It begins at the atlanto-occipital joint, passes through the foramen magnum, and exits at glabella. The occiput is therefore deeply connected to use of the inner eye, and head and neck positioning greatly affect inner-eye functioning.[11]

The posterior aspect of the atlanto-occipital joint is the location of an acupuncture point called Wind Palace (Governor Vessel 16[12]). Wind is the energy of the spirit, and the palace is the highest physical embodiment, or architectural location, of this energy. Wind Palace is the posterior pole of the channel of the inner eye. (In the Sufi system, the seventh chakra is located here, at Wind Palace.) You can use finger pressure and directed energy work to help open, then optimize the channel of the inner eye. It is an almost magical realm, and makes learning the anatomy worthwhile.

### Trauma and Dysfunction

Restrictions in occipital motion are involved in "compression head." The occiput may be affected via atlanto-occipital trauma at birth, impact injury (usually from a blunt instrument, such as a policeman's nightstick,[13] but also from falling backward onto an unyielding surface like concrete[14]), and in schizophrenia.[15]

The atlantoaxial and atlanto-occipital joints are the deep source of motion and stability for the temporomandibular joint,[16] and as such most occipital techniques may be included in the treatment of temporomandibular joint dysfunction.[17]

A CV4 can be useful in approaching and diagnosing the viscerocranium, especially the parts directly articulating with the neurocranium. To do this, perform a CV4 with *kime* directed at freeing the frontal/ethmoid/vomer/sphenoid complex, paying particular attention to the status of the falx cerebri.

Whiplash injury[18] has become so common that its treatment occupies a substantial proportion of many craniosacral therapists' professional time. The occiput is frequently involved, and must be stabilized for normal temporal and sphenoid function to return. Releasing tension from the tentorium, which connects the occiput with the temporals and sphenoid, is one of the decisive factors in successful treatment. Care must be taken in using a CV4 to treat whiplash injury as the elevation of the head off the table may echo the head position during the moment of maximum strain during the accident, thus exacerbating the client's condition.

### Interconnectedness

The straight sinus is a large vein that sits inside the diamond-shaped tunnel formed by the confluence of the falx and tentorium. Sloping inferior and posterior, it carries used blood from the thalamus, limbic system, and midbrain to its attachment to the internal occipital protuberance, where the blood empties into the paired transverse sinuses from whence it leaves the head through the jugular foramina.[19] The occiput is connected to every other bone of the neurocranium through the falx and tentorium.

The occiput is also a key focus in any discussion of cranial mechanics, as the internationally recognized system of diagnosing cranial fault patterns is based upon the position and movement of the sphenobasilar joint.[20]

### Visualization

Visualize the reciprocal tension membrane attachments to the occipital squama whenever you work with the occiput, and remember that this includes the core link. Perceive the brainstem, cerebellum, and occipital cortex deep to your fingers. Feel the spongy resilience of the cerebrospinal fluid beneath your palms, and visualize the lozenge-shaped fourth ventricle with its three outlets.

## TECHNIQUES

### Occipital and Sacral Coupled Hold: Core Link Appraisal

This technique is concerned with detecting the fluid continuity of movement – or its absence, or alteration – between the sacrum and occiput.

Stand at one side of the table level with the client's diaphragm in order to place your non-dominant hand under the sacrum, either in a standard outside-leg contact or transversely. (The transverse contact is better, both for taller clients and in general, because it places both hands in the same transverse plane, which makes mechanical perception easier.) Then take your other hand and place your index and middle fingers transversely, posterior to the neck, and move them superior until your index finger makes contact with the client's occipital squama. Your contact will be immediately below the inion, although the exact location depends on how the client holds his head upon his neck. Your hand is palm upward, allowing the occiput to rest upon the table. Make a very gentle, ¼ ounce (7 gram) contact – not enough to restrict the natural movement of the occiput, but just enough to feel its movement. This will give you quite sufficient contact to gauge motility.

Tune in first to your sacral hand, as you will lose sensitivity there first, then to your occipital hand. Then allow the input from both hands to merge, so that you can compare and contrast the two patterns. Are the bones in synchronous motion, or do they move in opposite directions, but at the same time? Is there a torsion in the spinal cord? By discerning at what spinal level there is an impingement in the motion, you can diagnose disc injury, osteophyte impingement, or the presence of a tumor. If the movement is indeed synchronous and fluid, initiate a delicate intention and motion with both hands to facilitate the glide of the spinal dura within its canal. Move the spinal cord alternately toward the feet and crown. If you get a sense of free glide between the two extremities, the dura and core link are normal.

## Cranial *Prana Yama*

Ask the client to focus on his breath, breathing slowly and powerfully through his nose. Instruct him to raise his head about thirty degrees off the table whenever the respiratory urge causes him to take an in-breath; he lowers his head with each out-breath. As this pattern becomes comfortable to the client, the cranial wave and respiration will tend to mesh, so that flexion occurs in sync with the in-breath and extension with the out-breath.

Once the client is doing this correctly and comfortably, place your hands on either side of his head with your index fingers over the mastoid processes, your thumbs on the greater wings of the sphenoid, and the heels of your hands over the parietals. Hold this position as the client moves his head up and down with respiration until you are able to sense the cranial wave in each bone – temporal, sphenoid, and parietal. (As a learning tool, first "get" temporal motion, then add the other bones in one at a time.)

When you have a sense of the cranial wave, you begin to add pressures that accentuate the bones' flexion on the in-breath. That is, put medial pressure on the mastoid processes with your index fingers, follow the sphenoid into flexion with your thumbs on the greater wings, and use the heels of your hands to mediate inferior pressure onto the parietals where they depress slightly in flexion at the sagittal suture. Reverse your motion as the bones move into extension when the client breathes out and lowers his head. (As this motion of your hands in three locations is complex, it is useful to simulate it for practice – about an hour and you should have it down.) Continue this with the client's breath and head motions until his muscles approach exhaustion.

This technique tires the scalenes and sternocleidomastoids and thus encourages opening of the cranium. This is particularly useful as a prelude to other craniosacral work and as a preliminary technique in an air sinus protocol.

## Suboccipital Hold

The spirit of these techniques is lightening. The objective is to take superimposed loads off of the atlas (first cervical vertebra) and to separate it from the 12 to 15 pound (5 to 7 kilogram) weight of the head sitting above it.

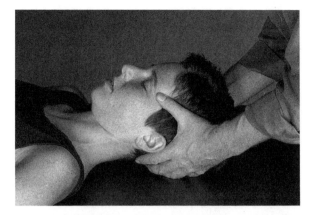

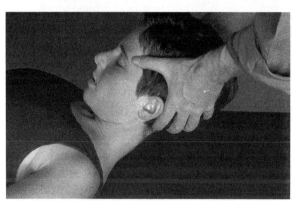

*Cranial* Prana Yama, *positions for out-breath (left) and in-breath (below)*

There are various ways of performing a suboccipital hold. One is to sit at the head of the table. Make sure the client's head is in the optimum position on the table vis-à-vis your forearm length. Slowly introduce your hands on either side of the occipital squama, moving them medial until they touch, lifting the head off the table. Now locate the tips of the mastoid processes, and slide medial and posterior from them until your fingertips lie posterior to the atlas. (An alternative way to do this is to lift the whole head off the table, into full flexion. This forward-bending motion exposes the transverse masses of the atlas. Retain contact as you lower the head back down upon the table.)

Keeping your index and middle fingers upon the posterior mass of the atlas, move your ring and little fingers superior between ¼ and ½ inch (.6 and 1.3 centimeters, or one atlas height) so that their tips rest on the occipital squama. Then flex your

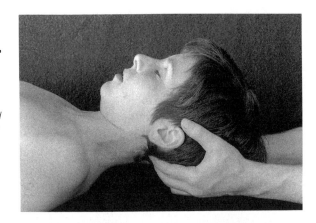

*Suboccipital Hold; in the second photo the model's head is rotated for clarity.*

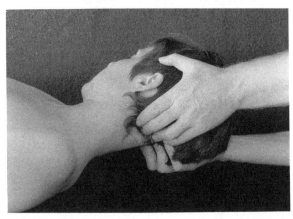

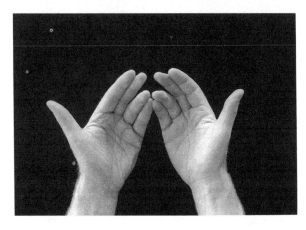

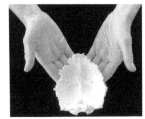
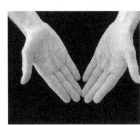

*Occipital Eight-Finger Hold, two views*

ring and little fingers slightly to better elevate the head. Your hands abut one another. Usually the head wants to migrate further cephalad and move into slight forward-bending as it does so, taking up slack from the entire neck; the location of your index and middle fingertips at the atlas allows you to ensure that maximum effective separation occurs there.

Begin to tune in to the behavior of the atlanto-occipital joint. You often have to tease it apart by adding extra traction, and micromovements, in whatever directions are indicated by the feel of the tissues as they perform their delicate dance. Stay present, sensing, until the atlas finally separates from the occiput – a point at which you may feel a definite tissue "sigh" as an inherent tension level suddenly subsides. Hold the position for a few more moments, as feels appropriate, before returning the head to the table and slowly withdrawing your hands. The client frequently feels as though he is 2 inches (5 centimeters) taller.

An alternative is to contact the axis (second cervical vertebra) rather than the atlas, and thus to free both the atlanto-occipital joint (this less specifically than with the preceding contact) and the atlantoaxial joint. Here there is no need to lift the head off the table, as you can palpate the axis with the client's head resting normally on the table. Take index- and middle-finger contact on the axis, and proceed as before.

## Occipital Eight-Finger Hold

Sit at the head of the table. Use the mastoid tips for landmarking. Rotate the client's head to the right, finding the left mastoid tip with your left index finger, then trace a line at least 2 inches (5 centimeters) directly posterior until you are ½ inch (1.3 centimeter) over the hair line. Then place the remaining fingers of your left hand on the occiput. Repeat on the other side, and make sure the fingers of both hands touch under the occiput. In this position, eight fingers are on the occipital squama – and only the squama – separating it from the table. Make sure the posterior aspects of your wrists are on the table surface, and that your thumbs do not contact the cranium but are instead held lightly off the head. Your fingertips are superior to the neck muscle attachments and at – or just below – the level of the inion.

This occipital contact is a very light, delicate hold; the 14 pound (6 kilogram) weight of the head rests on your finger shafts and pads, so there is no need to apply any pressure. The hand position reminds me of the one that wrestlers use at the beginning of a tournament: they open their hands to the referee to show that they have no concealed weapons. It is an open gesture, saying "I've got nothing to hide."

This occipital hold is primarily useful in diagnosing the movements of the occiput, in releasing neck and shoulder tension, and in beginning the process of freeing up the all-important sphenobasilar joint. Use it as a learning tool and as preparation for the CV4.

## The CV4

### Basic Uptake

Use the basic uptake for familiarization with the hold, then move on to learn the smooth uptake. Practice the smooth uptake at every opportunity as it delivers a far more professional feeling than the basic uptake, which feels very cumbersome in comparison.

Sit at the head of the table. Begin your familiarization with this technique by taking care with your landmarking. As in the occipital eight-finger hold, use the nearest available landmarks, the mastoids. After locating the mastoid tips, trace your index fingers 2½ to 3 inches (6.3 to 7.6 centimeters) directly posterior to find the contact area for the CV4. Place your thenar muscle there, preferably on the left side first, then the right, taking care to cradle the client's head securely and comfortably.

Crane your own head around, lateral to the client's mastoids, to inspect the location of your thenar eminences: they need to be directly posterior to the auricles of the ears. Ensure there is at least two, and possibly three, finger-widths between the posterior-most part of the helix of the ears and the start of your thenar eminences.

### Smooth Uptake

This technique gives you a way to smoothly lift the client's head off the table by rotating your thenar muscles into the optimum CV4 position. It has none of the fussiness inherent in attaining correct placement one side at a time, but it does require more practice.

Sitting at the head of the table, begin with your hands palms down on either side of the client's occipital squama. Make the hitchhiker's gesture with each hand, and insert your thumbs under the occiput, just superior to the acupuncture point Wind Palace (Governor Vessel 16). Repeat your mastoid landmarking to make sure your thenar muscles are in the right place, and move your hands cephalad until you establish firm osseous contact with the occiput. While the client is

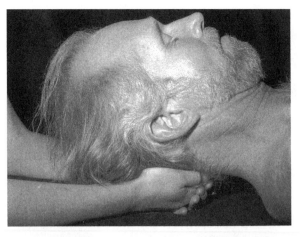

*The CV4, lateral view of the basic contact, with bony contact shown below*

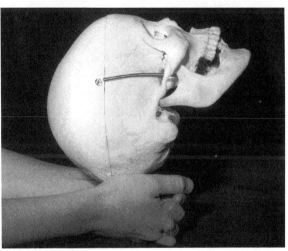

breathing out, brace your thenar muscles and smoothly and simultaneously rotate your hands and forearms outward (external rotation), rolling slightly inferior to slip under the occiput into the correct CV4 location. Once you are in position, make sure you are sufficiently posterior from the auricles (see above).

The CV4 is one of a handful of universal holds in craniosacral work: you can do almost everything with this one contact (see the end of this chapter for a list of its capabilities). Superb as a diagnostic tool, it permits an investigation of the entire reciprocal tension membrane, calvarium, straight sinus, and the status of cerebellar and cerebral tissues. It is one of the best techniques with which to induce a still point in the whole dreambody. The CV4 can also be useful in approaching and diagnosing the viscerocranium, especially the bones directly articulating with the neurocranium, such as the ethmoid and the frontal. To work with the neurocranium-viscerocranium juncture, perform a CV4 with *kime* directed at freeing the frontal/ethmoid/vomer/sphenoid complex. While you do this, pay particular listening attention to the falx cerebri.

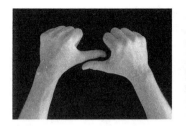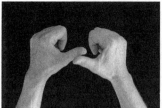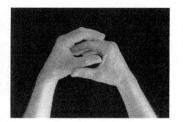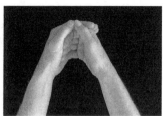

*Hand position sequence for smooth uptake of CV4*

Lao Tzu points out that the sage understands that nothing is ever perfect ... and that, seeing the imperfection of all things, the sage sees how perfect that is.[21] When you first take up a CV4, it never feels perfect, yet it is a hopeless pursuit to continue fussing and fidgeting in an effort to get an impeccable hold. The occiput is slightly different from the left to right sides, and your hands are slightly different. Accept that it feels slightly imbalanced, settle into it, and in a few minutes it will feel perfect – your proprioceptors will adjust to the imbalances to which your perfectionism cannot. Most bodyworkers need to train themselves not to dig their fingertips into the upper neck. The art is to leave your fingertips passive, acknowledging that there is no need to hurry. Let the body energy and motility patterns come to you. Do not be an aggressive hunter. Like Psyche, wait.

### One-Handed CV4

Use a smooth uptake of CV4 to begin the one-handed contact, but withdraw one hand as the hold becomes complete. Use the finger pads of your index, middle, and ring fingers of the remaining hand to take the place of the missing thenar eminence. Be sure to keep the head midline and centered. This one-handed contact allows you to use your free hand for three-dimensional, asymmetrical work elsewhere on the head or upper body. Sutherland is reputed to have originally taught the CV4 as a one-handed technique. Finding that his students had difficulties with it, he instituted the two-handed CV4 to take its place.

### Occipital Approach to the Transverse Sinus

Sit at the client's head and contact the occiput with the tips of four fingers of each hand lateral to the inion. This places your fingertips external to the transverse occipital sinus, which is where the tentorium splits before attaching to the endosteal dura – the part of the dura mater that is tightly adherent to the inside of the cranial bones. Compression here seems to facilitate venous drainage from the brain.

Lift the head off the table, balancing it on your fingertips. The weight of the head acting on your fingertips causes a slight deformation of the transverse sinus, accelerating venous blood flow out of the head. At first this technique feels like a juggling act, but persevere. Once you have the head balanced on your fingertips, wait for a sense of softening to come through, as congestion in the venous sinus becomes palpable. This technique may be effective in reducing or relieving headaches which are not responsive to a CV4. It may also be useful in teasing out neck tension. It is one of several components in the venous sinus protocol, which assists drainage of all the venous sinuses.

### Occipitofrontal Cant Hook Technique

You may perform this technique from either side. For the sake of clarity, I describe it from the client's left side. Sit facing the left side of the client's head. To take up the Occipital Cant Hook technique with your left hand, place your fingers except your thumb under the occiput, then place your thumb in contact with the asterion area of the left parietal bone. Your left thumb now points toward the ceiling. Make a similar contact with your right hand on the frontal bone, finger pads comfortably in contact with the right superior temporal line, at the point where it meets the orbital ridge. Your right thumb pad touches the left side of the frontal at the intersection of the temporal line and orbital ridge, pointing toward the floor.

Once you can feel the cranial wave – especially torsional patterns of the head – begin to tease open the sutures of the far side of the cranium, using your thumbpad contacts as fulcrums and your fingertips as gripping points, as openers. Your objective is to free the coronal, sphenotemporal, squamosal, and lambdoid sutures on the right side, which allows the right side of the tentorium and falx to begin unwinding, which you will feel with both hands.

This is a sophisticated technique that needs to be performed with sensitivity to the sutures you are compressing – in this case, the left coronal, sphenotemporal, and lambdoid. They may require some decompression upon completion of the Cant Hook work.

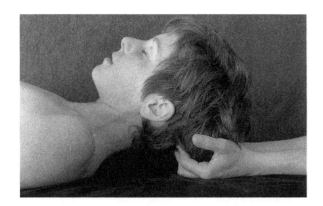

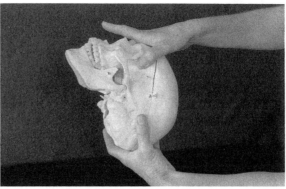

Use the Cant Hook for lateroflexion lesions at the sphenobasilar joint and to correct the results of impact injury to the occiput or one side of the head. It is well worth practicing this compound, coupled, interactive technique until you understand its full capabilities.

## Other Techniques that Can Affect the Occiput

■ Lumbar to Vertex Sweep
■ Sphenobasilar Decompression
■ Sphenoid and Occiput Cup and Straddle
■ Frontal Anterior Decompression
■ Mandible unwinding
■ Whole-body unwinding: head, shoulder, and arm techniques
■ Oral Coronal Shear Test
■ Auditory Tube Twist
■ Scalene muscle release work
■ Work with the Windows to the Sky points at the neck
■ Inner-eye work which accesses Wind Palace (Governor Vessel 16)

## The Fourteen Capabilities of the CV4

Study of this list after reading the chapters on the central nervous system, reciprocal tension membrane, and the sphenoid and occiput will help you deduce why the CV4 can have these varied effects.
Use the CV4 for the following:

■ To unwind the neck, atlanto-occipital joint, and cranial base
■ To unwind and balance the membrane system (reciprocal tension membrane)
■ To induce a still point in the movement and molding patterns of the occiput
■ To correct all types of headache (except those arising from a cerebrovascular accident or a brain tumor), employing different aspects of these fourteen capabilities

■ To redistribute cerebrospinal fluid throughout the spinal and cranial regions, and assist its evacuation from the fourth ventricle
■ To diagnose the difference between a "normal" and a "traumatic" head by sensing wave cadence, and subtle changes in membrane system tension and "feel"
■ To diagnose and locate the presence of a heretofore undiscovered cyst or tumor within the neurocranium, by sensing shifts in reciprocal tension membrane "feel"; through using the CV4 as a kind of sonar, bouncing pressure-wave echoes within the cranial enclosure; and by using the psychic art known as "psychometry" while performing a CV4
■ To optimize the relationship of the neuro-cranium to the viscerocranium
■ To reduce body temperature by approximately 1.4 degree Fahrenheit (one degree Celsius)
■ To interrupt and release a constant-on engram that is exacerbating muscle contraction headache and temporomandibular joint dysfunction
■ To induce whole-body relaxation (the rolling wave, or "magic carpet" effect) via compression of the pyramidal tracts of the medulla oblongata which especially affects the neck, pectoral muscles, pelvic girdle, and lumbar spine
■ To vector force and awareness within the neurocranium, with which many sutures can be mobilized, notably the coronal
■ To correct some sphenobasilar lesion patterns, notably lateral and vertical strain lesion patterns
■ To facilitate channel-changing assisting the client's movement into altered states of consciousness, such as the hypnagogic, through subtle electrical field changes to the Windows to the Sky points[22]

# 24
# The Sphenoid

1 Body, or clivus

2 Jugum

3 Greater wing

4 Lesser wing

5 Chiasmic groove

6 Sella turcica

7 Hypophysial fossa, hollow occupied by hypophsis, or pituitary

8 Anterior clinoid process

9 Posterior clinoid process

10 Dorsum sellae, or rear of the saddle

11 Carotid sulcus for internal carotid artery

12 Sphenoidal crest for articulation with perpendicular plate of ethmoid

13 Rostrum, an extension of sphenoidal crest

14 Apertures for sphenoid air sinus

15 Optic foramina

16 Superior orbital fissure

17 Cerebral surface

18 Temporal surface

19 Orbital surface

20 Zygomatic margin

21 Frontal margin

22 Parietal margin

23 Squamous border

24 Infratemporal crest

25 Foramen rotundum

26 Foramen ovale

27 Foramen spinosum

28 Sphenoid spine

29 Pterygoid, or vidian canal

30 Pterygoid processes

31 Lateral pterygoid plate

32 Medial pterygoid plate

33 Pterygoid hamulus, formed by the pull of the pterygomandibular raphe

34 Pterygoid notch

35 Sphenoid articulation with occiput, "Sphenobasilar Joint"

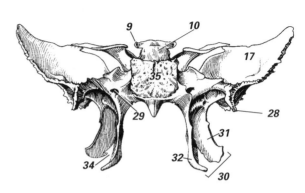

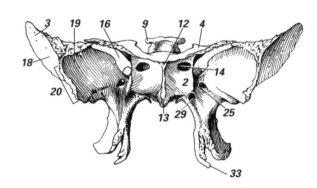

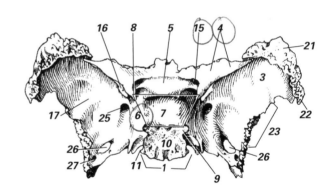

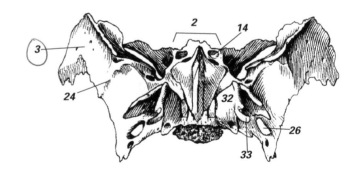

## Embryology and Osteology

Like the occiput, the sphenoid has its origins in vertebrae, but in its case the fusion of two embryonic vertebrae, not just one.[1] The anterior portion of the body of the sphenoid evolves from one vertebra, developing from six ossification centers. It is known as the jugum, and the lesser wings attach to it. The posterior of the two embryonic vertebrae forms the rear of the sphenoid body, known as the clivus, which develops from eight ossification centers. The clivus contains the sella turcica and forms the anchor for the attachment of the pterygoid processes, and for the greater wings. Both the greater and lesser wings of the sphenoid are evolutions from once-diminutive transverse processes.

These two "vertebrae" are joined not by an intervertebral disk, but by a peg and socket joint, anatomically described as a gomphosis.[2] The sphenoid body is in its two vertebral parts until eight months after conception, at which point the gomphosis fuses.[3] The greater wings are separate from the sphenoid body at birth; they unite by the end of the first year. Thus, the sphenoid is in three parts at birth: one body and two greater wings. The sphenoid air sinus does not begin to develop until the third or fourth year of life.

## Anatomy

The sphenoid is a delicate, intricately formed bone – the most spatially and visually complex bone of the cranium – that sits in the very center of the head. It is an extraordinary sight, appearing to be a cross between a butterfly, a dragonfly, and a bat. It is known as "Cho Kay Hotsu," the butterfly bone, in Japanese. (A Rolfer I visited in New York City had a sphenoid, mounted on a four-foot high pedestal, on display in his waiting room.) The more you look at it, the more you see.

Draw the sphenoid – you will be rewarded with a better spatial appreciation of both its delicacy and complexity. Three or four hours of drawing from at least four different angles, will help you to envision it with sufficient accuracy to really benefit your craniosacral work.

### Structure

The sphenoid is composed of an admixture of diploic and cortical bone. It has four wings, a recess for the pituitary, an array of foramina and fissures, and an air sinus. Its core structure is the sphenoid body, which appears robust from above, the sides, and below, but is in fact entirely hollowed out to house the air sinus. From the body spring two sets of wings. Imagine a dragonfly in an ivory color; the anterior, or lesser, wings are smaller, the very size of dragonfly wings; the posterior, or greater, wings are much larger and more robust, swinging upward like hands held together at the wrists and opening as if to receive the light of the sun from above. The pterygoid processes are suspended from the underside of the roots of the greater wings, close to the sphenoid body, and are therefore much narrower – by about half – than the superior-most aspect of the greater wings.

## Location

The greater wings are located at the temple. The anterior portions of the lesser and greater wings of the sphenoid form the rear of the eye sockets. The hamuli ("little hooks"), located at the most inferior part of the medial pterygoid plates, are palpable inside the mouth, about one tooth width posterior to the eighth upper tooth, and half a tooth width medial.

### Landmarks

Sphenoid landmarking is determined anteriorly by the location of the eyebrow and eyelid. The best area for palpation of the greater wings lies between two lines – one drawn posterior from the apex of the eyebrow and another drawn posterior from the lateral canthus of the eye. The wings go no further anterior than the zygomatic portion of the eye socket and no further posterior than the anterior margin of the sideburn hairline. The sphenobasilar joint lies in the same horizontal plane as the temporomandibular joints, but is situated slightly anterior to them.

## Sutures and Articulations

The sphenoid articulates with every bone of the neurocranium:

- The basilar portion of the occiput
- The temporals at both the petrous portion and the temporal squama posterolaterally
- The parietals at pterion (a variable – it may not articulate here)
- The ethmoid anteriorly
- The palatines inferiorly (unless they are absent)
- The frontal anteriorly, with articulations of both the lesser and greater wings
- The ala of the vomer inferiorly
- The zygomae anterolaterally

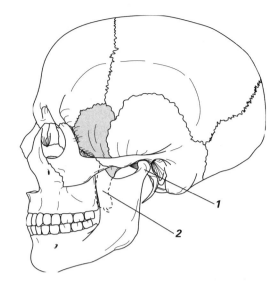

*Lateral view of the skull showing location of sphenoid and relationship of lateral pterygoid plate to condyle of mandible*

1 Condyle of mandible
2 Lateral portion of lateral pterygoid plate

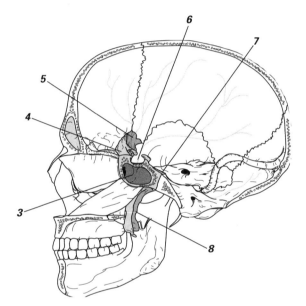

*Midsagittal view of the skull, showing articulations of the sphenoid and its air sinus*

3 Sphenoid sinus
4 Lesser wing
5 Greater wing
6 Sella turcica
7 Spheno-basilar joint
8 Medial face of lateral pterygoid plate

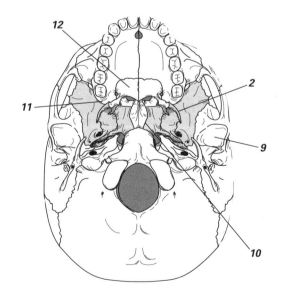

*Inferior view of the cranial base, showing location of the sphenoid and relationship of the pterygoid processes to the alveolar ridges of the maxillae*

9 Glenoid or temporomandibular fossa
10 Schyndelesis of sphenovomerine articulation
11 Alveolar ridge of maxilla
12 Palatine bone

Very rarely, when the palatines are absent,[5] the sphenoid articulates directly with the maxillae via the inferior aspects of the sphenoid body and the pterygoid processes.

Thus, the sphenoid articulates with twelve bones: the occiput, the vomer, the ethmoid, both palatines, both zygomae, both temporals, both parietals, and the frontal.

## Weight

A medically prepared disarticulated sphenoid weighs ½ ounce (14 grams).

## Detailed Anatomy and Musculature

The sphenoid lies slightly anterior to the center and base of the brain. At its center lies the sella turcica, with four clinoid processes forming vertical projections like a saddle with four pommels, thus the meaning of its Latin name – "Turkish saddle." The pituitary nestles in the center of this saddle.

The superior parts of the vertical portion of the greater wings are, strictly speaking, part of the vault of the neurocranium – much as the temporal squama are also part of the vault, even though the petrous portions of the temporals are part of the cranial base.

The dorsum sellae ("the rear of the saddle") is a small, quadrilateral plate of bone oriented almost vertically, at whose superior and lateral margins the posterior clinoid processes protrude upward. At its inferior margin, the dorsum sellae ends at the superior border of the sphenobasilar joint. It is slightly concave, a contour caused by the immediate presence of the anterior bulge of the brainstem structure called the pons.

The palatines interface with the inferior surface of the sphenoid body at a small, flat, gliding joint surface; this is lateral to the main articulation between the sphenoid and vomer, a joint classified as a "schindylesis," or tongue-and-groove articulation.

Six of the twelve cranial nerves pass through or over the sphenoid, a remarkable number that helps explain the panoply of possible symptoms from a faulted or injured sphenoid.[6] Five of them – the second, third, fourth, fifth, and sixth cranial nerves – pass through the sphenoid into the eye socket, and all of them except the second pass through the superior orbital fissure.

| Sphenoid Anatomy | |
|---|---|
| 4 surfaces | Cerebral, temporal, maxillary, and orbital |
| 4 aspects | Described colloquially as brain, temple, throat, and eye |
| 7 margins | Zygomatic, frontal, parietal, temporal, ethmoidal, vomerine, and palatine |
| 10 foramina | The 3 paired rotundum, ovale, spinosum, optic, and the vidian canal |
| 2 fissures | The supraorbital fissures |
| 4 grooves | Carotid sulcus, optic sulcus, and the grooves formed by the presence of the auditory tubes |

■ The first cranial nerve, the olfactory, passes just superior to the lesser wings.

■ The second cranial nerve, the optic, passes through the roots of the lesser wing. (The optic chiasm, where many of the optic nerve fibers cross over, rests on the optic sulcus, which is located on the superior aspect of the sphenoid body, just anterior to the sella turcica.)

■ The third cranial nerve, the superior division of the occulomotor nerve, passes through the superior orbital fissure.

■ The fourth cranial nerve, the trochlear, passes through the superior orbital fissure.

■ The facial branch of the fifth cranial nerve, (the lacrimal, frontal, and nasociliary branches of trigeminus) passes through the superior orbital fissure.

■ The mandibular branch of trigeminus passes through foramen ovale; the maxillary branch of trigeminus passes through foramen rotundum.

■ The sixth cranial nerve, the abducens, passes through the superior orbital fissure.

■ The vidian nerve, which receives a branch from the fifth cranial nerve (trigeminus), passes through the pterygoid roots in a tiny tunnel called the pterygoid canal, just inferior to the sphenoid body.

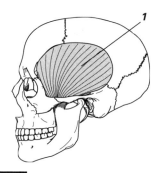
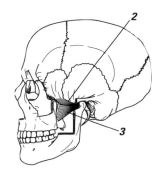
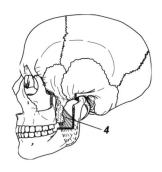

The temporalis muscle is covered by a tough fascia[7] that splits into a double-walled arrangement at eyelid level. From there to its fascial attachment to the zygomatic arch, it is usually drumskin-tight. Notice how tight the fascia feel at your own temple area immediately above the zygomatic arch, then move your fingers superior to the eyelid level and note how the fascia suddenly becomes markedly softer. This is the optimum location to palpate the energy, static position, and movement of the sphenoid.

### Musculature

The muscles attaching to the greater wings consist of the:

- Temporalis

The muscles attaching to the orbital (eye socket) portion of the greater wings consist of:

- All external muscles of the eyeball (arising from the common annular tendon) with the exception of the inferior oblique muscle
- Levator palpebrae superioris (also attached to the common annular tendon) which helps activate the upper eyelid

The muscles attaching to the internal pterygoid plate consist of the:

- Pterygomandibular raphe, the attachment for buccinator and superior pharyngeal constrictor
- Tensor veli palatini
- Levator levi palatini

The muscles attaching to the lateral pterygoid plate consist of the:

- Medial pterygoid
- Lateral pterygoid

## Physiology

The sphenoid plays vital roles in eyesight, neurological and hormonal function, and the functioning of the cranial "mechanism." The lateral and medial orbital rectus muscles are especially active in Rapid Eye Movement (R.E.M.) sleep.[8]

### Eyesight

The optic nerves pass through the roots of the lesser wings of the sphenoid. The optic chiasm (where most of the optic nerve fibers cross over to the opposite cerebral hemisphere) forms a slight depression (the optic sulcus) on the superior part of the sphenoid body, immediately anterior to the sella turcica. The three cranial nerves that control the external muscles of the eye (the third, occulomotor; the fourth, trochlear; the sixth, abducens) pass through the superior orbital fissure, which separates the lesser from the greater wing.

### Neurology

The frontal lobes of the brain rest on the superior face of the lesser wings; the temporal lobes rest in the scalloped posterior and inferior surfaces of the greater wings. The hypothalamus lies immediately superior to the sella turcica. The pons rests on the dorsum sellae.

The foramina and fissures of the sphenoid admit or exit the internal carotid artery, all three branches of the fifth cranial nerve, the middle meningeal artery, and the vidian nerve.

The olfactory tracts (the first cranial nerve) run across the superior aspect of the lesser wings. The inferior aspects of the sphenoid are host to shallow grooves formed by the presence of the cartilaginous auditory tubes, whose apertures to the nasopharynx are anchored to the medial pterygoid plates.

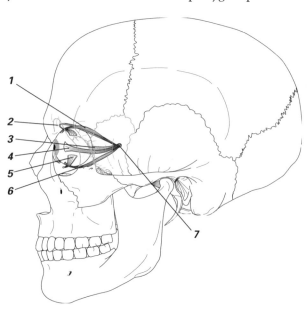

### Hormonal Functioning

The sella turcica creates a secure nest for the pituitary, which is cinched into place by the "roof" of the tentorium. This portion of the tentorium is called the tentorium of the sella turcica. Normal sphenoid flexion and extension movements act to "milk" the pituitary of its excess venous blood, optimizing hormonal function.[9,10]

The temperature of the pituitary must be kept within one degree Fahrenheit (0.6 degree Celsius) of optimum for normal body functioning to occur. One degree over, and fever begins, with the resultant loss of mental acuity. One degree under and we become a little sluggish; three degrees under and we enter hypothermia – we become "numb and dumb."

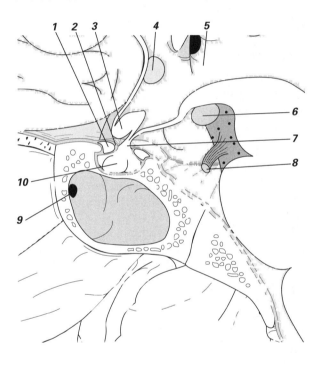

To achieve this necessary temperature stability in one of the hottest, deepest areas of the head, we have developed an extraordinary series of physiological strategies. First, the brain itself is kept slightly distant (⅛ inch, or 3 millimeters) from the pituitary itself by the pituitary stalk, thus helping to keep heat away. Second, cerebrospinal fluid circulates between the brain and the pituitary in the cisterna interpeduncularis and cisterna chiasmatis, high-roofed caverns in the subarachnoid space, helping dissipate and carry away unwanted heat.[11,12] Third, the pituitary sits on the paper-thin roof of cortical bone that encloses the air sinus of the sphenoid, which is cooled by a fluctuating circulation of air during nose-breathing (the air pressure changes dramatically from in-breath to out-breath, an action that is accentuated during *prana yama*). Last, the internal carotid arteries are routed well away from the pituitary and the all-important

hypothalamus, passing through the middle of the cavernous sinus, a network of webbed, bulbous caverns full of venous blood,[13] that keep the pulsating stream of hot arterial blood at a small but decisive distance. We instinctively splash cold water on the face in order to feel better when we are overheated; it is the pituitary and hypothalamus we are seeking to comfort, not the face. Cold water or a cold, wet cloth applied to the face cools the facial veins, whose venous blood moves posterior and inferior with gravity, to the cavernous sinus, thus helping to cool the pituitary.[14]

The pituitary is a light-sensitive gland. It senses moment-to-moment changes in light intensity, and adjusts the body economy according to the time of day it recognizes. Light reaches the pituitary through the eye sockets, and in a straight line from the nostrils – via the sphenoid air sinus. The suprachiasmic nucleus, located immediately superior to the optic chiasm, serves as the master clock of the human time-keeping mechanism. This mechanism allows us to set our biological clocks and circadian rhythms[15] according to the relative intensity and proportions of daylight and darkness.

### Mechanical Functioning

The sphenoid's extensive sutural articulations ensure that it is mechanically interrelated with every cranial bone, whether directly, through an intermediary bone (such as the palatines), or via the membrane system. When the sphenoid is faulted, the whole head tends to be faulted. Further, the sphenoid's muscular attachments to the mandible play an important role in temporomandibular joint conditions, and most forms of headache. Last, the small but strong zygomae, which articulate with the greater wings, can act as strong controllers of the sphenoid, inhibiting it from returning to normal after a trauma.

## Axis of Rotation

In the classical osteopathic model, the sphenoid's axis of rotation is said to pass horizontally and in the coronal plane through the middle of the sphenoid body. In the liquid-electric model, the sphenoid is regarded as moving in response to the floating spherical surface of the brain, particularly of the temporal lobes, nestled inside the greater wings of the sphenoid. It has no axis of rotation. The cranial wave motion of the sphenoid is modified by the status of both pterygoid muscles (particularly the lateral), temporalis, and masseter muscles and receives minor but important inputs from the external muscles of the eye.

**Far Left:**
*The pituitary in the sella turcica*

*1 Intercavernous sinus*
*2 Tentorium of sella turcica*
*3 Optic chiasm*
*4 Suprachiasmic nucleus*
*5 Third ventricle*
*6 Mamillary body*
*7 Pituitary stalk*
*8 CN III: occulomotor*
*9 Sphenoid sinus aperture*
*10 Pituitary*

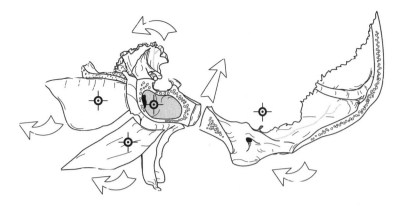

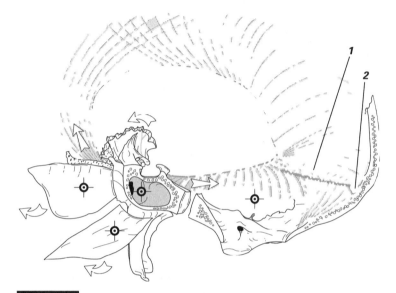

*Sphenoid motion in flexion*

**Above:**
*Flexion*

**Below:**
*Flexion, showing bone and membrane micro-movements*
*1 Straight sinus*
*2 Transverse sinus*

## Motion

### Osteopathic Model

In the osteopathic model (similar-motion model), as the sphenoid rotates (nose-dives) in true flexion, its body moves very slightly inferior, permitted and accompanied by the slight cephalad bowing of the sphenobasilar joint. Therefore, as the sphenoid flexes, the root of both lesser wings and the optic chiasm move anterior and inferior. The articulation for the ethmoid spine also moves antero-inferior (see above).

This motion means that the pterygoid processes circumduct in a posterior direction. Since they are slung below the body of the sphenoid, and are paired structures, they rotate externally in flexion. This widens the posterior part of the nasal fossa and the nasopharynx. (Remember this in the treatment of tinnitus, rhinitis, sinusitis, and nasal congestion.) The greater wings are considered to rotate externally in flexion, capable of this due to intra-osseous pliancy at their attachment to the body of the sphenoid.

In simple terms, the sphenoid tends to move into flexion (the fetal curl) on the in-breath. The sphenobasilar joint moves cephalad and, technically, the sphenoid is allowed to nose-dive by gliding off the parietals and by the slight slackening of the attachment of the tentorium to the anterior clinoid processes.

In terms of developing your perceptive skill, the challenge is to envision sphenoid motion not just in terms of the sphenoid itself, but also in terms of Sutherland's fulcrum, as this gives the basis for a full understanding of cranial mechanics. Sutherland's fulcrum[16] is an imaginary line drawn straight down the middle of the straight sinus (which lies at the junction of the falx and tentorium, running anterior and superior from the I.O.P.), which minutely changes position and shape with every movement of the sphenoid.

### Liquid-Electric Model

In the liquid-electric model, the sphenoid is regarded as moving in response to the fully-floating sphere of the brain, with the greater wings moving in opposite-motion (alternating) patterns.

This liquid-electric motion needs to be seen in relationship to the sphenoid's cardinal neighbors, the occiput, temporals, and parietals. As the left greater wing moves anteriorly during liquid-electric flexion, the left temporal bone rotates externally (this movement is also known as flexion, but more accurately and usefully as "external rotation" when describing the movement of paired bones; this is especially pertinent when describing temporal and zygomatic movements). In external rotation, the left temporal bone flares laterally and rotates very slightly anterior at the superior aspect of the squamous suture. During left temporal external rotation, the left greater wing of the sphenoid moves into flexion and inferior torsion – in other words, it moves inferiorly. As the temporals externally rotate they draw the tentorium both inferiorly and laterally.

To investigate other bone movements that occur during sphenoid flexion, let us begin with the occiput and consider what happens during left temporal external rotation. As the occiput circumducts and moves to the left in flexion, the falx is pulled posteriorly, inferiorly, and slightly left laterally. The falx is thus moved toward the straight sinus, pulling on the parietal bones and deflecting their movement. The combination of these movements causes the parietals to move laterally at the squamous suture, inferiorly at the sagittal suture, and into very slight internal rotation. As the left side of the sphenoid nose-dives in flexion, it glides anteriorly off of the parietals, which are rotating in the opposite direction. The pattern fluidly reverses in extension.

## Diagnostic Considerations

### Energetics

The sphenoid is the home of light-consciousness.[17] It is the visionary bone, seat of the inner eye.[18] The left eye is part of ajna, the inner-eye soul, the right eye part of sahasara, the crown soul. The glabella portion of the frontal and the entirety of the ethmoid are also part of the inner eye, but the sphenoid is its home. In Kriya Yoga the sphenoid is Christ Consciousness: "If thine eye be single, thine whole body be filled with light."[19]

The Chinese sage Xu Yin noted that on the fifty-sixth day of a meditation retreat, "Again my vision cleared, and I could see through walls."[20] Miyamoto Musashi declared "Vision is weak, perception is strong."[21] Mirabai noted that "My eyes flash through every obstruction."[22] The American equivalent of Xu Yin's achievement is Superman's inner eye, his X-ray vision. Something "catching our eye" or "catching our attention" is body language for inner-eye perception. Timothy Leary, still an active social commentator at age seventy-two, thirty years after the acid age, pointed out in 1993 that whoever controls your eyeballs controls your mind.[23]

The inner eye represents insight and has the ability to see what troubles everybody.[24] The inner eye allows an idiot savant the ability to see, instantly, the number of matches that have spilled out of a box onto the floor, or to solve complex mathematical problems faster than a supercomputer.[25] It is used by the academic genius who can calculate at lightning speed.[26]

A healthy sphenoid dreams with perception, clarity, and revelation, and may be clairvoyant. When faulted, the sphenoid dreams of death and dying. The sphenoid is occasionally represented in dreams by the image of a windshield.

### Trauma and Dysfunction

When traumatized, the sphenoid readily produces symptoms ranging in intensity from mild headache to severe personality disorder. Specific sphenobasilar lesion (fault) patterns are outlined below.

Optimizing the motility of the sphenoid can help in seasonal affective disorder (SAD, also called winter depression).[27] SAD can also be cured with light therapy, with the disorder usually disappearing within five days of exposure to five to six thousand lux of light shone either onto the patient's face, or a reflective surface in front of him as he reads a book, for three to four hours a day. Six thousand lux is less than one-tenth of midsummer sunlight, but is sufficient to have this remarkable effect. Perhaps the pituitary and pineal glands and the suprachiasmic nucleus[28] – the three cardinal regulators of our internal clock – all benefit from this suffusion of light. Night-shift workers' internal clocks were successfully reset for the first time in 1991 by ensuring two things: that their work place was lit with a similar five to six thousand lux luminescence, and that their bedrooms were in total darkness.[29]

## Sphenobasilar Lesion Patterns

The highest form of lesion pattern detection is a kind of passive unwinding. Contact the greater wings with a technique of your choice, perhaps with the Oral Coronal Shear Test (it is advantageous if the hold has both sphenoid and occiput contacts, allowing you to palpate directly the motion of both bones, and therefore of the sphenobasilar joint). Reduce hand tension to a minimum, establish energetic contact and communication, and then wait. As soon as you detect the spirals and forces acting through the sphenoid, follow them: let the sphenoid take you away. It will promptly move into its fault pattern, and all you have to do is follow it.

By doing this you can deduce where the sphenoid does not want to go – those directions will feel like a "no," a hard, emphatically resilient sense of "keep out." Remember the importance of waiting, waiting and listening. If the movements of the cranial bones come to a standstill, stop, and release your contact once movement begins to seep in again, after the still point.

The dreambody generally prefers this non-intrusive diagnosis of fault patterns to the alternative, which is to go through each pattern step-by-step. It is the high art, doing non-doing. People's heads are often "energetically hungry" for such work (I have come across this most often in older clients, whose heads seem to be starved of touch). In some people, however, this energetic approach will not work. The input you receive may be muddled, jumbled, confused, full of mixed messages. In this case, move to the analytic model, and begin to work through the eight sphenobasilar lesion patterns outlined below. As you study the itemization, refer to the flow chart and illustrations of the lesions and, ideally, have a sphenoid, occiput, and model of the reciprocal tension membrane (see p. 181) at hand to imitate the faults with the bones themselves.

Before you begin hands-on work, get present. Then enter an "open field" channel of consciousness so that you are working without any preconceived ideas of what you will find. Remember that the eight lesion patterns are simplified guidelines, and somewhat abstract. In real life people have

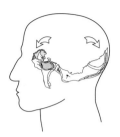

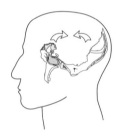

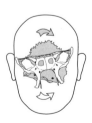

some admixture of patterns; for instance, a client will have a flexion lesion as their dominant movement, but with components of side-bending and torsion movements present as well. The value of the nomenclature is that it gives standard reference points so that patterns can be accurately described. These lesion patterns are also useful in making a technical diagnosis, one that has a universally agreed-upon format.

Treatment of the sphenobasilar lesions is best accomplished by considering the ten interactive options presented in Chapter 12, Modus Operandi, as well as the eleventh option, unwinding. Possible contacts include those listed in the techniques section below under The Six Sphenobasilar Holds (Vault and Base), or one of the "direct" sphenoid contacts in the itemization of sphenoid direct and indirect techniques that appear beginning on page 280. The following itemization of sphenobasilar fault patterns is summarized in flow chart form on pages 270–271.

### Flexion Lesion

***Definition and diagnosis*** A flexion lesion exists when the sphenoid moves more easily into flexion than extension. It is not evaluated according to the amount of movement, just the ease of movement. This lesion pattern is best detected with the Sphenoid and Occiput Cup and Straddle, the Oral Coronal Shear Test, or the Sphenoid and One-Handed CV4 technique (see Techniques, below).

***Ask yourself*** "Does the sphenoid nose-dive with greater ease than it returns in extension?" Your second question, refining your evaluation would be, "Does one greater wing nose-dive more easily than the other?"

***Symptoms and experiences*** People with flexion lesions tend to get simple dull headaches, frontal headaches, sinusitis,[30] and low-back pain. Flexion lesions[31] tend to occur in the plump (endomorph) to middle (mesomorphic) body types. These people tend to be ebullient, outgoing types whose more extreme representatives have no compunction about telling everyone their symptoms in public places. They may energetically pursue many different forms of treatment. Their head type is a lateral-expansion one, and they tend to lead expansive lives. In terms of the body language of the sphenoid's motion, however, the sphenoid with a flexion lesion is downcast. Inwardly, when alone, they may move into depression.

### Extension Lesion

***Definition and diagnosis*** An extension lesion exists when the sphenoid moves more easily into extension than flexion. (Again, not the amount of motion, just the ease.) Assess the sphenoid for this lesion using the Sphenoid and Occiput Cup and Straddle, or the Oral Coronal Shear Test, or the Sphenoid and One-Handed CV4 technique (see Techniques, below).

***Ask yourself*** "Does the sphenoid climb back superior with greater ease than it nose-dived?" Your second question, refining your evaluation, would be "Does one greater wing climb back up more easily than the other?"

***Symptoms and experiences*** Extension lesions lead to more severe headaches, including migraines. People with this pattern tend to be of the thin (ectomorphic) body type, intense people who are often moody and compulsive, and may lead driven lives. Extension head people prefer to live alone, with short periods of togetherness. They often love to run or jog, or follow a similarly energetic daily exercise regimen. They are introverted,[32] keep their symptoms to themselves, or share them with only a select few trusted intimates; they do not seek out treatment. They will say things like "This migraine proves to me that I have to go on a diet, exercise more, and clean up both my act and my desk. No thank you, I don't need any help, I can manage this perfectly well on my own."

With such a response pattern when stressed, their weakness is a tendency to lead a narrow life. And they will tend to have a narrow head – the long, thin, tall extension cranium. This may have formed at birth and been consolidated by a thousand subsequent life experiences whose interpretations produce the attitudes typical of the extension head type.

In terms of body language, in an extension lesion the sphenoid is looking up, as if aspiring to heaven. Extension head people look to God – either an inner or an outer one – for their support. They tend to be reclusive, mystic, and visionary. Krishnamurti, who endured many years of excruciating migraines,[33] exemplifies this tendency.

### Torsion Lesion

***Definition and diagnosis*** Named after the motion of the greater wing, where one side moves more easily and further cephalad. Thus, if the sphenoid is in a torsion lesion, one wing will be torqued more cephalad. If it is the right wing, the pattern is called a right torsion lesion, and vice versa. Take up a sphenoid and occiput contact, and then take one greater wing caudad while you move the other cephalad. At the same time, rotate their occiput in the opposite direction. Note the ease or reluctance with which one greater wing moves cephalad. Then repeat the test by taking the other wing cephalad. The best simple way to envisage torsion is to think of wringing out a wet towel: one hand (the sphenoid) goes one way while the other hand (the occiput) goes the other way. Maximum torque occurs at the sphenobasilar joint itself.

*Ask yourself* "On which side does the greater wing move cephalad more easily?" Note that, unlike flexion and extension lesions, which are evaluated solely according to the ease of motion, torsion is diagnosed according to the ease of motion *and* the amount of motion – the wing will move more cephalad, and more easily, to the side of the lesion.

*Symptoms and experiences* Dyslexia[34,35] is the most important symptom of a torsion lesion.[36,37] When dyslexia is due to a torsion lesion (and when the foundational or overlying emotional components have been resolved), correction of the lesion results in the immediate and permanent resolution of the dyslexia in children and young adults. In older people its treatment is more time-consuming and less dramatically successful. Other motor problems of the eye,[38] such as abducens failure, tracking disabilities, or depth-of-field deficits may also be the result of sphenoid torsion compounding psychological states. People with torsion lesions can also suffer from spinal scoliosis and associated neck and back pain. They say things like "Sometimes my body feels like a wet towel that has been twisted up by wringing the ends in opposite directions." Torsion lesions also affect the temporomandibular joints, and can change the bite.[39,40] Badly finished dental fillings or poorly fitting orthodontics can perpetuate a torsion lesion pattern.[41]

Emotional and psychological components are often intertwined with torsion lesions. Sphenoid torsion is body language for "being all twisted up" or "torn apart" by conflicting loyalties. This often occurs in children whose parents are fighting; the child, for security reasons, wants to take a side, but cannot because of conflicting feelings of loyalty to both parents. Imagine the child's head looking first at mom, then at dad, then at mom, then at dad....[42] The bone has no peace. Something has to give, and the sphenoid ends up being torqued to one side.

Working with dyslexic children, I have come across a consistent finding: they perceive stress within the parental bond, but try not to "see" it. This denial of perception twists up their fast-growing heads.[43] One child, plainly intelligent and perceptive, was suffering badly at grade school, as many children do.[44] While her sphenoid was in a torsion lesion pattern, it was not the result of physical trauma. Rather, she could see that her parents had no love left for each other, even though they attempted to hide it. Out of the need to continue living in that environment, her field faulted her sphenoid (perhaps through the intermediary of the lateral pterygoid muscles, and tooth clenching) and this acted as her blindfold. (The periphery – the social environment – altered the center, acting as the unified field.[45]) Unfortunately it "blindfolded" her at school too. I broached the subject with both mother and daughter, and then used craniosacral touch to correct the lesion pattern. The child was transformed within days. "What have you done with Jenny?," her schoolteacher inquired of the parents a week later, "This is not the same child."

Margaret Atwood describes a scenario for the psychological component in torsion lesion in her novel *The Robber Bride*. Tony, an only child, is sitting mutely at the dinner table, in the aftermath of a terse discussion between her warring parents:

*After that there is a silence, which fills with the sound of chewing. Tony has spent a good deal of her life listening to her parents chew. The noises their mouths make, their teeth grinding together as they bite down, are disconcerting to her. It's like seeing someone taking their clothes off through a bathroom window when they don't know you are there. Her mother eats nervously, in small bites; her father eats ruminatingly. His eyes are fixed on Anthea as if on a distant point in space; hers are narrowed a little, as if aiming.*

*Nothing moves, although great force is being exerted. Nothing moves yet. Tony feels as if there's a thick elastic band stretching right through her own head, with one end of it attached to each of them: any tighter and it would snap.*[46]

### Side-Bending Lesion

*Definition and diagnosis* Named for the greater wing that moves farther and more easily anterior on one side, creating a greater convexity on one side of the head. The best way to envision a side-bending lesion is to imagine the sphenobasilar joint viewed from above, with the joint hinged like a door and diverging to one side. The side where the gap is created is the side of the side-bending lesion. Thus, if the right side moves more fluidly and further anterior, creating a gap on the right side of the sphenobasilar joint, it is a "right side-bending lesion." The Oral Coronal Shear Test or

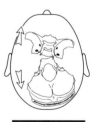

*Side-Bending Lesion*

## Sphenoid Lesion Patterns

| Lesion | Axis | | Symptoms |
|---|---|---|---|
| Flexion A, * | Paired, horizontal, coronal | | Simple dull headaches, sinusitis, low-back pain; occurs in mesomorphic or endomorphic body types; seek treatment; expansive heads means expansive lives |
| Extension A, * | Paired, horizontal, coronal | | More severe headaches, migraines; tend to be moody, compulsive/obsessive, loners; runners; often refuse treatment and seek aloneness<br><br>Ectomorphic body types<br><br>Narrow heads means narrow lives |
| Torsion B, ! | Single, horizontal, midsagittal | | Tend to spinal scoliosis; head, neck, and lumbar pain; motor problems of the eyes; dyslexia; scoliosis means torn apart by conflicting loyalties ("all twisted up")<br><br>Depicted: left torsion |
| Side-Bending B, * | Paired, vertical, sagittal | | More severe symptoms than torsion; mild personality change; rotatory conditions of the neck, especially hypermobile C1-C3; often ambivalence<br><br>Depicted: left side-bending |
| Lateral Strain C, # | Paired, vertical, sagittal | | Severe, chronic pain symptoms, eye motor and visual dysfunction, learning disabilities, personality disorders; semi-illiterate through dyslexia; cluster headaches<br><br>Depicted: left lateral strain |
| Vertical Strain C, # | Paired, horizontal, coronal | | As for Lateral Strain; if there is a flexion or extension component, add those symptoms; cluster headaches, possibly manic depression or schizophrenia<br><br>Depicted: vertical strain sphenoid superior ("high") |
| Lateroflexion C, > | Single, midsagittal | | Feelings of disassociation from the world; "plate of glass inside my head"; chronic depression, ongoing low-level headache, pressure within the cranium; abject dependency, and amorphous body pains<br><br>Depicted: left lateroflexion |
| Compression Head C | No axis, no movement or severely degraded movement | | The most severe condition; any combination of the above conditions or dysfunctions; may be present with a vertical or lateral strain lesion; morbid thoughts, suicidal depression, dreams of death or dying; absence of the suckling reflex in the newborn; check for atlanto-occipital impaction with all compression heads |

A = "Normal" dysfunction, i.e., not from severe trauma. A trauma may be emotional, spiritual, or physical. A trauma is an arrested action.

B = Usually from physical trauma

C = Almost always severe physical trauma, rarely from severe emotional trauma

\# = Opposite motion non-divergent lesions

\* = Opposite motion divergent lesions

! = Opposite motion, contra-rotating lesion

> = Similar motion, non-divergent lesion

| Diagnosed by | Named for | Techniques |
|---|---|---|
| Sphenoid moves more easily into flexion but amplitude is the same | Sphenoid moves more easily into flexion: "Flexion Head" | Hold sphenoid at limit of flexion, or assist into extension; use Sphenoid Four-Finger Hold, Sutherland's Grip, or Oral Coronal Shear Test |
| Sphenoid moves more easily into extension, but amplitude is the same | Sphenoid moves more easily into extension: "Extension Head" | Hold sphenoid at limit of extension, or assist into flexion; use Sphenoid Four-Finger Hold, Sutherland's Grip, or Oral Coronal Shear Test |
| Greater wing moves more easily and farther cephalad on one side | The side the greater wing goes most superior: "Left/Right Torsion Head" | Use Sutherland's Grip, Sphenoid and Occiput Cup & Straddle, Sphenobasilar Decompression, Oral Coronal Shear Test, or Sphenoid Four-Finger Hold |
| Greater wing moves further and more easily anterior on one side | Side where a gapping is created at sphenobasilar joint": Left/Right Side-Bending" | Use Sutherland's Grip, Sphenoid and Occiput Cup & Straddle, Sphenoid Four-Finger Hold, Sphenobasilar Decompression, Cant Hooks, or Oral Coronal Shear Test |
| Asynchronous rotation of both sphenoid and occiput as seen from above | The side where the greater wing makes a convexity ("side of the bulge"): "Lateral Strain Left/Right" | Use Cant Hooks, Sphenoid and Occiput Cup & Straddle, Oral Coronal Shear Test, or Sutherland's Grip |
| Sphenoid has moved vertically superior or inferior relative to the occiput | Whether the sphenoid has sheared cephalad or caudad at the sphenobasilar joint: sphenoid sheared superior or "Vertical Strain Sphenoid High" | Use Oral Coronal Shear Test, Sutherland's Grip, Sphenoid and Occiput Cup & Straddle |
| Sphenoid and occiput both move synchronously into torsion | The side that the sphenoid and occiput have both moved superior: "Lateroflexion Left/Right" | Use Oral Coronal Shear Test |
| Severe degradation, or complete absence of motility | The absence of motility, possibly compounded by being in compression while in vertical strain or lateral strain: "Compression Head" | Use CV4, all decompressive techniques Sphenoid and Occiput Cup & Straddle, Sutherland's Grip, Cant Hooks; treat the atlanto-occipital joint |

Sphenoid and Occiput Cup and Straddle are the best to discern this, but the Sphenoid Four-Finger Hold or the Ethmoid and Sphenoid Oral Thumb-Based Perpendicular Plate Release may also be used. Using the Sphenoid and Occiput Cup and Straddle, introduce anterior decompression on one side of the greater wings, bring the bone back to neutral, then repeat on the other side.

*Ask yourself* "On which side does the greater wing go anterior the easiest?"

*Symptoms and experiences* Side-bending lesions tend to produce more physical incapacitation than torsion lesions. Physically, these center around rotatory lesions of the cervical and lumbar spine, especially hypermobile vertebral segments at the first, second, and third cervical vertebrae. These are the clients who have seen a chiropractor twice a week for two years for neck adjustments, yet their necks are still unstable. The neck cannot balance because the spinal dura is rotating the vertebrae and forcing them into an abnormal "seating."

Psychologically, side-bending is associated with mild personality change, such as irritability in the previously easy-going, or the kind of short-duration depression that does not interfere with working abilities. During their side-bending lesion, these people tend to exhibit ambivalence, a kind of shrug-the-shoulders, couldn't-care-less attitude to life. Thus does their loss of purpose manifest. In body language terms, when the sphenoid is bent off to one side, life is put out of joint, it goes "off the rails." People feel "all out of kilter."

### Lateral Strain Lesion

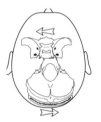

*Lateral Strain Lesion*

*Definition and diagnosis* This pattern is a shearing, or strain, of the sphenoid in a lateral direction across the sphenobasilar joint. The lesion is named according to the side of the head on which the sphenoid creates a convexity. (In a right lateral strain lesion, there will be a very slight convexity formed on the right side of the head as viewed from above, the result of the sphenoid displacement to that side.) Imagine the head as a watermelon. Cut the watermelon in half and hold the front and back halves in your hands with the cut in the vertical plane. Now "squidge" the front of the melon to the right while holding the back half stable. This imagery represents a right lateral strain. The sphenoid has been forcibly and traumatically displaced in a lateral direction, and thus "sticks out" on one side of the cranium; unable to dance its healthy spherical dance, it shuttles laterally and medially instead. It *does* move, which is good, but it does not move normally, which produces symptoms. There may be no trace of the normal flexion

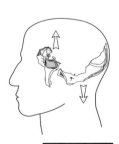

*Vertical Strain Lesion*

and extension pattern. Compared with the patterns described already, this is a more severe category of lesion, where there may be little or no trace of a normal axis of rotation. Consider using the Oral Coronal Shear Test or Sphenoid and Occiput Cup and Straddle to assess this lesion pattern.

*Ask yourself* "Which side is the sphenoid crawling out to?" or "Which way is the occiput going, which way the sphenoid?" Then dissect your answers into their component parts and, perhaps with your hands off the client's head and out of his field, imitate his pattern with your hands in space, cupping and straddling an imaginary head. Figure out what is happening at the sphenobasilar joint, and to the reciprocal tension membrane.

*Symptoms and experiences* Lateral strain is a serious fault pattern; some of the symptoms it produces are similar to those of other lesions, yet they are more serious in nature, as this is a more unnatural lesion and much less readily corrected. Symptoms include visual deficits and motor problems of the eyes, such as dyslexia (there is some similarity here to the torsion lesion); headaches, but cluster headaches rather than the migraines of the extension lesion; and the manifestation or exacerbation of chronic personality disorder (in side-bending there is only mild personality change). The lateral strain lesion may push a borderline personality into schizophrenia or manic depression. If the lateral strain occurred at birth, or through childhood violence, then the sufferer may be not only dyslexic as an adult, but illiterate, or semi-illiterate, even though plainly an intelligent being.

### Vertical Strain Lesion

*Definition and diagnosis* Vertical strain lesion is a shearing, or strain, of the sphenoid in a superior or inferior direction relative to the sphenobasilar joint. Like lateral strain, it is almost always induced by trauma from outside the head. As looked at from the side of the head, the sphenoid will have been displaced superiorly (perhaps from a blow to the underside of the mandible, such as from a boxer's uppercut) or inferiorly (from a blow under the occiput, such as from an impact from a policeman's nightstick swung upward). To use the watermelon analogy of the last lesion pattern, the rear half of the melon is displaced upward in a vertical strain, sphenoid low lesion. In simple terms, the sphenoid can be considered as moving in a vertical plane, vertically up (cephalad), or vertically down (caudad); either movement is vertical strain. The former would be called vertical strain, sphenoid high, which is reminiscent of an extension-like movement of the sphenoid. The latter, sphenoid low, would be the opposite, reminiscent of a flexion movement. However, because the lesion is caused by trauma, which overwhelms the normal integrity of the joint, the joint may not behave in tidy flexion- or extension-like movements at all, although remnants of such movement may be present. To test for this lesion, use the Oral Coronal Shear Test or Sphenoid and Occiput Cup and Straddle.

***Ask yourself*** "Is the primary sphenoid motion in a vertical plane, and does it move further and more easily in a cephalad or caudad direction?" Again, take your findings to their component parts and perhaps imitate the pattern off the client's head. Figure out what is happening at the sphenobasilar joint, the straight sinus, and throughout the reciprocal tension membrane.

***Symptoms and experiences*** The symptom picture is very similar to lateral strain, including cluster headaches, manic depression, and schizophrenia. Both vertical and lateral strain lesions are often accompanied by varying degrees of other lesion patterns, such as some torsion and some extension. The symptoms and the suffering therefore become compounded.

### Lateroflexion Lesion

***Definition and diagnosis*** This lesion is named by the side on which both the sphenoid and occiput are more superior. Lateroflexion is similar to a torsion lesion of the sphenoid, with an important difference: the occiput, instead of moving in the opposite direction (as it does in torsion), moves in the same direction as the sphenoid. Thus, both bones rotate around the same midsagittal axis, and both move superior on the same side at the same time. The watermelon (the analogy of the last two lesion patterns) is cut in two, but both the front and rear halves rotate the same way, disturbing sensitive brain structures, cranial sutures, the inner ear, and the neck. Lateroflexion is only caused by severe physical trauma, often by completely unexpected blows to the side of the face. By far the best technique to diagnose and correct this lesion is the Oral Coronal Shear Test. The Sphenoid and Occiput Cup and Straddle may also be used. Sutherland's Grip is less comprehensive since it neither stabilizes nor allows interactive work with the occiput, but its decompressive capabilities may be an asset.

***Symptoms and experiences*** This lesion is typified by a sense of separation from the world, often with the client using phrases like "a plate of glass" to describe his disassociation and malaise. In one six-month period in the early 1990s I worked with three people suffering from severe lateroflexion lesions, and this psychological pattern as well as

severe physical symptoms can be seen in their experiences.

In one case, the client had attempted to intervene in a marital dispute and was hit by the husband with an open-handed slap to one side of her face as she remonstrated with the wife. She did not see the blow coming – it was a complete surprise. She heard a sharp *crack* inside her head and sensed a light going out. Within forty-eight hours, she seemed to be a different person; she moved into what was to become chronic depression accompanied by an incessant pressure headache. When I first saw her six months later, she was still depressed and in pain. Nothing was right in her life, and she described how she felt by saying it was as if she was separated from the world by a sheet of glass that surrounded her a few feet out from her body.

In a second case, an Italian man was greeting his friend with the customary enthusiastic embrace and quick kiss to both sides of the face. But in their gusto they miscalculated when moving from one side to the other, and the sides of their heads clashed with sufficient force that one man broke his eardrum. He described how his head felt later, by saying he experienced a sensation as if he had a plate of glass stuck at an oblique angle through his head, separating one side of it from the other.

The third client, a psychology student, also described feeling as if he had a plate of glass in the middle of his head: everything was out of order, and he felt morose and eerily disconnected from the world. When his sphenoid corrected, he noted that an enormous weight lifted from his being; he realized he had been depressed for months and said that he laughed and smiled almost nonstop for two days after the treatment.

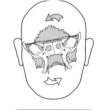

*Lateroflexion Lesion*

### Compression Head Lesion

***Definition and diagnosis*** Compression head is either the complete absence of the cranial wave in the head, or a severely degraded cranial wave, caused by jamming of the sphenobasilar joint so that it has no movement, or severely minimized movement. Again using our watermelon image, in compression head the two halves of the melon are jammed together so hard that they lose all ability to move independently of each other. In compression head the atlanto-occipital joint is almost always also compressed, particularly in the newborn.[47,48] Compression head is only caused by severe trauma, usually physical, rarely emotional. Any of the sphenoid greater wing contact techniques can be used to confirm this diagnosis. Sutherland's Grip and the Oral Coronal Shear Test are both particularly useful because they can be used for both diagnosis and treatment. As you

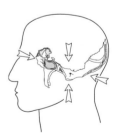

*Compression Head*

treat, "listen" for any sense of freedom returning to the sphenobasilar joint. Modulate and vary the vectors you are using for physical decompression, and track what you are doing with your own intention to obtain release.

*Ask yourself* "Is there any movement at all in this head? Does it feel stone-like and inert, or is there only the faintest filament of freedom?" Both situations indicate the presence of a compression head lesion.

*Symptoms and experiences* Compression head rarely occurs neatly, with the sphenobasilar joint tidily compressed in its neutral position. It occurs as the result of extreme violence to the cranium,[49] and tends to exhibit symptoms of whatever other displacements are also lodged into the cranial bone and suture architecture, such as vertical strain and flexion components. As such, this lesion pattern can display all and any of the symptoms or experiences itemized in the seven patterns mentioned previously, but it is chiefly characterized by severe, unremitting headache and the complete loss of functional ability at work and in relationship. Even morphine-derived medication cannot totally relieve the headache pain.

One client, Nigel, typified compression head. One day he and a workmate were moving heavy oak tabletops downstairs, one at a time. Nigel went first, walking backward. The stairs spiraled tightly, only just allowing them to negotiate the curve. When they had almost finished, they picked up two tabletops instead of one; tired and getting a little careless, they decided to take them both at once. As Nigel began walking backward down the stairs, the upper tabletop slid forward, toward his head. He tried to stop it with his fingertips, but it was too heavy. He instinctively moved his head backward in an effort to avoid the heavy piece of wood, but the back of his head hit the stairwell. An instant later his forehead was impacted by the accelerating tabletop and he heard a *crack* inside his head. Agonizing pain began within a few seconds.

Later that day Nigel went to see his family doctor, who referred him for an X-ray, which showed nothing abnormal. Prescription painkillers did not entirely remove the pain in his head, which became so severe that he could not work, or even sit still. He went back to his doctor, was given stronger medication and, when that did not work,

was referred to a neurologist. Finding no source for the pain, the neurologist referred him to Stanford University's Pain Clinic, but as there was a one-month wait, Nigel's girlfriend contacted me to ask for an appointment.

I saw Nigel almost a month after the accident, and he had been in unremitting pain the whole time. He looked miserable, and was depressed and at his wit's end. Meditating with him before working on his head, I perceived a torsion lesion of his sphenoid. I employed Sutherland's Grip to reduce the torsion lesion, and found to my surprise that not only was he in torsion, but in compression too – that is, his head had no cranial wave at all. It felt like a solid piece of cold and confused cast iron. This made perfect sense, given the nature of the impact: his coronal suture and sphenobasilar joint had been massively compressed.

It took twenty minutes of strong anterior decompressive traction with Sutherland's Grip for the maxillae, frontal, and sphenoid to release and begin a little tentative and reluctant unwinding. Then Nigel's face changed to a healthier color, and a tear rolled down his cheek. "How do you feel now?," I inquired. In a soft voice, seemingly from very far away, he answered "I feel *so* good!"

A few days later his girlfriend said that when he came home from the session he smiled for the first time in three weeks. The pain abated, but was by no means gone. He went to Stanford and spent more than a week in the pain clinic, but nothing worked as well as the craniosacral session had, so his consultant, acknowledging this, recommended he continue "that work you had in Carmel." It took several more months of patient work for his head to return to something like normal.

### Shear Planes

The above outline completes a review of the eight sphenobasilar lesion patterns. There are other faults that the sphenoid is heir to, however, notably from trauma that displaces or compresses sphenoid sutures, or sutures affecting the sphenoid – such as the zygomaticomaxillary sutures, which are particularly vulnerable to impacts from certain angles. There are two principal shear planes in the head – the sagittal and coronal – and heads tend to fault through (across) these sutural planes, which represent areas of potential structural weakness in the absorption of physical impact.

In the coronal shear plane, the front half of the head may fault vertically superior at the coronal suture when a person falls face-first on a sidewalk

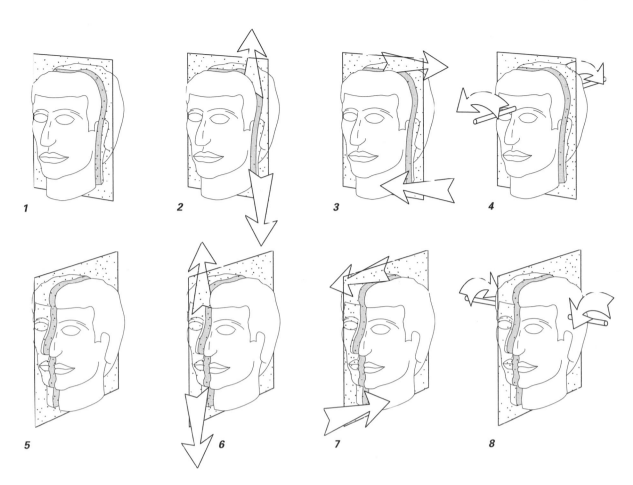

and catches the blow on the chin. The front half of the head seems to move upward, while the rear half seems to stay where it was. The head could fault vertically inferior when a person stands up suddenly in a confined space and hits the top of his forehead on a beam. A blow to the side of the head by a baseball bat or hockey stick may shear the frontal bone laterally (a more common injury at the coronal shear plane) away from the impact, the shearing again taking place at the coronal suture.

Sagittal shear plane faulting occurs with an impact to one side of the face, causing that side to displace posteriorly along a line of weakness extending from the sagittal suture and falx superiorly, down through the perpendicular plate of the ethmoid, the vomer, and the median palatine suture.

Techniques that encompass both sides of the shear plane are most effective in rectifying faults across it. Thus, for coronal shear faults, use the Oral Coronal Shear Test or a Cant Hook technique that will successfully engage, release, and balance the coronal suture. For sagittal shear faults, consider using the Temporal Palming technique.

## Interconnectedness

The sphenoid is the very definition of interconnectedness. Thirteen bones articulate directly with it; it is the anterior pole of attachment of the tentorium (Sutherland's "anterior inferior pole"). The optic nerves pass through it, and cross over on it, and more cranial nerves pass through, over, or under it than any other bone in the head. Energetically, the sphenoid is both sight (our dominant sense) and perception.

## Visualization

The sphenoid, as the inner eye, is where we see the world. In order to perceive the client's sphenoid, look at its physical location (encompassing the eye socket, temple, and roof of the mouth) and also begin to sense its presence as an energy field. Using your own inner eye, let your eyes move into soft-focus, wide-angle vision. Sometimes, either immediately or within a minute or two, you begin to sense it; at other times it may help to imagine a shape over the location of the sphenoid and see if that "starter" image helps you to see what is really there. You might:

- Imagine a dragonfly, and give it an ivory color.
- Imagine a bat, and make it fly at dusk with its legs hanging down (noting which movements it is good at and which not).
- Imagine a lunar landing module, incredibly complex, shimmering gold, its fine external wires the cranial nerves (noting how it hovers and where it is a little unbalanced).

Flesh out the details of the temporal lobes, optic chiasm, olfactory tracts, and pterygoid muscles. Make the sphenoid three-dimensional and alive.

## TECHNIQUES

Remember to consider the status of the jaw and cervical musculature in any assessment of, or work with, the sphenoid. Learn to palpate the sphenoid with the client supine, sitting, and prone, just as you would the atlas (first cervical vertebra). Prone palpation is of limited effectiveness, however, because of the compressive forces acting on the sphenoid through the frontal and viscerocranium, or whatever parts of the head are resting on the table.

The primary six techniques – the six sphenobasilar holds, listed first below – represent the most effective evaluation tools for sphenobasilar lesion assessment. Some are more suited than others to gauge the particular lesion type at the sphenobasilar joint – consult the flow chart of lesion patterns for specific recommendations. For treatment, remember your ten interactive options, as well as unwinding. The three most effective holds for treatment of the sphenobasilar lesions are, in order of effectiveness, the Oral Coronal Shear Test, the Ethmoid and Sphenoid Oral Thumb-Based Perpendicular Plate Release, and Sutherland's Grip. The Oral Coronal Shear Test is the best single technique to treat all eight sphenobasilar lesions.

**Far right:**
*Sphenoid Four-Finger Hold; only the index and middle fingers actually touch the head.*

## The Six Sphenobasilar Holds (Vault and Base)

The six basic sphenobasilar holds for assessing sphenoid-occiput behavior, status, and position are outlined below in order of simplicity. It is wise to start with one hold and practice it often enough

that you become comfortable with it and begin to build up a database – that is, you feel enough different heads that you know what normal is and can thus recognize non-normal. As soon as you are comfortable, introduce a second hold, and use these first two until you feel competent before adding a third, and so on until you are proficient with all six. Once you have mastered all six, learn to recognize which techniques will serve you best in different cases, helping you to assess the particular pattern(s) you suspect are present, based on the client's symptoms and your perception and visualization.

### *Sphenoid Four-Finger Hold*

This contact, with two fingers on each greater wing, is a beautifully delicate hold, as if you were measuring the wingspan of a butterfly. Sit or kneel at the head of the table. With the client laying supine the greater wings of the sphenoid are horizontal; landmark them at the temple and take up contact with the index and middle fingers of each hand in a very delicate palpation, aligning your fingerpads horizontally with the greater wings. Place your forearms on the table with internal rotation so that your pisiform bones touch the table surface – this places the acupuncture point Spirit Gate (Heart 7) in contact with the table and gives you the minimum unsupported "throw," or spanning distance, between the unmoving table surface and the client's motile sphenoid. The contact pressure is very light – about ⅕ ounce (5.6 grams). You are palpating through the temporalis muscle, so be sure the client's jaw is relaxed and his upper and lower teeth not touching. Palpation is the forte of this technique; without an occipital contact, it is less effective for the treatment of sphenobasilar lesions. Still, you can use it for gentle decompression, unwinding, or exaggeration (one of the ten interactive options).

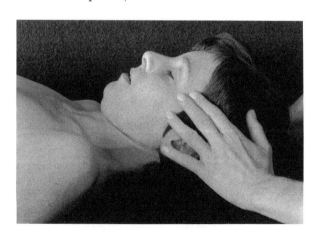

### Sphenobasilar Decompression

Again sit or kneel at the head of the table. Place eight fingers on the occiput (no need to interpose them between the client's head and the table surface), then place your thumbs over the greater wings so that their shafts point toward each other at a forty-five-degree angle anteriorly and medially. Avoid any other bony contact of your hands with the client's head. The contact pressure is light – about ⅕ ounce (5.6 grams). Tune in to your thumb contacts and assess the motility patterns, the "signature," of the sphenoid. Then "listen" to the occiput with your other eight fingers. Once you have a sense of the movement of the sphenoid and occiput individually, let the separation go and see how much information you can gather about the relationship between the two. Since they meet at the sphenobasilar joint, this technique gives you a chance to determine its functioning.

As a second stage, follow palpation with thumb-based decompression of the sphenobasilar joint to tune in to the tissues that lie between your sphenoid contact and your occiput contact. Use the human ability to see in vectors to palpate, visualize, and then unwind specific target tissues, in this case the sphenobasilar joint and reciprocal tension membrane. To introduce decompression of the sphenobasilar joint, first take out all skin slack under your thumbs so that you have a firm purchase over the wings themselves – not on the supraorbital ridges or the orbital portions of the zygomae. Then gradually increase thumb pressure on the greater wings, monitoring the status of the sphenoid, the occiput, and the sphenobasilar joint as you gently and fluidly introduce decompression.

It is possible to distinguish the six levels of tissue separation from first contact to final completion, as follows: (1) Releases in the skin, scalp, and fascia when you take out the skin and subcutaneous slack with your thumbs. This separation occurs relatively easily and fluidly. (2) Muscular release, chiefly of the occipitofrontalis and temporalis; this feels somewhat slower, more reluctant, sometimes begrudging – the muscles may take some time to let go. (3) Sutural separation, which feels quite sudden and of short amplitude when (and if) it occurs. The feeling is akin to prising apart a magnet from a piece of metal – first there is resistance, then suddenly none, all within a very short distance. (4) Dural release, which feels altogether more resilient, like elastic bands reluctantly giving way, fighting with you like a miniature tug of war as the reciprocal tension membrane unwinds and seems to make up its mind how much to let you win by. (5) A freeing up of cere-

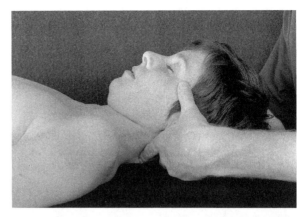

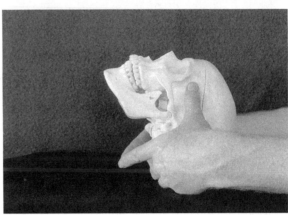

*Sphenobasilar Decompression, showing bony contact below*

brospinal fluid circulation and a movement of the fluid into areas that previously felt compressed, unavailable to its access. With this release, the movements of the whole head suddenly feel oceanic, tidal, and expansive – you have all seven seas in your hands. This is the domain of optimized cerebrospinal fluid. (6) Energetic release – here there is not so much movement as the experience of light and energy, and the tactile sensation of chemical/electrical fire unrolling and spreading outward in waves under your fingers.

While using your thumbs to propagate the sphenoid anteriorly at the fourth level (reciprocal tension membrane release), begin to move the sphenoid anterior, tracking the effects of both the actual movement, and your intention, at the occiput. Maintain the fluid progression of your lift until you sense the separation unraveling under your fingers. Wait, monitor, and tease the mechanism into balance and equanimity. Wait again, then come back to it and check that the change has taken hold. Diagnose whether any restriction is sutural, or in the reciprocal tension membrane, and localize and determine the vector of intention necessary to clear the mechanism. Feel and visualize the effect your treatment is having on the whole reciprocal tension membrane, and especially the tentorium (via the clinoid processes).

It is important to visualize the effect of the decompression on the sphenobasilar joint. This technique allows mobility, spaciousness, and normalization to return to this central joint. It facilitates a return to oceanic consciousness, however briefly, in those who are ready for it. Such illuminative experiences can be quite transformational.

### Sphenoid and Occiput Cup and Straddle

This technique (not illustrated) cups the occiput while straddling the greater wings of the sphenoid. Sit or kneel at the side of the table adjacent to the client's head and place one hand underneath the head, limiting your contact, as much as possible, to the occiput. Make sure that your hand acts as intermediary between the head and the treatment table. Tune in to your supporting hand until you are satisfied that you have an imprint of the occipital motility pattern, then move your free hand to span the forehead straddling the greater wings (the thumb on the wing closest to you, and whatever finger or fingers can reach on the other). Once you have established deep contact, sense what the tissues need from the ten interactive options and/or unwinding.

*Far right, top:*
*Sutherland's grip for palpation*

*Far right, middle:*
*with hooking contact*

*Far right, bottom:*
*hooking contact with model*

*Right:*
*Sphenoid and one-handed CV4*

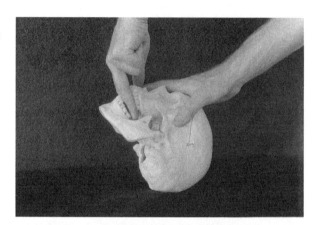

### Sphenoid and One-Handed CV4

In this hold you take a CV4 contact under the occiput then span the greater wings with the other hand. The One-Handed CV4 gives you a thenar eminence contact with the occipital squama and elevates the head 2 to 3 inches (5 to 7.6 centimeters) off the table. The greater wing contact allows you to sense with great delicacy how the sphenoid is moving in relationship to the occiput. This technique allows compound interactive diagnosis of all eight fault patterns of the sphenobasilar joint. (See one handed CV4, p. 258.)

### Sutherland's Grip

Sutherland's Grip, wherein you span the greater wings and have two fingers on or posterior to the maxillary teeth, is the finest technique for working with the sphenopalatine ganglion in the treatment and interdicting of an oncoming migraine. It is also one of the best treatment techniques for sphenobasilar lesions and for releasing the palatines from traumatic compression injury. Because you have no contact with the occiput, however, it is not adept at sphenobasilar lesion diagnosis. Stand to one side of the table and place the index and middle fingers of one hand on the biting surface of the upper teeth, as far posterior as the final teeth,

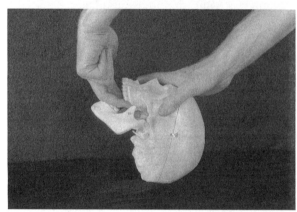

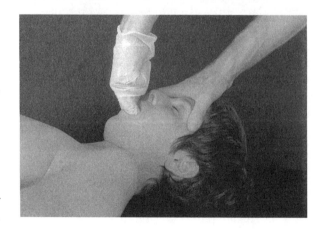

or even to the end of the alveolar ridge of the maxillae. The other hand straddles the sphenoid's greater wings. You are aiming to gauge any alteration from the normal sphenoid movement pattern.

The second stage of the technique involves an anterior decompression of the maxillae, achieved by hooking your fingertips deftly posterior to the eighth teeth and the end of alveolar ridges, freeing up the pterygoid processes of the sphenoid and allowing the sphenoid to move more freely in the event of there being an impaction between the maxillae, palatines, and pterygoid processes.

To correct lesion patterns with this technique, use exaggeration, compression, or the opposite of normal motility to obtain release. Sutherland's Grip is very useful in traumatic impaction of the viscerocranium in general, and of the maxillae and sphenoid in particular. It is also useful for obtaining a reading of the vomer and ethmoid.

### Oral Coronal Shear Test

This is a very capable and potentially powerful grip, designed to free the head at the coronal and sphenobasilar shear plane. Sit to the right of the client's head and use your left hand to cup the occiput, with your forearm and hand arranged parallel to the falx (i.e., in the sagittal plane, fingertips pointing toward the coccyx). The right takes up a straddle contact. First the little finger is placed inside the left side of the mouth just cephalad to the buccal surface of the alveolar ridge of the maxilla, then the next three fingers are placed on the left side of the client's face, up to and including the greater wing and the frontal supraorbital ridge. Your right thumb monitors and then may modify movement of the right side of the client's face with contact on the greater wing. It is very effective for the deeply traumatized head.

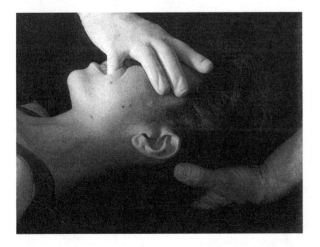

### Composite Lesion Testing

### Stacking

"Stacking" refers to a specific testing and treatment module chiefly used to treat sphenobasilar lesions. As this is an advanced procedure, do not attempt to master it until you have enough experience to be thoroughly familiar with the testing and treatment of individual lesion patterns. You may use any of the six vault and base holds itemized above. Sit at the client's head and – while you are gaining familiarity with stacking – take up a simple vault hold, such as the Sphenoid Four-Finger Hold, the technique where you place two fingers on each greater wing. Test for flexion – that is, once you can feel the sphenoid's motion pattern, discern that part of its motion most like flexion and follow it into flexion. Then follow it back into that part of its motion most like extension and note which of the two motions is easier, or seems preferred by the sphenoid.

Hold the sphenoid at the limit of the direction to which it moves the most easily, either flexion or extension, then test for a torsion lesion by taking the greater wings superior and inferior sequentially. Hold at the limit of the side the greater wing moves more superior most easily.

Now, while holding the flexion or extension and torsion patterns at their limits, continue to work through the sequence of lesion patterns, from side-bending through lateral and vertical strain and including lateroflexion, stacking them until each is held at its limit. *Note: Do not take the sequence beyond side-bending (that is, beyond the first four patterns), in a client who has no symptoms indicating the presence of one of the latter four lesions.* Hold "the mechanism" there until you feel it soften, and let go softly but suddenly. Immediately come straight off the greater wings in a pure lateral fashion. With this preparation, the sphenoid will naturally correct itself, in cases of mild to moderate faulting. It is unlikely to be successful in the kind of severe faulting that results from extreme trauma.

### Coupled Holds

These coupled holds are where craniosacral work lives. They give you the capability to "wield" and "mold" the head in almost magical ways. You cannot do this in ordinary "little me" consciousness.

*Far Left:*
*Oral Coronal Shear Test*

### Sphenoid External Coupled Contact with Mandible

Stand to one side of the client's head and use two hands to straddle both the mandible and sphenoid. Balance the greater wings with the external surface of the mandible, first perhaps in the anteroposterior plane with compression/decompression (taking care not to compress the sphenopalatine ganglion), followed by the cephalad-caudad plane.

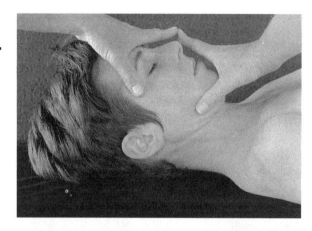

*Sphenoid External Coupled Contact with Mandible*

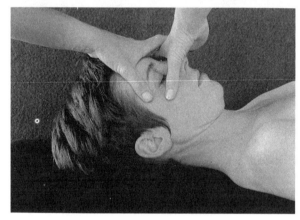

*Sphenoid External Coupled Contact with Zygomae*

### Sphenoid External Coupled Contact with Zygomae

As with the last technique, this is an interactive unwinding contact. The contact and considerations are similar on the zygomae, which act as strong "governors" of the sphenoid. I use this over and over again to correct sphenoid and temporal trauma. The success of the technique hinges on visualization of the structural interface and anatomical contents of the sphenoid and zygomae. This is a very useful hold for all sphenoid-related conditions, and for working with facial trauma and sinusitis.

Stand to one side of the client and take up a straddle contact with the sphenoid's greater wings, being sure to get the base of your index finger on glabella. Now contact the lateral aspects of the zygomae with your other hand, using a thumb and

middle finger contact and taking out a little of the skin slack, in order to establish firmer osseous contact.

Visualize the structural interfaces. The spheno-zygomatic suture, a highly variable, slightly serrated suture, forms part of the posterior and lateral composition of the orbit. Tune in to one hand first; when you have found the motility pattern, move your focus to the other hand. As you begin to sense the zygomae release with gentle interactive work, decompressing, or unwinding, the sphenoid may suddenly move more freely. Stay with the sphenoid until you sense it move into a deep still point.

## Sphenoid Air Sinus Drainage

Sit or stand to one side of the client and apply a spanning contact over the frontal bone and the greater wings with your cephalad hand. Place the index or middle finger of your caudad hand in an oral contact on the hard palate no further posterior than the level of the fifth to sixth teeth (this is to stay well anterior of the transverse palatine suture, which typically lies in the interspace between seventh and eighth teeth), and vector pressure and intention superior and posterior at the sphenoid air sinus. During flexion, accentuate the movement of the frontal and sphenoid into true flexion. At the same time, begin to very gently increase the pressure you are administering through your oral

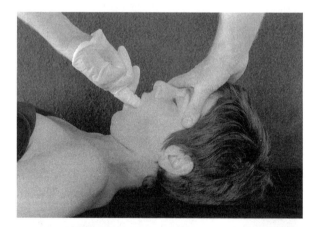

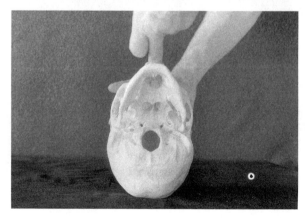

**Far right:** *Sphenoid Air Sinus Drainage, showing bony contact below; note the left forearm angle.*

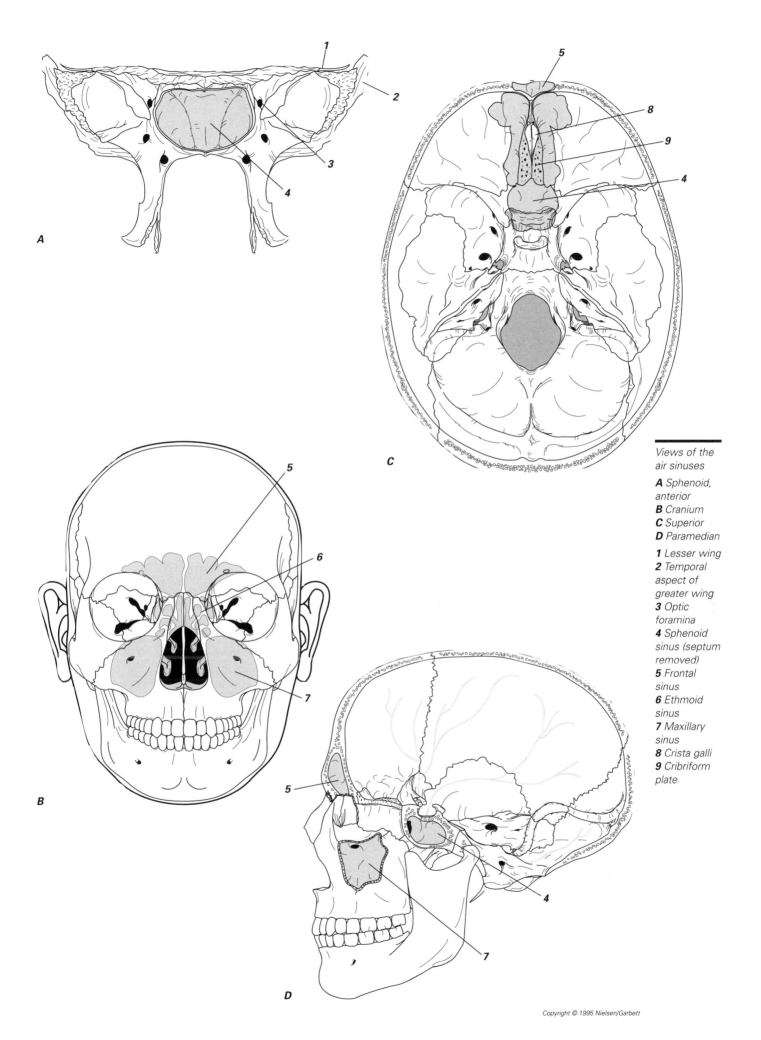

Views of the
air sinuses

*A* Sphenoid,
anterior
*B* Cranium
*C* Superior
*D* Paramedian

*1* Lesser wing
*2* Temporal
aspect of
greater wing
*3* Optic
foramina
*4* Sphenoid
sinus (septum
removed)
*5* Frontal
sinus
*6* Ethmoid
sinus
*7* Maxillary
sinus
*8* Crista galli
*9* Cribriform
plate

finger, so as to compress the vomer; this will effectively move the vomer opposite the way it moves during sphenoid flexion (that is, you are moving the vomer opposite of physiological motion). Your intent is to gently drive the vomer toward the air sinus of the sphenoid. Successfully done, this will cause an oblation of the sphenoid air sinus, and if continued in each flexion cycle will promote mucous drainage of the sinus.

This is the kind of technique best learned in a tutorial setting, not from a book. In my experience, it is meaningless to give a pressure value to the oral finger's exertion – after all, how many people really know what 2 ounces (57 grams) of pressure feels like? The pressure must be effective, yet non-invasive, and people's heads respond so differently, with such varying pain thresholds. It is thus far more important to stay sensitive to "the mechanism" and to the present moment. The wisest course is to keep your pressure to a level where you can still feel the cranial wave formations. If you lose touch with the wave, you may have overwhelmed it by pressing too hard.

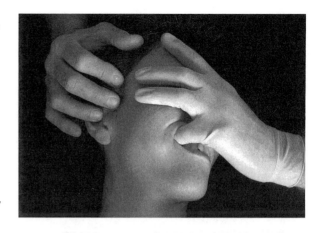

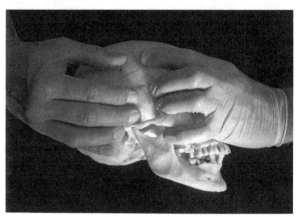

## Sphenotemporal Oral Correction

Since the sphenoid and temporals are so often twinned in trauma, here is a technique to balance their relationship. It can be used first on one side of the head and then the other, or only on the affected side; this example uses the right side.

Sit on the client's left and rotate his head to his left. Use your left hand to take up the oral maxillary and external sphenoid contact used in the Oral Coronal Shear Test. Now place your right hand gently over the exposed right temporal bone as follows: ring finger into or slightly posterior to the ear canal, fifth finger lateral to the mastoid process, middle and index fingers on the temporal bone portion of the sideburn hairline (to make this quite clear in class, I call this the "Elvis Presley sideburn line"), just ¼ inch (6 millimeters) from the middle and ring finger of the sphenoid hand. Now use these two contacts to work gently and carefully, sensing and visualizing asymmetrically and three dimensionally. This is very much the domain of the tentorium, so keep checking in on it with finger-feel and visualizations.

Consider ending with either a CV4, Temporal Palming, or Sutherland's Grip to leave the tentorium balanced, especially if you have worked on one side only.

## Cant Hook Techniques

Cant Hook techniques are especially good for the kind of frontal traumas seen in car accidents that result in dashboard impaction. In these cases the challenge is to tease the frontal back off its compression into the coronal shear plane.

### Sphenofrontal Release at Lesser Wing

This technique is to free the anterior surface of the lesser wing at its articulation to the cortical plate of the frontal. There may be an impaction at any point in the length of the suture; or, in compression head, the whole suture may be, or appear to be, impacted.

If you perceived impaction at one lateral extreme of the lesser wing, then you would sit opposite that side as it is usually easier to focus more sensitivity on a lesion further from you by using your fingertips. This example has you sitting to the client's right, with the assumption that the lesion is on the left. Place your caudad and cephalad thumbs on the greater wing nearest you and your caudad middle and ring fingers on the opposite greater wing. Your cephalad index finger is then placed on the frontal bone opposite you, contacting it at the junction of the superior temporal line and the supra-orbital ridge.

The primary objective is to stabilize the sphenoid while applying Cant Hook leverage to the opposite frontal, gapping the suture of the lesser wing with the frontal. Visualize this. Take the

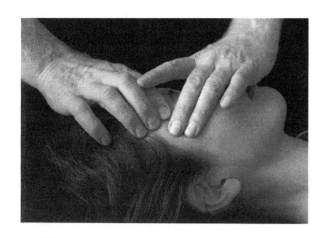

sphenoid into extension while taking the frontal anterior. Work interactively, and move into unwinding when the pattern starts to release.

### Sphenoid and Viscerocranium Release

This application of the Cant Hook technique differs in its focus and contact points from the technique described above.

Sit or stand at the side of the table adjacent to the client's head. Take up one spanning contact on the greater wings and a second over frontal, zygomae, maxillae, or mandible, pointing your frontal thumb toward the floor. Stabilizing with your thumbs, use the leverage possibilities of fully flexed wrists to begin mediating to these structures. Think in terms of balancing in a rotational plane with a vertical midline axis of rotation running through the anterior sutures of the sphenoid (visualize them all), or the sphenobasilar joint, depending on where you discern opening to be needed.

One interesting specialty is to work interactively with the maxillae with your caudad spanning hand, using an oral contact of the little finger cephalad to the buccal surface of the alveolar ridge. (In most people, oral contact encourages viscerocranial release.) There are two primary planes to consider working in: the vertical, taking the maxillae either anterior or posterior, or the horizontal (coronal), taking the maxillae either inferiorly or superiorly.

## Indirect Work

### Wrist and Elbow Corrections of the Sphenobasilar Joint

This is the most advanced of the sphenoid techniques. Of the two arms, the left wrist and elbow seem to present the best indirect access to the sphenoid. Stand to the client's left and take a comforting, handshake contact of your left hand with the client's left hand. Cup your right hand and use it to support his elbow, which acts as the proxy for the sphenoid. Take out the tissue and joint slack,

visualize the sphenoid as floating, and wait for the tissue and joint slack to be taken up by gentle traction. Wait for the sphenoid to come out to you before asking it what it needs. Only then can you begin unwinding. One student observed that "he touched my elbow, and it all came out … everything I needed to see."

## Other Techniques That Can Affect the Sphenoid

- Clear the Confusion (Unwinding the Falx)
- Lateral Pterygoid Release
- The CV4
- Cranial *Prana Yama*
- Ethmoid Oral Index-Finger Maxillary Approach
- Temporal Auricle Decompression and Temporal Palming
- Zygomatic decompressions
- Maxillary Lateral Decompression of the Median Palatine Suture
- Palatine Evaluation and Palatine Compression/Decompression
- Frontal Anterior Decompression
- Vomer Thumb-Based Tripod Technique
- Corrective dental work
- SAD treatment using five to six lux of light for thirty minutes per day

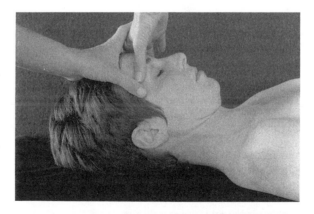

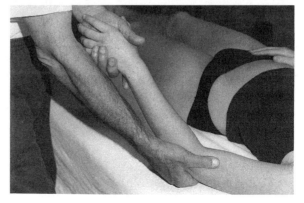

*Far Left:*
*Cant Hook: Spheno-frontal Release, showing finger placement (technique from left side)*

*Cant Hook: Spheno-frontal Release, showing thumb placement (technique from right side)*

*Indirect access to sphenoid through the left wrist and elbow*

# 25
# The Temporals

**Etymology**

**Temporals** *from the Latin tempus,
meaning time, as in temporary
and tempus fugit, (time flies)*

**Mastoid** *from the Greek for nipple*

**Petrous** *from the Greek for a stone,
as in Peter, the rock*

**1** *Temporal portion of mastoid suture,
"margo occipitalis," articulates with
occiput*

**2** *Mastoid process*

**3** *Apex of petrous part connected to body
of sphenoid by apical ligament*

**4** *Carotid canal, transmits internal
carotid artery*

**5** *Auditory canal for auditory tube (inferior)
and tensor muscle of tympanum (smaller
and superior)*

**6** *Anterior surface of petrous part, or
pyramid*

**7** *Trigeminal impression, formed by
trigeminal ganglion*

**8** *Superior margin of petrous part*

**9** *Groove for superior petrosal sinus,
formed between ridges of attachment of
tentorium cerebelli*

**10** *Internal acoustic meatus, transmits
CN VII and VIII, facial, vestibulococlear, and
intermediate nerves*

**11** *Jugular notch forms temporal margin
of jugular foramen*

**12** *Jugular fossa, for bulb of superior
jugular vein*

**13** *Styloid process, vestige of second gill
slit visible in human embryo at four weeks*

**14** *Stylomastoid foramen, transmits
CN VII, the facial nerve*

**15** *Tympanic ring*

**16** *External auditory meatus*

**17** *Suprameatal spine*

**18** *Squamous part of temporal bone*

**19** *Parietal margin, temporal portion of
squamous suture*

**20** *Parietal notch*

**21** *Sphenoid margin, temporal portion of
overlapping sphenotemporal suture*

**22** *Zygomatic process of temporal bone*

**23** *Mandibular or glenoid fossa, temporal
component of temporomandibular joint*

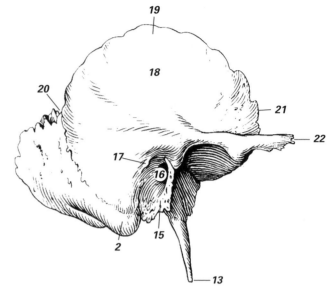

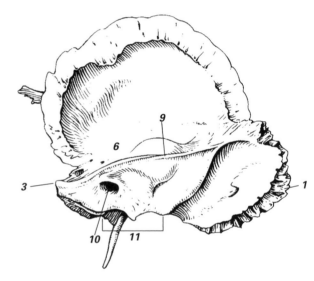

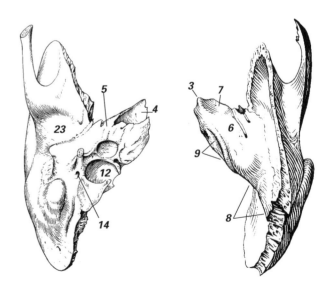

## Embryology and Osteology

The temporals ossify from ten different centers beginning in the seventh week after conception (compared with just one for the more extensive but plainer parietals) and are still in three component parts at birth: squamous, petrous, and tympanic ring. At birth the mastoids are formed only in cartilage.

The continual efforts of the infant to raise his head bring on, or "force," the ossification of the mastoid via the sternocleidomastoid muscles. A healthy infant can hold his head up unassisted by six months, at which point the mastoids have ossified.

## Anatomy

### Structure

The temporals are compound, complex bones that form the most decisive lateral structure of the cranium. They are composed of diploic bone, which takes several different forms:

- A thin fan-shaped upper portion called the squama
- A flying buttress formation that joins with the zygomae
- An anvil-shaped petrous portion whose cone-shaped extremity articulates with the sphenoid
- A cone-shaped mastoid that is formed by traction from the sternocleidomastoid

## Location

The temporals are located posterolateral to the sphenoid, inferior to the parietals, and anterior and lateral to the occiput.

### Landmarks

The temporals are readily located by the auricles of the ear, which are wholly attached to them. The squama extends some ½ inch (1.3 centimeter) superior to the apex of the helix of the auricle, but does not reach above the apex of the eyebrow line. The sphenotemporal suture can be felt at the sideburn hairline. The temporozygomatic suture can be felt on the inferior border of the zygomatic arch approximately halfway between the ear canal and the lateral border of the eye socket.

## Sutures and Articulations

The temporals have complex sutures. They present a highly variable, delicate, ballerina-on-points suture with the zygomae; a rolling overlap, or squamous suture with the parietals; a modified and

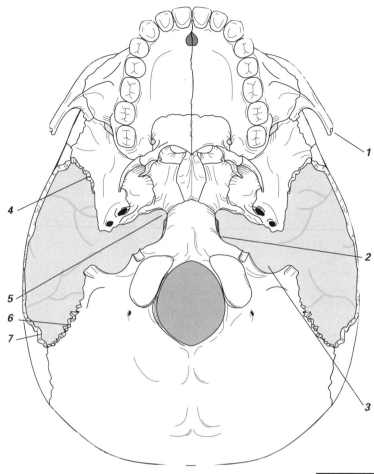

robust interdigitated suture with the occiput; a modified harmonic (plain) suture with the sphenoid; and an open, no-contact border with the condylar and basilar portions of the occiput at the cranial base.

The temporals are the most superficial of the four bones that meet at pterion. They are one of three bones that form asterion, where they meet the occiput and the parietals.

Each temporal articulates with a maximum of five bones:

- The sphenoid
- The occiput
- One parietal
- One zygoma
- The frontal (a variable articulation)

## Weight

A medically-prepared, disarticulated temporal bone weighs ⅘ ounce (22.7 grams).

*The cranial base with temporals removed to show the fjords into which the petrous portions of the temporals fit*

*1 Zygomatico-temporal suture*
*2 Location of inferior petrosal sulcus*
*3 Posterio-medial border of jugular foramen*
*4 Spheno-temporal suture*
*5 Location of foramen lacerum*
*6 Mastoid suture*
*7 Squamous suture*

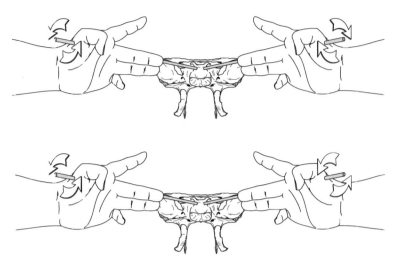

***Above:***

*Six gun
imitation of
temporal
similar
motion (left
and right
temporal
flexion)*

***Below:***

*Six gun
imitation of
temporal
opposite
motion (left
flexion, right
extension)*

## Detailed Anatomy and Musculature

I use a modified "six-gun" finger configuration as an aid to visualizing temporal anatomy and motion. Put one hand into a "six-gun" configuration, just as you did playing cowboys and Indians as a child. Modify this slightly by pointing your middle and ring fingers together at a forty-five-degree angle into flexion from the palm, while keeping the tip of your little finger in full flexion, touching the palm. In a similar way bring the cocked thumb into flexed contact with the base of your index finger. You now have a passable imitation of a temporal bone. The thumb represents the squama, the index finger the zygomatic portion of the temporal, the middle and ring fingers the petrous portion, and the little finger the mastoid. Now make the same configuration with both hands, and place the tips of your middle fingers ½ inch (1.3 centimeters) apart, articulating with an imaginary sphenoid body in the center of the head.

Note the three repetitions of forty-five-degree angles: the angle between the petrous portion and the superimposed squama; the angle of the petrous portion as seen from above, as it moves medially and anteriorly to its articulation with the sphenoid; and the angle between the petrous portion and the styloid process.

The petrous portion angles anteromedially to approximate to, or articulate with, the posterior portion of the clivus of the sphenoid at the infero-lateral border of the dorsum sellae. The mastoid lies inferior to the lateral-most part of the petrous portion of the bone. Superior to the petrous portion, the temporals change from what is technically a cranial base bone into a cranial vault bone, giving rise to the thin, seashell-like squama, which offers its scalloped articulatory surface to the lateral surface of the parietals. The squama can be regarded as a triangular upward growth of the petrous portion and is known as its apex.

The middle and ring fingers of your six guns, imitating the anterior anvils of the petrous portions, fit into long tapered fjords formed by the basilar and condylar portions of the occiput posteriorly and the inferior portions of the greater wings of the sphenoid anteriorly. The temporals may present a fibrous, pointy union with the sphenoid, called the petroclinoid or apical ligament.

The border separating the temporals from the occiput begins at the jugular foramen, remains open throughout life, and is not properly an articulation at all but a kind of elongated crevice. The inferior petrosal sulcus sinus runs along it. It is remarkable that at the very center of the cranial base (where the greatest weight-bearing and stress occurs) two of the prime bone structures do not articulate along part of their common border – an arrangement that maximizes malleability and therefore shock absorption. Lacking the mutual bracing of a suture, the bones themselves (basilar and condylar portions of the occiput, and the petrous portions of the temporals) are more robust, to make up in independent strength what they lack in mutual support.

The temporals vie with the sphenoid in complexity. While the sphenoid holds the pituitary, the temporals holds the organs of hearing and balance in the inner ear. The seventh cranial nerve (the facial nerve) weaves through the petrous portion, making two right angles. The eighth cranial nerve (the vestibulocochlear nerve) passes through the same foramina, the internal acoustic meatus.

Additional temporal landmarks worth noting include the foramen lacerum (shared with the sphenoid), the jugular foramen (shared with the occiput), the temporomandibular fossa and its saddle joint architecture, and the styloid process (whose attachments form a small but important ingredient in temporal motility).

A variety of muscular inputs, as listed below, can affect temporal status. The sternocleidomastoid and temporalis are the most powerful and important muscles that directly affect the temporals.

### Musculature

The muscles that attach to the temporals consist of the:

- Sternocleidomastoid
- Temporalis
- Longissimus capitus
- Splenius capitus

## Physiology

The temporals are highly complex bones. The occiput, parietals, sphenoid, and zygomae articulate with the temporals, as well as the dynamically decisive mandible, which hangs from them. Each temporal bone rotates around the long axis of the petrous portion, as exemplified in the six-gun analogy used above to describe its shape. There are also some eccentric inputs from surrounding structures.

The temporals are effective "governors" of the sphenoid; think of them as inseparable and mischievous[1,2] twins – whenever you access one, remember to consider the other. I also look to the mandible whenever the temporals are affected, and thus have four bones to consider: both temporals, the sphenoid, and the mandible.

Styloid and mastoid ligamentous and muscular attachments add further potentially disequilibriating forces. The tugs, tears, triturations, and traumas of the teeth, and the action of the muscles of mastication, all affect the temporals. They do this through the temporomandibular joint, the lateral pterygoid muscles, the retrodiscal ligaments, the sphenotemporal ligaments, the stylomandibular ligaments, and the most powerful neck muscles of all, the sternocleidomastoids.

Alderman's ear is a curious phenomenon, elicited through cold-water stimulation of a recurrent branch of the tenth cranial nerve (the vagus nerve), which curls up behind the ear. Hundreds of years ago, during ceremonial banquets in London, satiated aldermen would summon a well-trained waiter to pour a discreet trickle of cold water just behind their ears; this caused contraction of the tissues around the recurrent branch, simulating the same nerve impulses as does an empty and contracting stomach. Hunger was stimulated; the aldermen could satisfy decorum by going on eating, and became very obese.

Thirty percent of all people who swim more than twice a week (e.g., many surfers, all swimming instructors) develop a bony overgrowth, called an exostosis, inside the ear canal.[3] The exostosis seems to be a protection for the drum, both from the increased water pressures of diving and the increased acoustic delivery of the watery medium. This protective mechanism must have been used in fairly recent evolutionary times (less than one hundred thousand years ago?) to be elicited so readily. It is, after all, a bone growing in response to the relatively gentle pressure of surface water, not the gross physical loads that we are used to seeing bone change under, such as the enlargement of a javelin thrower's wrist.[4,5]

A highway patrol officer in Florida noted that he caught speeding motorists using radar, laser, timed quarter miles, aircraft, and human behavioral clues. Among the latter, he noted that those guilty of speeding almost always scratch a "little pointy-shaped bone" just behind their left ear while protesting their innocence.

## Axes of Rotation

The axes of rotation for the temporals in the classical model run from the anteromedial tip of the petrous portions in posterolateral directions at forty-five-degree angles to spots ⅛ inch (3 millimeters) posterior to the tympanic rings of the ear canals.

## Motion

The petrous tip is anchored to the posterolateral corner of the body of the sphenoid by the (variable) petroclinoid ligament. This structure helps create the axis of rotation and maintains a pinpoint articulation between the petrous tip and the root of the posterior clinoid process.

To better understand temporal motion, place your hands in the modified six-gun configuration outlined above and mimic the movements described below.

### Osteopathic Model

The classical motion pattern (similar-motion model) consists of both temporals moving into external rotation (flexion) at the same time. Simulate this with your hands by rotating your middle fingertips around the imagined point of contact between them – the clivus of the sphenoid (posterior part of the sphenoid body). Rotate your wrists externally and note how the different parts of the simulated bone move.

### Liquid-Electric Model

Motion in the liquid-electric model differs in two ways: first, that the temporals do not conform to the classical axis but rather move in response to propulsive inputs from the fully-floating spherical surface of the brain, and the cranial wave inputs from the temporalis and sternocleidomastoid muscles. Second, the temporals move in "opposite motion," that is, they alternate their flexion and extension cycles, thus, as the left temporal is externally rotating (flexing), the right is internally rotating (extending). This is the pattern that I have found in some 90 percent of my clients once they are in a meditative state.

In the liquid-electric model, as one temporal bone rolls out into external rotation (flexion) along the midline of the petrous portion, the temporal squama moves anteriorly, laterally, and slightly inferiorly and the mastoid process moves medially, inferiorly, and posteriorly. This motion draws the tentorium on the same side inferiorly and laterally (able to so because the opposite temporal is moving into extension, thus "paying out the slack" in the tentorium).

## Diagnostic Considerations

### Energetics

Gerda, age sixty, had suffered occipital and mastoid pain for many years – when asked how many, she answered "Ever since I can remember ... well, since I was twenty anyway." While I worked with the Square Ashtray hold, she had a realization of the origin of the pain, and recounted the following experience:

*I saw my mother lying down. Suddenly I was anxious. Now I saw a doctor holding a newborn baby too hard with a grip across the mastoids, and it hurt me. This is the first time that I've felt the pain and simultaneously seen its origin.*

Energetically, the temporals are part of the throat soul center, which is concerned with verbal expression, flexibility in life, the absorption of love and the digestion of new experiences. The temporals and sphenoid are located at the temples – quite literally a holy place that needs to be approached with reverence. (As the voice commanded Moses from the burning bush: "Put off your shoes from your feet, for the place on which you are standing is holy ground."[6])

The temporals are also about balance in life, which is eloquently described by Robert Fulghum in his book *All I Really Need To Know I Learned in Kindergarten:*

*Share everything.*
*Play fair.*
*Don't hit people.*
*Put things back where you found them.*
*Clean up your own mess.*
*Don't take things that aren't yours.*
*Say you're sorry when you hurt somebody.*
*Wash your hands before you eat.*
*Flush.*
*Warm cookies and cold milk are good for you.*
*Live a balanced life – learn some and think some and draw and paint and sing and dance and play and work every day some.*
*Take a nap every afternoon.*
*When you go out into the world, watch out for traffic, hold hands, and stick together.*
*Be aware of wonder. Remember the little seed in the Styrofoam cup: The roots go down and the plant goes up and nobody really knows how or why, but we are all like that.*
*Goldfish and hamsters and white mice and even the little seed in the Styrofoam cup – they all die. So do we.*
*And then remember the Dick-and-Jane books and the first word you learned – the biggest word of all – look.[7]*

The heavy scheduling of modern life can remove this balance, our "organizers" serving to over-organize our lives. One symptom of the loss of balance in life – vertigo – can be seen as the client saying "please pick me up." Tereza, the heroine in Milan Kundera's *The Unbearable Lightness of Being*, suffered from vertigo, and Kundera observes that vertigo is "please pick me up."[8] The lines impressed me. Since then, every time I have been presented with a client with vertigo, they have rung true.

Tinnitus is "I don't want to hear it anymore!"[9] It is often a symptom with a strong causative emotional component. (One of my students, a newly married Italian man, noted with great candor that "When I lust after another woman, it brings on my tinnitus.") In tinnitus and deafness, people cut themselves off from the world; through hearing we assimilate our environment, or choose not to. The temporals are often involved in withdrawal.

Renaissance dissectionists believed that the auditory nerve was composed of three pathways. They concluded from cadaver evidence that the brain was meant to hear at three distinct levels. To one pathway they ascribed the hearing of the mundane conversations of the everyday world. The second, they surmised, was designed to interpret and absorb all art and higher learning. The third existed so that the soul might hear the guidance it needed.

Cutting-edge research in hearing-aid work turns on the use of probes that can pick up the strength of the electrical signals reaching the sound-interpretation centers of the brain. Using this apparatus, Swiss researchers found that a hearing-impaired person attenuates the electrical activity produced by words that, for him, carry a negative association, while transmitting affirmative, positively association words unimpaired. Thus the word "kitchen" may be found to be attenuated in a man with a negative complex of feelings toward his mother. Such weakening of the signals begins with a few words, but eventually crosses the audible spectrum and ends in deafness.

By discovering which words are attenuated, the researchers can train the client to stop his emotions from changing his nervous system. He can continue to have confused feelings about his mother, but now he *feels* them, rather than trying to wall himself off from the feelings by not hearing key works. Then the feelings no longer block his auditory cognition. With such biofeedback-like training, clients' hearing returns to normal within a few weeks. One Swiss researcher[7] whom I met believes this work may make almost all hearing aids redundant within ten years.

Psychogenic states – especially anger, suppressed rage, anxiety, and tension – play an emphatic role in temporal bone balance.[10] These emotions are mediated to the temporals through the temporomandibular joints and sternocleidomastoid and temporalis tension.

### Trauma and Dysfunction

Clients feel quite out of sorts when their temporals are faulted. They may suffer from disequilibrium or vertigo and short-term memory lapses. You may observe personality changes and short-term emotional problems as well. Temporal disequilibrium is a frequent side-effect of automobile whiplash injury.[11] Treat the temporals exceedingly carefully, and never leave the bones abruptly in an unbalanced position – check for the "neutral" or flexion phase, and only then lift off.

Schoolteachers all over the world used to punish children by yanking their ears in an abrupt and repeated oscillatory fashion. This strange, obviously instinctive ritual form of punishment (it is probably tens of thousands of years old) may guarantee feelings of malaise and repentance in the unfortunate child by displacing and altering the energetic field of his temporal bones.

The open architecture of the jugular and petrous portions makes the cranial base portion of the temporals susceptible to displacement,[12] especially in low-impact trauma, such as falling onto grass while running, and low-speed whiplash injury.

Muscle contraction headaches[13] provide a rewarding case study of the mechanisms through which the muscular components of stress affect cranial and temporal structures. In treatment, find ways of keeping the client's jaw open (use a ¼ inch [6 millimeter] dowel placed transversely between the teeth in a particularly tight-mouthed individual.) Encourage him to place the tip of his tongue on his hard palate so that his teeth are separated yet he can still breathe normally. Encourage spaciousness and freedom in the stomatognathic system (the cranial, neck, and upper thorax muscles, bones, and ligaments involved in biting, chewing, and swallowing).

The seventh cranial nerve (facial nerve) makes two right angles as it weaves through the petrous portion of the temporals: it is almost as if the nerve is trapped in place. If the temporal bones displace (due to ongoing stress mediated to them through posture or muscular tension) or lose their inherent mobility, the nerve can be faulted. If the nerve is compressed or put under tension, acute peripheral facial paralysis, or "Bell's Palsy" can result.[14] This serious condition typically takes three to nine months to heal, with 75 to 90 percent of suffers recovering to a "cosmetically acceptable level."[15] However, 16 percent are left with major defects.[16] The highest incidence of Bell's Palsy occurs in the third trimester,[16] which may be due to altered mediastinal influence upon the cranial base, or increased tension in the sternocleidomastoid muscles, or both.

The very short auditory tubes of infants quite readily allow bacterial infections to spread from the nasopharynx into the inner ears or mastoid air cells. (Breast feeding can help to reduce ear infections in the newborn by up to 50 percent.[17,18]) Craniosacral work with children in these cases focuses on draining the space between the ramus of the mandible and the mastoid process of the temporal bone.

Tinnitus is challenging, an area of craniosacral work[19] where success is variable: sometimes treatment works, and at other times, for no apparent reason, it does not. Possible treatments in craniosacral work would encompass normalization of the atlanto-occipital joint and gentle upper neck decompression and unwinding to optimize the position and motion of the atlas.[20,21,22] Focusing on the Window To The Sky acupuncture point Small Intestine 17, with the intention of allowing the point time to close, may help.[23] Investigate the need to work to normalize the lateral pterygoid muscles; and the following techniques: Auditory Tube Twist;[24] Auditory Tubes: Direct Digital Approach; Temporal Auricle Decompression; and Temporal Palming. (Tinnitus can also be treated through acupuncture; Ericksonian hypnosis; eliminating sugar and dairy foods from the diet; the homeopathic remedy gingko biloa; and blood thinners when the tinnitus is caused by arterial pressure in close proximity to the vestibulocochlear nerve).

## Interconnectedness

The temporals are functionally wedded to the sphenoid and mandible, forming the vital central unit of function in craniosacral work.

The temporal bones' connection to the tentorium is immediate and extensive. Temporal faulting always involves the tentorium, which therefore tends to implicate the other bones that attach to the tentorium – the sphenoid, occiput, and the other temporal bone. The core link[25] means that the sacrum and ilia may also be affected, or be affecting the temporals.

Temporal status and motility seem to echo the other main lateral joints of the body, the shoulders and hips. The mastoid processes have an energetic connection to the ischial tuberosities.

## Visualization

Begin your visualization with the modified six-gun shape of the temporals, then flesh out the image with the tentorial attachments to the petrous ridge, and the apical ligament connecting the apical tip to the clivus of the sphenoid. The cerebellum lies beneath the tentorium, the temporal lobes of the brain above. The ganglia of the largest cranial nerve, the trigeminus, rests on the superior aspect of the petrous portions, where it leaves a slight depression. Lastly, add the seventh and eighth cranial nerves passing into the temporals through the internal acoustic meatus.

## TECHNIQUES

### Temporal Three-Finger Contact

Sit or kneel at the head of the table and ensure that the entire length of your forearms can rest on the table surface. This technique uses a contact with the auricles, or external ears, to gauge temporal motility. The thumb is placed inside the anti-helix, or inner curvature of the external ear, opposed to the index and middle fingers, which are gently curled external to the auricles, contacting their posterior surface. (There is no direct contact with the temporal bones.)

The petrous portions of the temporals – the inferior anvils – angle anteromedially in toward the sphenoid at a forty-five-degree angle. For palpation, apply ⅕ to ⅓ ounce (5.6 to 9.5 grams) of decompression at the same forty-five-degree angle, this time posterolaterally.

This technique has universal capabilities – you can use it as diagnostic and therapeutic tool for a wide range of temporal conditions, such as whiplash, tinnitus, and headache, as well as for tentorial unwinding in cases of "compression head."

### Temporal Auricle Decompression

Stay with the above contact on the external ear. Your ⅕ to ⅓ ounce (5.6 to 9.5 grams) of mild decompression has taken out the skin slack, and you can now begin to fluidly increase your traction to move into temporal decompression. Ensure that your forearms are parallel, and maximize your wrist flexion. Visualize the forty-five-degree angle of the petrous portions and decompress at that angle, increasing your traction to 1 to 2 ounces (28 to 57 grams) if necessary. The traction must be sufficient, and you must be able to continue to sense the cranial wave, otherwise you are "out of touch" and simply working by rote. The spirit of your movement is disengagement and freedom: to disengage the apex of the petrous portion from its articulation (through the apical ligament) with the clivus of the sphenoid.

Forty-five degrees is the nominal. Sense, by making fine micromovements of your fingers, the actual angle at which each temporal will decompress. You are unwinding the tentorium with this technique, so visualize it, listen to its dance, and end when you sense it moving into a deep still point.

Use this in working with tinnitus, vertigo, nausea, hearing impairment or loss, autism, and to help correct personality changes after a whiplash injury. It is also a major euphoric, and therefore useful in working with depression.

## Scalene and Temporal Hold, Head Turned to One Side

This technique works on one temporal bone and the anterior triangle of the neck on the same side. Sit or kneel at the head of the table. Rotate the client's head to one side and arrange both of your hands palms down, one more inferior with a spanning contact on the exposed scalene muscle, clavicle, and upper pectoral muscle and the other mediating to the exposed temporal, zygoma, and mandibular bones as well as the overlying muscles. Sense the motility in both places of contact, and let your hands be drawn to whatever specific areas and directions the tissues take you in.

This technique enables you to work with thoracic outlet conditions, such as the nerve impingement of shoulder-arm-hand syndrome, by working both with the local area and the involved cranial structures. It also enables you to balance and unwind the bulk of the stomatognathic system, one side at a time. Consider using it for clients with headaches and whiplash injury. It is a very elegant technique.

## Temporal Palming: Lateral Structures Quad Spread

This is mildly compressive temporal and lateral structures technique that perfectly complements the mildly decompressive Temporal Auricle Decompression described above.

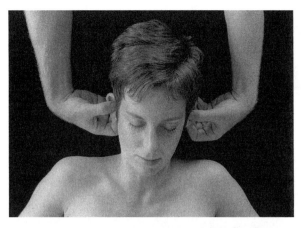

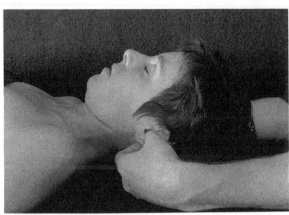

*Temporal Three-finger Contact, two views; note wrist and forearm angles.*

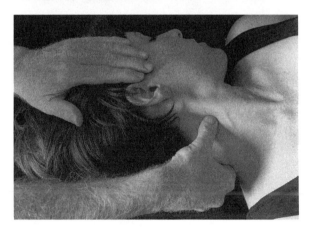

*Scalene and Temporal Hold, head turned to one side*

Sit or kneel at the head of the table. Place the auricle of the ears neatly in the palms of your hands so that you completely cover the external ears (no part visible). Check that the shafts of your thumbs cover the greater wings of the sphenoid and the zygomae, your palms are completely over the external ear, your central three fingers are lateral to the transverse process mass of the neck (or just anterior in those with stout necks), and your fifth finger is in contact with the lateral occipital squama. Your touch to the lateral aspects of the head with the outer margins of your palms should be very light, your contact with the greater wings firm, but still light.

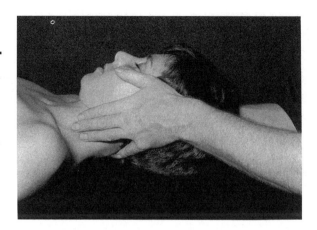

*Temporal Palming: Lateral Structures Quad Spread, showing bony contact below*

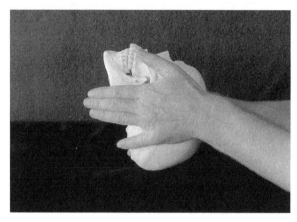

## Square Ashtray

This is a very definite, strongly interactive bilateral mastoid contact. A heavy-hitter of a temporal technique, at the opposite end of the pressure spectrum from the delicate Temporal Auricle Decompression, it should not be used in those who have no symptoms of cranial dysfunction.

The name "Square Ashtray" refers to the shape of the basic cradling position taken by your thenar eminences as they support the paired mastoid bones. It dates from the early 1950s, when a majority of men smoked and, lacking sufficient numbers of real skulls, osteopaths-in-training practiced the technique by cradling a square ashtray between their thenar eminences while walking around the classroom in a wide circle. The tutor made corrections to the thumbs and ashtray as each student paused respectfully in front of him.

Support the cranium off the table, taking care to be sure you are using only thenar contact. Finger contact with the posterior part of the neck must be very light. This position allows you to monitor the motility patterns of the temporals with a high-pressure contact that offers considerable leverage over the bones. It is like an extra-wide CV4, but differs in three respects:

■ The thumbs are lateral to the neck, not posterior
■ The fingers are aligned vertically, with the little fingers touching the table surface and the

Wait. Soon you will be able to begin to feel, like trees emerging from the mist, the tentorium. It is under slight compression from your contact, which softens its normal tensility and allows you freedom to correct imbalances – in the temporal bones and in life – that are not accessible to decompressive work. Gently clear any imbalances once you have a definite sense of the patterns involved. Once the tentorium is normalized, check the straight sinus with the Occipital Approach to the Transverse Sinus or a CV4, and check the falx with a Frontal Anterior Decompression, or with the Auditory Tube Twist.

The Temporal Auricle Decompression tests the temporals in one plane; with Temporal Palming we are now beginning to check all of the planes of motion sequentially. This enables us to tease out the last threads of adherence or imbalance in the temporals' structural interrelationships with the neurocranial bones and mandible. Thus, Temporal Auricle Decompression – which is decompressive, working in a plane that the palming contact cannot fully access – is the natural partner to the mildly compressive nature of Temporal Palming. In most cases, begin with the decompression before moving on to the palming.

**Far right:** *Square Ashtray, showing bony contact below*

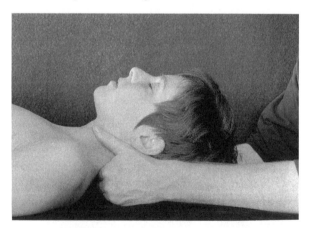

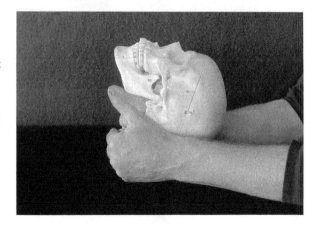

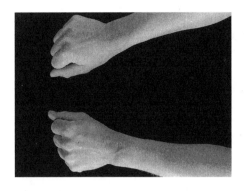
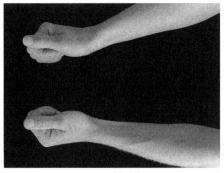
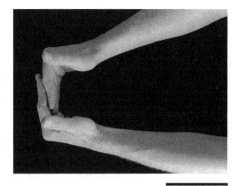

index fingers directly vertical to it, touching the posterior aspect of the client's neck
- The contact area is on the posterior ramps of the mastoids, not the occipital squama

The Square Ashtray is designed to use the weight of the head, in conjunction with the distance of the mastoid from the temporal axis of rotation, to give the healer sufficient mechanical advantage over an impacted temporal bone, or bones, that she can skillfully correct them. It excels at lateral separation of the temporal squama from the enclosed parietals, achieved through medially directed pressure, fluidly applied to the posterolateral aspects of the mastoid processes. Keep the basic contact – thenar muscle contact on the posterior ramps of the mastoids – impeccable as you do this.

You can also use this hold for a profound balancing of the temporals and tentorium in severe head injuries. Its leverage and pressure advantages are useful to unwind the temporal bones, the tentorium specifically, the entire membrane system in general, and the cervical spine. A rapid high-velocity, low-amplitude medial compression of the mastoids can be used as a resuscitation technique *in extremis.*[26]

Consider using the Passive-Interactive Square Ashtray (below), a less pressure-intensive version – for clients who have recently suffered a cerebrovascular accident (stroke) or have a brain tumor, when the use of the square ashtray is contraindicated.

### *Smooth Uptake*

The smooth uptake to assume the Square Ashtray contact is very similar to that for the CV4. Sit at the head of the table with the palms of your hands face down and your fingers lightly curled into your palms. Place the lateral border of your thenar muscles into contact with the posterior ramps of the client's mastoid processes, keeping your thumbs in against your index fingers (unlike the hitchhiker gesture used in the CV4 uptake). Wait a few seconds until you are breathing in time with your client, then externally rotate your forearms as he

breathes out, maintaining an even pressure on the mastoids with your rotating thenar eminences. In this way, by the time you have rotated your forearms halfway to supination, the head will be held in the Square Ashtray position.

### Passive-Interactive Square Ashtray

This is a soft way to interact with the mastoids, which gives a different perspective for temporal work from the Temporal Auricle Decompression, or Temporal Palming. The hold is the position used at the start of the smooth uptake for the Square Ashtray contact – that is, your lightly curled fists are lateral to each mastoid and your forearms in full pronation, resting parallel to each other on the table surface. Stay in this position and tune in to the client's head, sensing the temporals, tentorium, and whole head.

This is excellent as a tuning-in, low-pressure contact. It introduces minimal structural impact since, unlike the full Square Ashtray, the head remains resting on the table. Like all very delicate techniques, it is nonetheless powerful. Use it to correct flexion-extension imbalance patterns where you do not wish to raise the head and use high contact pressures – for example, for clients with brain tumors, or who have had recent cerebrovascular accidents. This technique, like a full Square Ashtray, has the capability to interact with the tentorium, but is less invasive.

### Temporal Oscillation

This technique is based on the Square Ashtray, but instead of harnessing the mastoids as a listening post, or using them for steady-state molding work, you introduce an oscillation designed to "lubricate," then free, the squamous sutures. Use this technique with extreme care, since the possibility of destabilizing the normal pattern – which would cause a loss of balance in life – is immediate and pronounced.

*Hand position sequence for Square Ashtray Smooth Uptake; note differences to the final CV4 location (see p. 258, photo on top right).*

Temporal Oscillation is the treatment of choice for locked and immotile temporals (whether caused by physical or emotional trauma) and for autism. Consider using it in whiplash injury that has not responded to more subtle temporal work, and for the interactive method known as "opposite physiological motion" (where you take a bone into flexion as it moves into extension).

## Directed Energy to the Mammillary Bodies

This technique uses the acupuncture point Ear Gate (Triple Warmer 21)[27] as its point of contact and focus. A gate is the way in, and Ear Gate is taught in some schools of shiatsu as the beginning and end point for facial work. It is a "hinge" point, or powerful opening place, for the head in both the coronal and horizontal planes.

Ear Gate is located where the helix – the outer curvature of the ear – joins the temple, immediately superior to the temporal portion of the zygomatic arch. Once you have found the point, use your middle fingers (the "fire" fingers in Ayurveda, and therefore the best to use for directed energy work) as energy transmitters. Point your middle fingers directly toward each other, through Ear Gate, toward the very center of the brain. Your target structures are the mammillary bodies, which are situated immediately posterior to the pituitary stalk, inferior to the hypothalamus, and anterior to

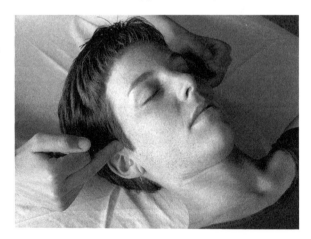

*Directed Energy to the Mammillary Bodies*

the pons. The mammillary bodies are involved in regulating our sense of well-being.

As you feel your energy begin to penetrate the client's head, begin to access your own energy field with quiet power breathing, or *chi kung*

techniques. Focus your energy on the mammillary bodies. Now bring in visualization. Imagine your energy as a straight rainbow, or a silver-white laser beam. See it reaching the mammillary bodies and lighting them up, like a Christmas tree. Continue to transmit light and energy, and an enhanced sense of well-being, to your client. Breathe energy into your four-chambered heart,[28] especially into clear heart and strong heart. It helps if you smile when you do this – a very different quality of energy will be transmitted. Often, as you smile unbeknownst to him, the client begins smiling too.

Because it enhances the client's sense of well-being, this technique is a treatment of choice for those suffering from depression, traumatized mechanisms, and emotional abuse.

## Temporal Cross-Check

Since the temporals are so easily faulted, it is a good idea to know many techniques to access and correct them. This technique is useful in situations where one temporal bone is either immobile or hypermobile while its partner is apparently normal. It can also be useful when balancing the affected side, say in tinnitus, seems to have no effect. Then use Temporal Cross-Check to discern whether the symptom-free side is, in fact, destabilizing the faulted side.

Sit at the client's head and take up a Temporal Palming contact on the traumatized or dysfunctional side. Rotate the head so that it rests in your palm, then use your free hand to test – and if necessary, mobilize – the bones that compose the lateral structures of the exposed side in this order: zygoma, sphenoid, frontal, parietal, occiput.

Use decompressive sutural release techniques to test and free the structures, and observe their interaction with the affected temporal; for this you can modify such techniques as the Temporal Squamous Suture Release and the Frontal Anterior Decompression. Find interactive or unwinding still points with one structure before moving to the next. You might also consider using Sutherland's Grip on the maxillae with your free hand, to further decompress the sphenoid, especially if it is in a forced-flexion lesion from an anteroposterior maxillary impact. This may free the temporal bone sufficiently for it to be able to normalize. (An example of this would be an automobile-related injury, where the maxillae impacts the padding of the dashboard. Automotive padding is of sufficient density to cause compressive impaction from relatively low-speed collisions.)

## Temporal Squamous Suture Release

This technique, designed to release the squamous suture, uses simultaneous pressure on a temporal bone and a parietal bone to tease them apart in both the superoinferior and mediolateral planes. Internal and external contra-rotatory motion may also be employed. It is excellent for practicing non-usual hand usage, and as you refine what F. M. Alexander, the founder of the Alexander Technique, called "the use of the self,"[29,30] your hands will gain more expertise at finger "feel."

Sit at the client's left, rotating his head to his right to expose his left lateral structures. Note before starting that the key to this technique is that your thumbs point in opposite directions, so that the fingers of one hand go down the postero-lateral aspect of the neck, while the fingers of the other lie over the lateral aspects of the face.

Your left hand makes a thenar eminence contact on the posterior margin of the temporal squama (on the temporal side of the parietal notch) with the thumb shaft medial to the superior portion of the auricle; contact the parietal with your right thenar eminence, laying your hand so that your thumb shafts parallel each other on either side of the squamous suture. Listen to the cycling rhythms of the cranium, and initiate separation of the squamous suture when it begins separating cephalad during extension: with your left hand stabilize the temporal bone and begin to take it caudad, and with your right hand perform a unilateral parietal lift to take it cephalad. Slightly flex both wrists in such a way that your thumbpads rotate internally to take up slightly more contact with the two bones.

## Other Techniques that Can Affect the Temporal Bones

- The CV4
- All leg and coxal bone techniques
- Stomatognathic system work, particularly release of the sternocleidomastoids
- Cant Hook techniques to the occiput, sphenoid, and frontal
- Auditory Tube Twist
- Cranial *Prana Yama*
- Frontal Anterior Decompression
- Suboccipital hold
- Oral Coronal Shear Test
- Sutherland's Grip
- Sphenobasilar Decompression

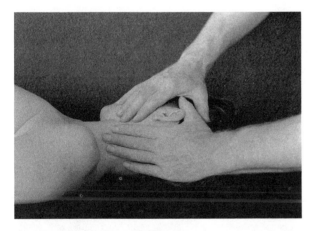

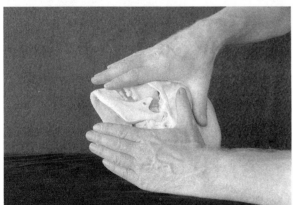

**Far left:**
*Temporal Squamous Suture Release, showing bony contact below.*

# 26
# The Parietals

**Etymology**

**Parietal**  from the Latin paries, the wall
(as in "partition")

**1** Left parietal bone, lateral view

**2** Right parietal bone, medial view

**3** Occipital margin, parietal portion of heavily interdigitated lambdoid suture

**4** Squamous margin, parietal portion of overlapping squamous suture

**5** Sagittal margin, where parietal bones articulate with each other at heavily interdigitated sagittal suture

**6** Frontal margin, parietal portion of interdigitated coronal suture, articulates frontal bone

**7** Parietal foramen, transmits parietal emissary vein from superior sagittal sinus

**8** Superior temporal line, formed by arcuate attachment of fascia overlying temporalis

**9** Inferior temporal line, formed by attachment of temporalis

**10** Groove for superior sagittal sinus, formed by pull of bifurcated falx cerebri

**11** Groove for sigmoid sinus

**12** Grooves formed by middle meningeal artery

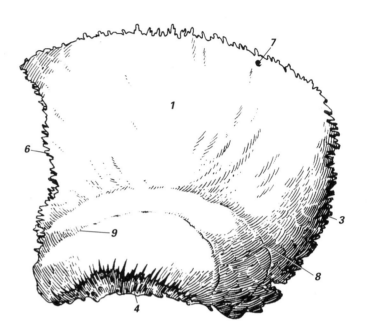

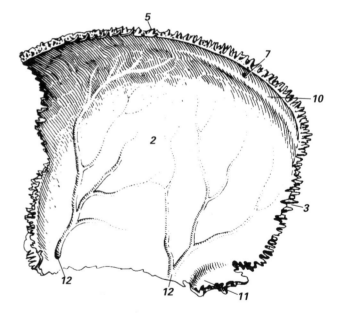

## Embryology and Osteology

As vault bones, the parietals are formed entirely from a membranous matrix. There is one ossification center for each bone, which begins to lay down bone cells seven weeks after conception. The centers are visible at birth, and throughout life, as the parietal eminences.

The parietals are fairly well formed at birth, although their angles remain in membrane for up to two years. This is because the ossification center is in the middle of the bone, and ossification spreads slowly centrifugally, reaching the angles last. This centrifugal pattern is ideal for producing round bones like femurs and vertebral bodies, and the cranial bones also use a "round bone" construction blueprint. The large bones of the cranial vault require a quadrilateral shape, however, so their corners – the fontanels, or the apertures left open in the cranial vault where circular ossification centers meet – remain open at birth. This allows several vital molding and circumducting maneuvers, which help permit the compression of the skull during birth.

## Anatomy

### Structure

The parietals are very simple diploic bones, quadrilateral in form, and clam shell-like in appearance. They are biconcave on their internal surface.

## Location

The inferior border of the parietals is at the apex of the eyebrow line. The parietals are superior to the temporals, beginning ½ inch (1.3 centimeter) above the most superior part of the helix of the ears. They are anterior and superior to the occipital squama, superior and posterior to the sphenoid, and posterior to the frontal bone.

### Landmarks

Each parietal is one of four bones (parietal, temporal, sphenoid, and frontal) that make up pterion, at which point the parietals are the third-deepest bone from the cranial surface. Each parietal is also one of three bones (parietal, temporal, and occiput) that make up asterion, located superior and posterior to the mastoid tip. At the sagittal suture, they are home to the crown soul center, which is located at bregma in Taoist and Hindu landmarking. Just posterior to the vertex of the head is the location of Bindu, an ancillary soul center in the Hindu cosmology, and the point where the spirit leaves the body shortly after death to join the soul.[1]

## Sutures and Articulations

Three of the parietals' four suture lines are simple interdigitated sutures: the sagittal suture with the opposite parietal, the coronal sutures with the frontal, and the lambdoid sutures with the occiput. The fourth, the sutures on their inferior aspects, are the "rolling overlap" or highly specialized squamous sutures with the temporal bones.

Each parietal bone articulates with (at most) five bones:

- The partner parietal
- The occiput
- The sphenoid (a variable articulation)
- One temporal
- The frontal

## Weight

A disarticulated, medically prepared parietal bone weighs 1½ ounces (42.5 grams).

## Detailed Anatomy and Musculature

The parietals are quadrilateral bones. They present two surfaces (the lateral-most one nearly vertical), four borders, and four angles. They are the least specialized – simplest – large bones in the entire cranium.

The parietals offer attachment to temporalis and auricularis superior. Temporalis[2] arises from a long, arc-shaped face of bone known as the inferior temporal ridge (or line), located on the lateral parietal surface and the temporal fossa inferior to the ridge. (Temporalis inserts into, and causes the shape of, the coronoid process of the mandible, where it is palpable in the jaws-open position.) The fascia of temporalis arises from the superior temporal ridge, separates into a double-walled layer ½ inch (1.3 centimeter) above the zygomatic arch, and then inserts into the superior border of the zygomatic arch. Tap yourself here – the double-walled fascia can be as tight as a drumskin, which is why it is easier to palpate the sphenoid when your fingers are superior to the double-walled area of the fascia.

Each parietal articulates with up to five bones: the partner parietal, the occiput, one temporal, the sphenoid, and the frontal. Occasionally there is no articulation with the sphenoid, in which case there is an articulation with a posteriorly extended frontal bone.

It is easy to assume that the parietals extend much further anterior than they in fact do, so note how far posterior the coronal suture is. The coronal suture represents a flap-like opening allowing easy lateral glide of the parietals. On the internal surface of a disarticulated bone, look for the small pit-like depressions – called granular foveolae and often widely distributed inside the top of the head – caused by the arachnoid granulations. They are by no means limited to the location of the superior sagittal sinus. The internal aspect of the bone is also marked by the deep furrows formed by the middle meningeal artery.

Externally, look for the superior and inferior temporal lines formed, respectively, by the fascial attachment of the temporalis muscle and by the muscle itself. Above these lie the more roughened external surface of the bone, which is covered by the aponeurosis of occipitofrontalis. Posteriorly, look for the highly variable parietal foramen, a needle-sized aperture to allow exit to an emissary vein. The cranial landmark known as obelion is located at the sagittal suture between the parietal foramina.

(The aponeurosis of occipitofrontalis [the scalp] passes over the superior halves of the parietals, but does not attach to them – it glides over them.)

### Musculature

The muscles attaching to the parietals consist of the:

- Temporalis
- Auricularis superior

## Physiology

The compound curvatures of the parietal bones are essential for cranial motility. Parietal bones have undergone enormous changes in both size, curvature, and sutural alignment in the last three million years. (The *Homo sapiens neanderthalis* coronal suture was almost horizontal 125,000 years ago.[3]) Their curvatures have also received an inordinate amount of "man-made" attention,[4,5] such as in the cranial molding of the Paracus culture of ancient Peru.

## Axes of Rotation

In the classical model, the axes of rotation for the parietals run in an anteroposterior plane approximately two-thirds down the parietal wall.

## Motion

Studies that utilized tightly compressed dial gauges pressing onto the scalp of immobilized monkeys showed parietal motion to be in the range of ten to twenty-five microns.[6] With sensitive fingers (which do not diminish osseous motility like the points of dial gauges do) palpating the larger human head with its more extensive sutural area, the movement discerned is greater.[7]

### Osteopathic Model

The classical (similar-motion) model has the parietals displacing slightly inferiorly at the sagittal suture during flexion.

### Liquid-Electric Model

In the liquid-electric model, the dominant motion comes from brain motion, modified by temporalis and occipitofrontalis muscle movements and tonicity.

As the left side of the greater wing of the sphenoid nose-dives in flexion, it glides anteriorly off of the parietals, which are rotating in the opposite direction. (The superior surfaces of the sphenoid's greater wings are a mildly roughened surface for articulation with the parietals, permitting easier motion.) As the left greater wing moves anteriorly during flexion, the left temporal bone rotates externally, flaring laterally at the squamous suture. As the occiput circumducts and moves to the left, the falx is pulled posteriorly, inferiorly, and slightly left laterally, moving toward the straight sinus and pulling on the parietal bones, deflecting their movement. The combination of these movements causes the parietals to move laterally at the squamous suture, inferiorly at the sagittal suture, and into very slight internal rotation.

The movement toward the straight sinus allows some potential "slack" where the tentorium attaches to the posteroinferior angle of the parietal bone. This is variable – the tentorium does not always attach to the parietals – but in any case the adhesion of the endosteal to the internal wall of the parietals ensures compliance with temporal motion. Thus, the posteroinferior angles (the parietal notches and asterion) of the left parietal move lateral – kick out – because of the "slack" produced in the tentorium by left temporal external rotation (flexion).

A pivoting occurs where the parietals change their bevels at their junctions with the lambdoid and coronal sutures. The sagittal suture shows deeper interdigitation posteriorly, which allows for greater separation. This is consistent with the liquid-electric model.

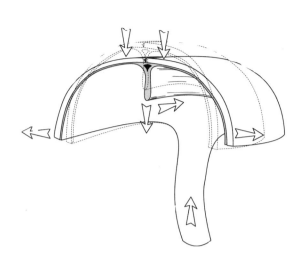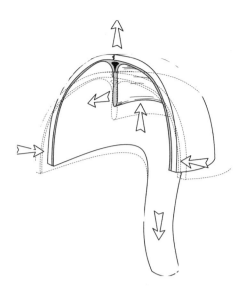

## Diagnostic Considerations

### Energetics

The parietals are the vault of our cathedral roof.
In the words of a student:

> When having the work on my cranium I went
> inward. Inward to my own cranium, which
> became a cathedral. The arches and special
> 'bones' all had a meaning in my cathedral. It
> was amazing to see the symbology in each spe-
> cial shape, its history, its origin. My own stark-
> white perfect cathedral within me!

In almost every way the parietals are plain,
rather uninteresting bones. But they are home to
the crown soul, which represents a transcendence
of all material fixations, needs, longings, and dis-
content, and makes them very satisfying structures
to dance with. Eastern religions honor the path to
spiritual enlightenment as life's primary purpose.
Let material worries go, focus on ascension. Sum-
ming this attitude up, the Hindu story "The Hum-
bling of Indra" has Shiva[8] say again and again "Life
is short, why build a house?"[9]

The crown soul is known in India as "the kundalini chakra"[10] and its Hindu symbol is the trinity
of Brahma, Vishnu, and Shiva. The Buddhist symbol of the crown soul is the thousand-petaled lotus.
In Oriental medicine, the vertex is the location of
the acupuncture point Hundred Meeting Places
(Governor Vessel 20). At the crown:[11]

- Nothing is good or bad except that
thinking makes it so.[12]
- There is no blame and no judgment,
no heresy and no dogma.
- Everything is exactly as it needs to be.
- There is timelessness.
- We are one another.
- We know, without thinking, what
troubles everybody.

The parietals also reflect anger, particularly at the
loss of spiritual equanimity as in the expression,
"He made me so angry I wanted to blow my top!"

### Trauma and Dysfunction

The parietals are wonderful: they hardly ever go
wrong. My only experience with a parietally mediated symptom that needed craniosacral work was a
traumatically induced loss of full visual field. This
loss cleared up after a parietal lift.

## Interconnectedness

The parietals are quiescent bones. While they are
obviously falx bones, they do not seem to interrelate with the ethmoid, frontal, or occiput in any
meaningful way. But they do "pass on the message" from the sacrum, spine and occiput to the
ethmoid and maxillae, by way of the falx.

## Visualization

Visualize the parietals like the giant clam-shell
doors of an observatory. Then put the superior
sagittal sinus, falx, arachnoid granulations nestling
into the granular foveolae, and middle meningeal
artery into your picture. Next add the motor and
somasthetic cortex, and come inferior down to
Broca's and Wernicke's Areas on the left side. On
the right side, visualize "the circuit board of mysticism,"[13] the right temporal lobe, where the cortical
component of transformational spiritual experiences seem to be focused. Cap it with the aponeurosis of the occipitofrontalis. Then change dimen-
sions and perceive the crown soul as it extends
from bregma to the vertex flaring out like a long
brilliantly hued natural-gas flare.[14]

## TECHNIQUES

### Basic Parietal Hold

This employs four fingerpads arranged in a horizontal plane about ½ inch (1.3 centimeters) cephalad to the squamous suture, which is, in turn, about 1 inch (2.6 centimeters) superior to the vertex of the helix of the external ear.

Sit or kneel at the head of the table. Begin by observing the height of the client's ear canals off the table, and place your middle fingers at the same height and ½ inch (1.3 centimeters) superior to the vertex of the helix. Note that all of the finger placements use pad contact. Place your thumbs on the head ½ inch (1.3 centimeters) further posterior, to ensure that they are posterior to bregma (which is directly superior to the ear canals). Make sure that your thumbtips are ½ inch (1.3 centimeters) apart, on either side of the sagittal suture. Now place your index fingers slightly posterior to the sideburn hairline, or palpate the sphenotemporal suture and be posterior to it. Place your little fingers on the table surface and sweep medially until you touch the head; this will still be parietal contact. Complete your contact by adjusting your ring fingers to be equidistant between your middle and little fingers.

*Basic Parietal Hold*

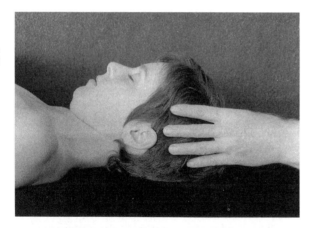

*Parietal Lift*

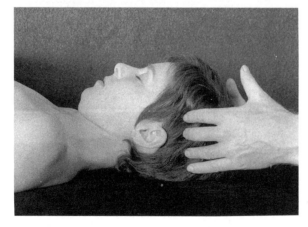

Healers with exceptionally large hands may need to place their thumbs onto the opposite parietal bones. The disadvantage of this is that it creates a crossover for the nervous system to compute, and hence makes analyzing movement patterns slightly more difficult.

### Parietal Lift

This technique uses the same contact as the Basic Parietal Hold, but its objective is more than palpation. It is designed to decompress the parietals superiorly, open the sagittal suture, and create space for the crown soul.

From the basic hold, begin to move your wrists, very gently, into slight flexion – about twenty to thirty degrees of flexion. Keep your elbows beside your chest walls (counter to habitual body use, which would have you move your elbows lateral rather than flexing your wrists). Your thumbs come off the head, and your other fingers change from pad to tip contact. Stay sensitive to the bones' motility patterns as you increase contact pressure (medial pressure) and begin to introduce superior decompression. Use enough medially directed pressure so that you do not slip, but not so much that the client feels it invasive, or distressing.

Modulate wrist flexion and purchase until you "link up" and feel the parietals begin to lift off. Track the lift through its overlapping stages of separation and movement; sense parietal flexion, and any restriction in it from muscular, fascial, osseous, or dural tissues. This completes the first phase of this technique – the technical.

The second stage is energetic, which brings with it the capability to open the crown soul. Understanding this energetic component is vitally important: the opening will not occur if the immediate environment is inimical, cold, and hard, so you must alter your own field to create an appropriate space. To prepare a warm, secure, and open environment for the client's crown soul to open into, breathe into your spiritual heart, find the still point at the top of your in-breath, and create some intercostal stretch pain to increase your awareness of the warm space of the cave of your heart. Expand your field into, and beyond, this space.

Now bring in an image of, or the feeling for, the one you love the most. This might be a spouse, child, religious figure, or a pet. (I remember fondly the student who stated, somewhat abashedly, at the end of this exercise that the image that arose for him was that of his horse. Looking sheepishly around the classroom, he wanted to know if this was okay. The totem does not matter; it is the spirit of the love inspired that has the power to unlock your heart.) Sense the opening of the client's crown soul, keeping your heart space open.

The medial compression of the parietals allows them to free from the clasp of the temporals, and once this has occurred the sagittal suture can open, and with it the crown. Tune in to the falx, which is the main midline structure impeding decompression; you may feel it unwinding. Sense how long the crown soul needs your physical and energetic focus; and soften your purchase and gently allow the parietals to return to their normal resting place on their own when you sense either a profound still point or when all tissue tension releases.

## Scalp Unwinding

Scalp unwinding is accomplished by gently teasing the scalp free of the parietal periosteum either by "crinkling" it with your fingerpads or comfortably pulling it via the hair. There is a curious difference between men and women that often becomes apparent with this technique. Women quite like firm hair pulling: men hate it.

## *Chi Kung* to the Crown Soul

*Chi kung*[15] refers here to the transmission of energy across space and tissue. Place your thumbnails back-to-back right on the sagittal suture at the vertex. (An alternative contact would be at bregma.) Then direct energy down your thumbs and through the straight sinus, with the intention of transmitting energy down the client's spinal cord to his coccyx, even to the soles of his feet, opening his channel to Mother Earth.

Clarity of intention is vital, as is previsualization of the target structures. "See" the falx, brain stem, spinal cord, and coccyx and direct energy, imagining it as red or silver light. Enter deep, power breathing and maintain your focus. Track borborygmus, facial expression, respiration, skin temperature, and rapid eye movement to stay present and therefore responsive to your client's level of consciousness.

The spirit of this contact is one of clearing the space between the hemispheres of the cerebrum and opening the Governor Vessel.

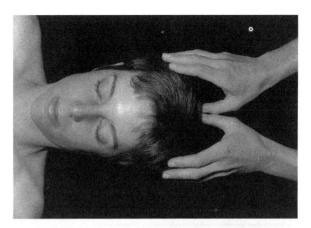
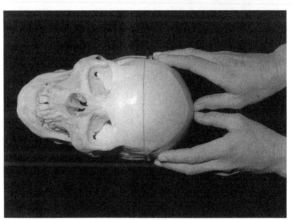

*Chi Kung to the Crown Soul, two views*

## Other Techniques that Can Affect the Parietals

- Anterior Frontal Decompression
- The CV4
- All temporal techniques
- Release of the Posterior Fibers of Temporalis
- Mandible Compression
- Auditory Tube Twist
- Cant Hook techniques to the occiput, sphenoid, and frontal
- All sacral techniques, which may be effective via a release of spinal dura tension, resulting in a reduction of falx contraction

# 27
# The Frontal

## Etymology

**Frontal**  from the Latin frons,
for forehead

**1**  Squama of frontal bone

**2**  Superciliary arch, or eyebrow ridge

**3**  Supraorbital margin

**4**  Glabella, a smooth area between
superciliary arches

**5**  Supraorbital foramen or notch, transmits
supraorbital artery and lateral part of
supraorbital nerve

**6**  Orbital part, or orbito-nasal plate, forms
vault of orbit

**7**  Ethmoidal notch, a fjord-like aperture
between left and right orbito-nasal plates
where ethmoid fits via plain suture

**8**  Nasal spine, articulates with nasal bones
via plain suture

**9**  Parietal margin, interdigitated frontal
portion of coronal suture

**10**  Zygomatic process, where frontal
articulates with zygoma via dentate suture

**11**  Superior temporal line, formed by
arcuate attachment of fascia overlying
temporalis

**12**  Frontal crest, double ridge of bone
formed by pull of bifurcated falx cerebri, in
middle of which is located superior sagittal
sinus

**13**  Foramen cecum, blind canal

**14**  Frontal air sinus, with openings on
medial and inferior surface for air circulation
into nasal cavity

**15**  Orbitonasal margin, where frontal
articulates with lesser wing of sphenoid

**16**  Aperture of frontal sinus

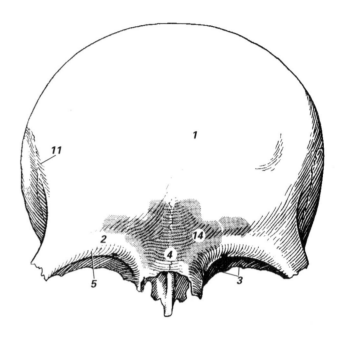

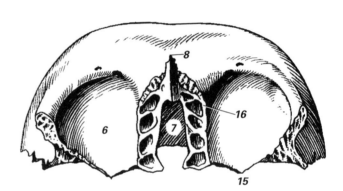

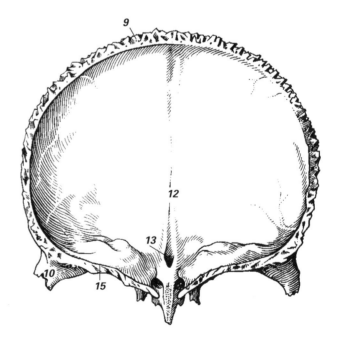

## Embryology and Osteology

Like all cranial vault bones, the frontal bone ossifies from a membranous precursor; the ossification
begins from two centers in the seventh or eighth
week of fetal development. At birth the bone is
still in two parts, separated down the sagittal midline by the metopic suture. This suture typically
ossifies between the seventh or eighth year,[1] but
less than 10 percent of people[2] have an open
metopic suture throughout life. The convention in
craniosacral work is to always refer to the frontal
bone in the plural, to honor the hinging that is said
to occur at the frontal midline during classical flexion and extension movements. However, since the
hominoid metopic suture largely disappeared 36
million years ago,[3,4] and more than 90 percent of
people have no suture here, I refer to the frontal
bone in the singular.

## Anatomy

The frontal is a very large, biconcave, prominently
domed bone. It forms part of the anterior pole of
attachment of the falx, forms part of the eye
socket, and houses the all-important frontal and
prefrontal lobes of the brain.

### Structure

The exposed surfaces of the domes of the frontal
are diploic bone, hollowed out at their inferior and
medial corners by the frontal air sinuses. The
frontal is very robust at the zygomatic sutures. The
portion of the bone that separates the frontal and
prefrontal lobes from the eyes is diploic bone anteriorly, but further posterior becomes a single delicate shelf of cortical bone the thickness of the
lesser wings at their articulations.

## Location

This is the most obviously hominid bone in the
human body. Four million years ago we had almost
nothing above or behind the eyebrows, but the
brain has since grown so rapidly into the frontal
region that our eyebrow ridges have almost disappeared. The high-domed cathedral of our frontal
vault is unique to *Homo sapiens sapiens*.

### Landmarks

The lateral extremities of the eyebrows mark the
sutures between the frontal and the zygomae, with
the frontal extending no further inferior than the
lateral eyebrow level. The sideburn lines mark the
posterior limit of the frontal at pterion; at the top
of the head, they do not extend posterior to a line

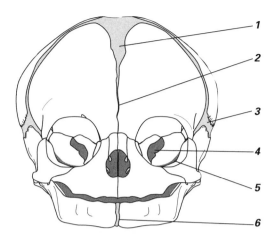

The metopic
suture at
birth
**1** Anterior
fontanel
**2** Metopic
suture
**3** Sphenoidal
fontanel
**4** Superior
orbital
fissure
**5** Inferior
orbital
fissure
**6** Symphysis
mentis

drawn vertically from the ear canals to the crown.
The frontal is the deepest of the four bones (temporal, sphenoid, parietal, and frontal, in order of
depth) that make up pterion.

## Sutures and Articulations

The frontal makes its articulations through many
different types of joints. The frontal has a heavily
interdigitated suture with the parietals; a mildly
interdigitated suture with the lesser wings of the
sphenoid; an uneven, highly variable plain suture
with the ethmoid (located in a fjord-shaped notch
that is narrower anteriorly); a recessed, slightly
interdigitated suture with the nasal bones; robust,
heavily interdigitated sutures with the zygomae;
and recessed, conical cave-like sutures with the
uppermost ramps of the maxillae. When the
metopic suture is present throughout life, it is
interdigitated.

The frontal bone articulates with as many as
fourteen bones:

- The sphenoid at the lesser wing
- The ethmoid
- Two parietals
- Two temporals (variable – they
may not touch)
- Two zygomae
- Two maxillae
- Two lacrimal bones
- Two nasal bones

## Weight

A medically prepared, disarticulated frontal bone
which has ossified at the metopic suture weighs
1⅔ ounce (47.3 grams).

## Detailed Anatomy and Musculature

The frontal is sometimes described as a cockle shell. For teaching purposes it is classically divided into a vertical or frontal portion, and a horizontal or orbitonasal portion. The supraorbital ridges act to provide orbital shading, protection, and the threat-signaling apparatus called eyebrows, but are also promulgated by the internal growth of the air sinuses – which can progressively collapse in the event of severe trauma to better protect the eyes, and the brain. This works in much the same way that modern cars protect their occupants by having a strong safety cell around the passenger compartment, and a more easily deformable fore and aft structure that allows for shock absorption upon impact.

The frontal forms the anterior-most portion of the neurocranial vault, and encloses the most recently evolved sections of the cerebral hemispheres, the frontal and prefrontal lobes. The frontal is marked anteriorly by the supraorbital ridges, which form the margin of the upper half of the orbital cavities; the right ridge is larger. At bregma the coronal suture marks the most superior and posterior margin of the frontal. It may be helpful in terms of approximate landmarking to consider that the anterior part of the auricle (the external ear) is approximately 1 inch (2.6 centimeters) posterior to the inferior border of the coronal suture at pterion.

Internally the frontal forms a tapering groove, more narrow anteriorly, into which the ethmoid fits. There is also a very sharp ridge on the internal surface of the vertical portion (just superior to the crista galli of the ethmoid) formed by the attachment of the falx. This ridge develops into a double-ridged structure within 1 inch (2.6 centimeters) of the tip of the crista galli due to the bifurcation of the falx, just before it attaches to the bone. (The superior sagittal sinus, which channels venous blood posterior, nestles in the curved pink tunnel that results from the double ridge.) This crest is functionally continuous with the crista galli of the ethmoid.

The crista galli is formed by the powerful pull the falx exerts upon the cribriform plate of the ethmoid. Note that the falx, just before terminating at the crista galli, leaves the internal surface of the frontal, causing a gap between membrane and bone at the anterior pole of the falx. However, the firm and extensive adherence of the endosteal dura to surrounding bone means that this anatomical detail has no functional effect.

### Musculature

The muscles attaching to the frontal consist of the:
- Temporalis
- Frontal portions of epicranius (occipitofrontalis)
- Corrugator supercilli
- Procerus
- Orbital part of orbicularis occuli

## Physiology

The frontal has some fascinating evolutionary attributes, such as the deep-diving reflex. Its motion pattern plays an important role in cranial mechanics and its extensive domed surface area means that it receives compound inputs from the movement of the brain, as mediated through the cerebrospinal fluid.

The deep-diving reflex is a relic of our time in the sea. There is a pressure- and temperature-sensitive patch in the glabella area that extends into the frontal air sinuses, whose single-walled structure allows the deep-diving reflex to sense bone deflection caused by increased water pressure more readily than diploic bone would. With every 33 feet (10 meters) of depth, water pressure increases by one atmosphere (760 millimeters of mercury, or 14.7 pounds per square inch).

Sperm whales dive more than 3,300 feet (1,000 meters), at which depth humans would be crushed to death by the increased water pressure. Whales, air-breathing, hot-blooded mammals like ourselves, survive at these depths through their version of the deep-diving reflex, which registers temperature and pressure change as they pass through each thermocline[1] and lowers their blood pressure to compensate. Reaching the colder, deeper thermoclines, the whale locks oxygenated blood in its brain, removing blood from less vital areas like digestion and reproduction. Photographs of sperm whales below 3,300 feet (1,000 meters) show progressive implosion of their rib cages. (Sperm whales dive the deepest of all the great whales.[5] When a sperm whales is injured, the others in its pod gather around it and align all their foreheads to touch the disabled whale, doing this until the disabled whale recovers. I imagine it as a kind of whale *chi kung*. This wonderful, compassionate practice proved devastating for the sperm whales when noted by the harpoonists on whaling ships – they realized that if they could deliberately injure but not kill one whale, they could draw in and kill the rest of the pod.)

Newfound knowledge of the deep-diving reflex saved one boy's life after he fell through thin ice during the harsh winter of 1986. The five-year-old

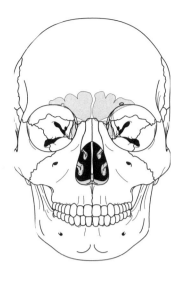

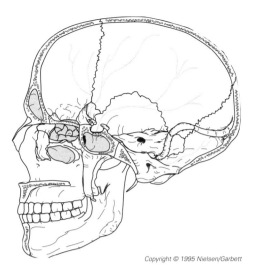

*Anterior and
lateral views
of the frontal
air sinus*

boy had been walking with his father and dog along the banks of one of the Great Lakes, and had thrown a stick onto the ice of the lake for the dog to chase. When the dog rushed for the stick and fell through the ice 30 feet (10 meters) from shore, the boy, before his father could stop him – chased after the dog in an attempted rescue, and also fell through the ice. The man knew better than to follow, and ran to telephone 911. Twenty minutes later two divers dropped from a helicopter through the hole left by the boy; it took them ten minutes with powerful searchlights to locate his body under the ice. When brought to the surface, the boy was clinically dead: quite blue in color, no heartbeat, no breath, body core temperature at eighty degrees.

Five years earlier his body would have been put in a body bag and sent to the morgue. In 1986, the emergency room physicians knew there was hope. Hooking the stiff body up to a kidney dialysis machine, they restarted his heart and breathing as the machine warmed his blood at a predetermined slow rate. Drugs were administered to keep him in a coma until his blood had reached the critical temperature where the deep-diving reflex could release its grip and the brain remain undamaged. Within a day the boy was awake and functioning normally, having transited the trauma intact even though irreversible brain damage normally ensues after five minutes of oxygen deprivation. He had been under water for at least thirty minutes, but the deep-diving reflex, stimulated by the freezing water, had locked richly oxygenated blood into his brain and the intense cold had helped forestall deterioration. From this and similar ice-water accidents,[607] we now know that the deep-diving reflex is present and fully functioning in children until about six years of age. It is a welcome relic!

The deep-diving reflex is also engaged when you splash cold water or place a cool cloth on your forehead – it is part of what makes you feel refreshed. The cooled venous blood of the facial

system then makes its way posterior to the cavernous sinus, a rich network of venous caverns that surrounds the pituitary – a gland calibrated to function properly only within a narrow one-degree temperature range. We immediately feel relieved.

The frontal air sinuses also play a part in voice, song, and sound production, and their rapid expansion at puberty is part of the voice change humans undergo at that time. A gifted opera singer knows how to direct sound and pressure waves inside his own air sinus network – a system of caverns, tunnels, and air cells. The result is a beauteous thing to be immersed in:

> *Jessye Norman's voice is an astonishing instrument. In a recital on Sunday night in Avery Fisher Hall, it seemed a grand mansion of sound. It defines an extraordinary space. It has enormous dimensions, reaching backwards and upward. It opens onto unexpected vistas. It contains sunlit rooms, narrow passageways, cavernous halls.*[7]

The air sinuses play a vital role in cetaceans' underwater communication, acting as acoustical mirrors to focus their sonar beams.[8] If you were to swim between two communicating whales, your air sinuses would vibrate, hum, and resonate according to the modulating vibrational frequencies of whale song, and the vibrations might reach the point of pain. Much of the whale's acoustic spectrum is outside our own – palpable, although inaudible. The air sinuses lighten the head, permitting very rapid rotation (a great asset in threat situations), and also help give it buoyancy in salt water.

## Axis of Rotation

In the classical model the frontal axis of rotation is aligned almost vertically, from the upper part of the dome close to bregma running through each side of the frontal inferior, anterior, and slightly lateral to pass through the middle of each eyeball.

## Motion

In classical craniosacral work, the metopic suture (midline of the frontal) is always regarded as being "open." Refine your skill to the point that you can feel the motility pattern in each cranium, and therefore discern which type of frontal bone exists – fused at the metopic suture, or paired. You can also palpate the area of the suture, and sense whether it is present.

### Osteopathic Model

The maxillae are regarded as "hanging" from the frontal.[9] The orbitonasal plate of the frontal that provides the fjord for the ethmoid and separates the frontal lobes from the eyes is regarded in traditional cranial osteopathy as the viscerocranial part of the frontal. In the osteopathic (similar-motion) model, the sphenoid is considered to "drive" the viscerocranium, including the orbitonasal plate of the frontal – that is, it is seen to provide the propulsive force from which all viscerocranial motion originates.[10] Since the sphenoid articulates with most of the facial bones, it has a strong and immediate influence on all of the viscerocranial bones. The falx is responsible for the remainder of frontal motion in this model: it moves posterior in flexion, thus pulling the midline of the frontal with it and opposing the anterior push of the sphenoid. The result of these opposing forces is that the frontal broadens laterally during classical flexion and move slightly posterior at the metopic suture line.

Seen the other way around, the maxillae and zygomae exert a strong effect upon the sphenoid. The frontal, on the other hand, rarely seems to do so; it only faults as the result of extreme trauma (see Diagnostic Considerations, below).

### Liquid-Electric Model

The liquid-electric model does not see the sphenoid as the driving force for the viscerocranium, but rather as a central unit of function with strong propulsive inputs from the brain. These impulses, in the optimum state, are absorbed by synchronous movements of the adjacent bones. The viscerocranial bones, including the frontal, of course have their own strong muscular attachments, notably of temporalis and occipitofrontalis. In this model, the viscerocranial bones are regarded as having enough motion in their normal state to "get out of the way" of the sphenoid, and thus not be driven by it.

In the liquid-electric model, the healthy frontal behaves much like the occiput, like its alternating flexion and extension cycle from side to side. Thus when the left frontal is in flexion, the right is in extension. The bone is drawn slightly posterior by the falx moving posterior and inferior in flexion. The lateral extremity of each side of the frontal moves further lateral during its flexion phase; that is, the bone widens. The ethmoid, acting as a sponge, absorbs the disparate motion of the frontal and resolves it into its own ethmoidal midsagittal torsion pattern, with minor flexion and extension components received from the oscillating sphenoid.

## Diagnostic Considerations

Compared with more volatile bones like the sphenoid or temporals, the frontal is not often involved in either symptom production or location. Its air sinus does become inflamed in chronic sinusitis,[11] but it drains with gravity in an upright posture, and even when recumbent (unlike the maxillary sinuses, which can only drain when the body is recumbent or inverted). The frontal is frequently impacted in automobile accidents, especially when the person is not wearing a seat belt and the frontal impacts the steering wheel or dashboard. It is also a frequent site of muscle contraction and migraine headaches.

*Energetics*

At glabella, the frontal is the exit point of the channel of the inner eye.[12] The frontal and ethmoid area becomes "cloudy" when an individual cannot see his way ahead, as if lost in a swirling mountain mist and out of touch with the rest of the world. The frontal itself gets into stubbornness when stressed, and the individual becomes pig-headed or bull-headed. Stubbornness is the negative shadow of perseverance. The frontal is invested with the energy of Aries the Ram. Sometimes it is exhilarating to push and shove in life, but when such behavior becomes obsessive we may end up butting our heads against a brick wall.

When the frontal represents determination, it tends to be "stupid" determination – the kind that says "what I need to fix this is a bigger hammer." The mandible and mentalis ("the thinker") represent "smart" determination, the kind that says "what we need to fix this is to sit down, have a cup of tea, and figure out where the release mechanism is."

The high dome of the frontal, in its positive aspect, also represents intelligence, wisdom, conscience, and ethics. It is symbolic of the evolved human's ability to choose not to follow instinctive behavior, that which separates us from our more instinct-ruled primate cousins.

*Trauma and Dysfunction*

In frontal impact injuries such as from a dashboard compression or surfing impact, sutural locking can be so severe[13] that decompressive techniques cannot release it. Months of patient Cant Hook or asymmetrical technique work (such as the Oral Coronal Shear Test) may be needed to tease the sutures apart sufficiently for cranial wave formations to again pass through them unimpeded.

A student described his experience of the first contact with his frontal bone in this way:

*"I know these hands," I thought as he touched my frontal bone. I felt an immediate sense of trust. After a few minutes of traction my left coronal suture suddenly opened, I felt cerebrospinal fluid rush into the space behind my forehead for the first time since the horse kicked me there. I feel now like I have a whole new head. My brain works again!*

The frontal and pre-frontal lobes of the brain help us make long-term plans, allow us to consider thoughts of life and death, conscience and ethics, and play an important role in working memory.[14] They may also play a role in the regulation of emotional behavior and mood.

The more venous congestion is relieved within the head, the more effective ensuing cranial technique will be. Relieving back-pressure is an asset in the tonsillitis and mastoiditis common in childhood, may help in parotitis and inner-ear infections, and is an important foundation treatment in working with adults with most forms of headache.

In the late 1980s a severely obsessive-compulsive man (he used to wash his hands hundreds of times a day and take showers continually), identified in medical literature only as "George," attempted to commit suicide by shooting himself through the frontal with a twenty-two caliber handgun. The literature referred to his attempt as "successful radical surgery" because, while very bloody, it did not kill him and in fact seemed to have cured his obsessive-compulsive behavior. His doctors noted that he had lost none of his I.Q., and that he went on to enter college. Dr. Thomas Ballantine, a psychiatrist at Massachusetts General Hospital, noted that "The idea that a man could blow out part of his frontal lobe and have his pathological symptoms cured is quite remarkable, but not beyond belief."

In acupuncture, frontal headaches are understood to arise occasionally when one or more organ systems suddenly come "on-line" at once. For instance, the large intestine organ system is at its strongest between five and seven in the morning, and a frontal headache that begins at this time may have large intestine involvement. The stomach system is at its strongest between seven and nine in the morning, and the kidneys between five and seven in the evening.

Further, there are strong reflexes from the liver to the right frontal eminence, and from the gall bladder to the left. (Liver dysfunction tends to give right-sided frontal headaches, right-sided migraines, right-sided sinusitis, and right leg pains.)

### Interconnectedness

*Far right:*
*Frontal*
*Anterior*
*Decompres-*
*sion, two*
*views*

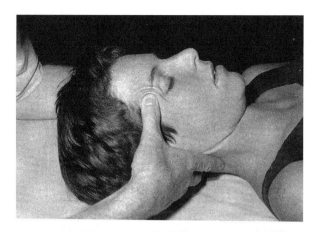

As we have seen, the viscerocranial bones (maxillae, mandible, nasals, ethmoid, palatines, and zygomae) are classically considered as hanging from the frontal. Coupled contacts, such as the Frontal-Mandible-Zygomae Triple Spread, allow you to balance the neurocranium – represented here by the frontal – with the viscerocranial bones.

### Visualization

With your client supine on the table, visualize the frontal as a hot-air balloon anchored to the ground only by the slightly elastic tether of the falx. Add to your visualization the delicate articulations of the frontal's orbitonasal plate to the lesser wings of the sphenoid, and place the olfactory bulbs over the cribriform plate of the ethmoid, wedged in the fjord provided for it by the frontal. Imagine the energy of the frontal and prefrontal lobes of the brain suffusing the frontal bone with chemical-electric fire, sending shimmers and heat-hazes dancing across its surface.

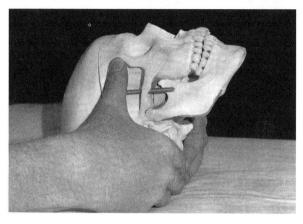

### TECHNIQUES

### Frontal Anterior Decompression

This decompressive technique is a good way to begin working with the frontal bone. The contact points are thumbtip-sized depressions formed by the intersections of the zygomae with the superior temporal lines, at the posterior and superior margins of the eye sockets. The contact points are located approximately ½ inch (1.3 centimeter) anterior and a little cephalad to the landmarking for contacting the greater wing of the sphenoid.

Sit or kneel at the head of the table. Flex your wrists and align your thumbs so that they point toward each other in the transverse plane and create a forty-five-degree anteromedial angle to the table surface. Take out skin slack with a scooping motion (this takes care of the first layer of release, that of the skin), returning to the precise contact area. Be sure that your thumbtips abut the posterior margin of the superior temporal line. Now gently and fluidly introduce anterior decompression while monitoring motility. Take the frontal lift through the five remaining layers of release – mus-

cular, osseous, dural, cerebrospinal fluid, and energetic. As a diagnostic tool, sense in which level there is an adhesion, contraction, or need for unwinding. Feel the separations and responses in each stage of the freeing-up process.

No craniosacral technique works all the time, with every client. This is a wonderfully euphoric technique – when it works. In optimum cases the client experiences an enormous sense of light and expansion inside his whole head. (When it does not "work," the client experiences no relief and no euphoria.) The Parietal Lift and Release of the Posterior Fibers of Temporalis may have the same euphoric effect. A Frontal Anterior Decompression is also one of the best techniques for unwinding the falx in the anteroposterior plane. When you are "driving" the frontal anterior and the sutures release, you can begin to unwind tension patterns in the endosteal dura deep to the suture and the falx cerebri in the midline; when contracted, both inhibit further anterior motion of the frontal.

## Clear the Confusion (Unwinding the Falx)

I learned this technique, designed specifically to clear the energy field between the cerebral hemispheres, from Betty Balcombe, a gifted psychic healer, in 1984. I have since evolved it into a technique that encompasses the whole body. Besides clearing the field, it is also a fine technique for unwinding the falx and, via the falx, the rest of the reciprocal tension membrane. Consider using it in frontal, falx, and "mask" area headaches (those that affect a band around the eyes 1 inch [2½ centimeters] wide).

For the basic form, stand at the head of the table, bring your thumbs together (lateral aspects of the thumbnails in contact) and place them midway up the anterior aspect of the nose, just where the nasal bones begin. Take up a firm and quite small (localized) contact using the tips of your thumbs, not the pads. At the same time rest your index and middle fingerpads on the contact area for the greater wings of the sphenoid. Wait until you have a definite energetic contact with both the nasal bones and sphenoid, and sense and monitor the activity of the deep cranial structures, specifically the anterior pole of attachment of the tentorium through the greater wings. Then begin moving your thumbs superiorly and posteriorly over nasion to glabella.

At glabella, pause and begin to increase the pressure of your contact, directing energy inside the head to access the falx's anterior pole of attachment at the crista galli of the ethmoid. Because of the thumbs' placement external to the falx, and the index and middle fingers' placement (at the greater wings) external to the tentorium, this technique can be considered a kind of anterior CV4.

Once you feel "hooked up" with the falx, begin moving superiorly along the metopic suture line. There is a distinct change of energy midway up the forehead (but, curiously, no acupuncture point here); pause there and tune in, way in. This point allows you to first access, and then stimulate, the hypothalamus. Then continue up the forehead to the hairline, where you reduce pressure so as not to pull the client's hair unpleasantly. (Many women like a mild degree of hair pulling, while men seem to hate it.) Continue along the line of

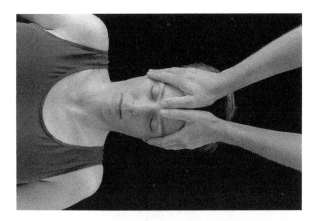

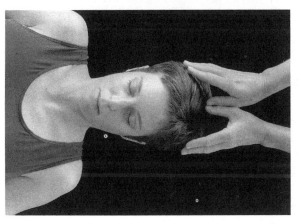

*Two stages of the Clear the Confusion Technique*

the sagittal suture until you reach the vertex. While you trace this path with your thumbs, your other fingers are acting as guides and lateral braces, passing from the greater wings to the parietal bones. At the vertex, move to thumbnail-tip contact and send energy down the spinal cord – the Red Road. Come off gently and respectfully, clearing your hands from the client's field before moving them in any other directions.

You may also begin Clear the Confusion at the chin, or the heart soul center in the center of the breastbone; at the feet is also possible, sweeping up the anterior aspects of the thighs, over the anterior superior iliac spines, and then along the midline of the body to the nasal bones.

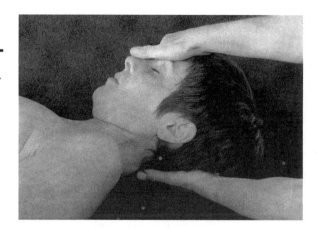

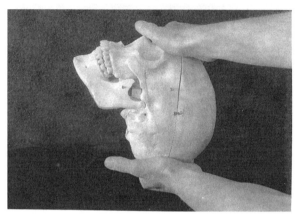

*Frontal Cup and Straddle, two views*

## Frontal Cup and Straddle

Sit to your client's left side and cup your left hand under his head to contact the occiput and part of the parietals; align your hand so that the "heart line" (the distal palmar crease) is directly posterior to the falx. Place your right hand over the frontal, straddling most of the bone with fingers and palm, and again aligned so that the "heart line" of this hand is directly on the falx line. Rest your thumb lightly on the nasal bones. Care with exact placement will be rewarded with enhanced sensitivity.

This technique has an altogether different "flavor" than other techniques that encompass working with two bones simultaneously, such as Sphenobasilar Decompression. It is more of a gentle, all-encompassing, sensitive hold designed to begin very delicate molding movements of the head. Although simple, it can take you to very advanced

capabilities. Among craniosacral techniques, it is one of the best to feel the movement of the brain within the cranial cavity. It is also wonderful for:

- Sensing the movement of the frontal, then frontal and occiput
- Sensing and unwinding the falx
- Working with traumas that have caused a displacement along the sagittal shear plane
- Sensitive palpation of the cerebrospinal fluid and oscillatory enhancement of its circulation
- Optimizing the position of the brain within the dural cavity

You will also begin to discern neck unwinding patterns, so it is a technique to consider for whiplash injury, neck sprain, and cervical spine arthritis. In whiplash injury, your objective is threefold: to balance the brain and spinal cord within the head and neck, to unwind the head from the neck, and to unwind the neck itself.

## Fronto-Occipital Drainage

This is a modified cup and straddle technique designed to facilitate vascular drainage of all the venous sinuses in the head. Use this technique in the opening stages of a treatment: once venous congestion in the head is relieved, the cranial mechanism will respond more favorably to subsequent work. Client cooperation is essential, so spend a few minutes demonstrating how the client should bring his spine and limbs into an extension movement.

Sit to one side, preferably the client's left. Place your left hand under the occiput and your right over the frontal so that both thumbs point inferiorly. Have the client breathe through his mouth to better promote mandibular release. Synchronize your breathing with his, and during the out-breath (cranial and body extension) take both the frontal and occiput into exaggerated extension. At the same time, instruct the client to bend his neck and thoracic spine slightly backward (using muscle force) while simultaneously introducing internal rotation to his arms and legs. Choose to either follow the cycle into flexion during the in-breath, or relax your contact pressure slightly so that the client can regroup his energy and concentration for the next extension cycle. Stay with your contact until you feel the resistance under your hands soften.

## Frontal-Zygomae-Mandible Triple Spread

Sit comfortably at your client's head and place the pads of your central three fingers on either side of the mental protuberance of the mandible. Place the bases of your fingers (metacarpophalangeal joints) on the raised prominence of the zygomae and the heels of your hands on the frontal, around the curvature of the forehead as it changes from the coronal to sagittal plane. Tune in to all six contacts – three bones with each hand – first sequentially, finally simultaneously. Then, with subtle alterations of pressure and timing, begin to balance the motion of the viscerocranium with that of the neurocranium.

This is an excellent fine-balancing technique, one that feels very tender and caring; it is especially useful in the completion stages of deep reconstructive work, such as the treatment of facial injury. It helps relax the eyes and readily induces altered states of consciousness, and is also useful to end a whole-body unwinding session. An apt metaphor for this technique is that it is like the jewelers' rouge used for fine polishing, once more robust work is complete.

## Other Techniques that Can Affect the Frontal

■ Auditory Twist Technique
■ Temporal Cross-Check
■ The CV4
■ Occipitofrontal Cant Hook Technique
■ All ethmoid and zygomatic techniques
■ Incisive Bone Decompression and Unwinding
■ "Cleansing diets," non-dairy diets, and *prana yama* breathing
■ Biofeedback techniques that educate clients in relaxing their occipitofrontal and temporalis muscles

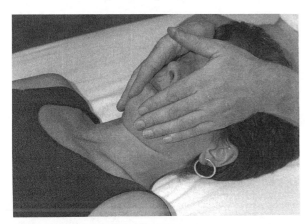

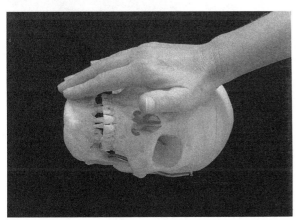

***Far right:*** *Frontal-Zygomae-Mandible Triple Spread; for clarity, only one hand is shown in contact in lower photo.*

# 28
# The Ethmoid

### Etymology

**Ethmoid** from the Greek, meaning a sieve

**Crista galli** Latin for a cock's comb

**Turbinates** from the Latin for a whirl

**Concha** from the Greek for a shell

**Cribriform** from the Latin, meaning sievelike

---

**1** Cribiform plate, thin horizontal bony surface perforated by apertures for transmitting olfactory fibers from olfactory bulb, CN I

**2** Crista galli, small bony crest formed by pull of falx cerebri

**3** Ala crista galli, paired forward-projecting wing-like processes, articulate via plain suture with frontal crest

**4** Perpendicular plate, vertical bony lamina projecting down from cribiform plate and forming anterosuperior portion of nasal septum

**5** Ethmoid labyrinth, collective term for ethmoidal air cell network located between orbit and nasal cavity

**6** Exposed ethmoidal air cells

**7** Orbital lamina, paper-thin bony plate forming part of medial wall of orbital cavity

**8** Supreme nasal concha, a vestigial turbinate bone

**9** Superior concha

**10** Middle concha

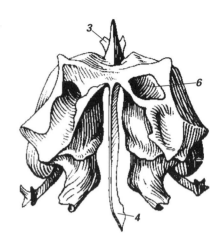

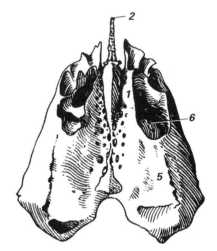

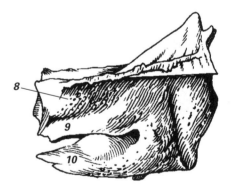

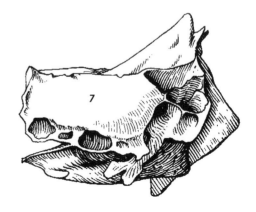

## Embryology and Osteology

The ethmoid develops from two minute ossification centers, one for each lateral mass (which will later contain the ethmoid air cells), beginning in the twelfth week of fetal development. At birth the ethmoid is half membrane, half bone – its bony portions consisting solely of two tiny lateral masses – permitting substantial deformation and compression during birth. Ossification of the perpendicular plate and the crista galli arises from one center in the vomerine cartilage and is complete by the age of one, joining with the lateral masses to complete the configuration of the ethmoid by the age of two. The honeycomb-shaped air sinus cells that fill out the lateral masses do not begin to form until age four, at which point the ethmoid begins to take on its mature form.

The ossification times of the lateral masses versus those of the perpendicular plate show how vital ethmoid malleability is during birth. Birth, and the bony accommodations necessary to get the large cranium through the small birth canal, dictate how the head behaves not just during birth but for the remainder of life. DeJarnette suggests that the ethmoid acts like a damp sponge, deforming readily in response to the motion of other bones. The fact that it is largely in cartilage at birth allows for the ethmoid to function in this way.

## Anatomy

The ethmoid is an exceedingly delicate, thin-walled pneumatic bone. Disarticulated, it looks like nothing more than the tiny head of a bird's skeleton, such as you might find under a bush after a hard winter.

### Structure

The ethmoid is almost entirely composed of paper-thin, single-walled cortical bone. The crista galli is formed by the powerful pull exerted upon it by the falx, and at ⅛ inch (3 millimeters) is the thickest part of the ethmoid.

## Location

The ethmoid forms the medial part of the eye socket. It lies anterior to the sphenoid, inferior and medial to the frontal, and posterior to the nasal bones. The ethmoid is superior and (partly) medial to the maxillae, and also superior and (partly) anterior to the vomer.

### Landmarks

The ethmoid lies posterior to nasion and glabella. It is visible in the skull as the gossamer-thin medial quarter of the orbit.

## Sutures and Articulations

The ethmoid has no heavily interdigitated sutures; it relies on its pliancy to accommodate to the motion of its larger neighbors. The ethmoid presents mildly interdigitated but delicate sutures of a thickness of ¹⁄₁₆ inch (1.5 millimeters) with the lesser wings of sphenoid; harmonic (plain) sutures with each maxilla; harmonic sutures with the frontal; harmonic sutures with the lacrimals; and a harmonic suture where its perpendicular plate meets the nasals.

The ethmoid articulates with nine bones:

- The sphenoid
- The vomer
- Both nasals
- Both palatines
- Both maxillae
- The frontal

## Weight

A medically prepared, disarticulated ethmoid weighs ¹⁄₁₈ ounce (1.5 grams).

## Detailed Anatomy and Musculature

The ethmoid and frontal form part of both the neurocranium and viscerocranium, and are therefore called "transitional bones." Sutherland did not regard the ethmoid as a speed reducer, although it absorbs motion in much the same way. His three speed reducers – the palatines, vomer, and zygomae – are pure viscerocranial bones.

The ethmoid is made up of four parts:

- A midsagittal vertical plate known as the perpendicular plate
- A horizontal plate called the cribriform plate
- Two lateral masses of air cells that form the upper three conchae (or turbinate bones)

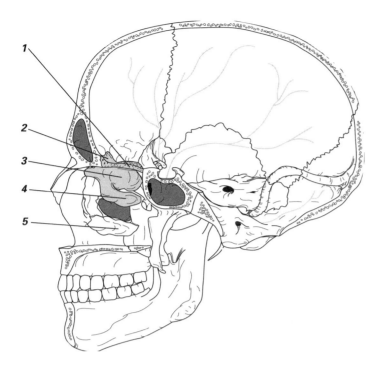

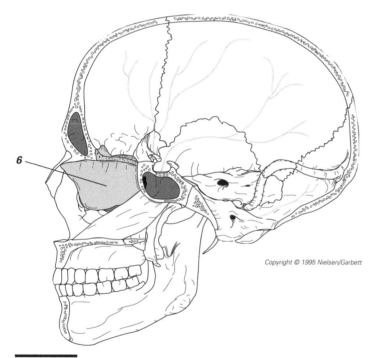

*Copyright © 1995 Nielsen/Garbett*

**Top:**
*Lateral aspect of right nasal cavity*

**Bottom:**
*Left side of nasal septum*

*1 Cribriform plate*
*2 Crista galli*
*3 Superior concha*
*4 Middle concha*
*5 Inferior concha*
*6 Perpendicular plate*

These conchae are part of the air sinus network that is functionally continuous from the frontal to the air sinus of the sphenoid.

The perpendicular plate of the ethmoid is a midline bone and part of the viscerocranium. The lateral masses, which contain the ethmoid's air sinus network of air cells, and form the upper three conchae, are part of the viscerocranium. Their most superior aspect, the cribriform plate, lies on either side of the crista galli, which derives its particular pointed shape from the anterior and superior tension of the sickle-shaped falx cerebri. Both the crista galli and cribriform plate are part of the neurocranium.

Mechanically speaking, the viscerocranium hangs from the ethmoid and frontal, with the falx acting as the suspensory ligament. The frontal provides the tapered fjord into which the slightly wedge-shaped ethmoid fits. At its inferior border, the ethmoid articulates with the triangular cartilage of the nose. The upper half of its posterior border articulates with the sphenoid crest, the lower half with the vomer.

The air cells articulate directly with the sphenoid air sinus through two apertures about ⅛ inch (3 millimeters) in diameter and approximate to the orbital processes of the palatines. The air cells are closed off inferolaterally at the articulation with the maxillae. You can see the honeycomb construction of the air sinus network on the medial wall of the orbit as you look into the eye socket of a medically prepared skull: the bone is as thin as paper here, and often broken inadvertently when handling the skull. If you shine a flashlight up the nose of such a skull, and look at its beam through the eye sockets, the honeycomb of the air sinus network is perfectly revealed.

### Musculature

The ethmoid has no muscle attachments.

## Physiology

While the ethmoid may lack muscle attachments, it does have one very important attachment – that of the falx. The powerful pull of the falx forms the crista galli, which shares (with the coronoid processes of the mandible and the mastoid processes of the temporals) the fusiform conical shape that results from muscle or membrane traction. The apex of the crista galli's triangular shape faces the direction of maximum traction, which is anterior and superior.

The ethmoid air cells and conchae warm and moisten the incoming charge of air on a cold morning. They moisten the super-dry air of aircraft air-conditioning as best as they can. The conchae, which used to be called the turbinates, are – as implied by the two names – conch shell-shaped bones, specialized parts of the ethmoid air-cell network that spin, expand, and therefore speed up the incoming flow of air. The air is spun outward to come into contact with more of the warm, wet mucous membrane than it otherwise would, helping to warm and moisten the incoming air to make it more amenable to the lungs. Continual movement of the ethmoid is vital for the normal drainage of mucous from within the air-cell network. Neanderthals had a more extensive ethmoid air-cell network than we do, which enabled them to excel in the cold, dry air of the last ice age.

The olfactory bulbs (first cranial nerve) sit atop the cribriform plate and drop some sixty small nerve fibers through each side of it. The fibers divide and spread out to innervate a small (1 square inch, or 2.6 square centimeter) patch of mucous membrane on the lateral and medial walls of the most superior part of each nasal cavity. There 25 million ciliated nerve fibers provide us with our sense of smell. (Wolves have an olfactory patch fourteen times larger than ours, and some biologists estimate that wolves can smell a hundred times better than humans.[1]) Our olfactory capability is upgraded with the help of odorant binding protein,[2] which the lateral nasal glands (opening through a discrete duct at the tip of the internal aspect of the nose) spray into the incoming charge of air in a fine mist. Odorant binding protein locks in with airborne odor molecules and facilitates their identification at the olfactory patches, especially when we take a "pheromone breath" (a breath into the cathedral roof in order to assess someone's hormonal compatibility with one's self[3,4]).

## Axis of Rotation

In the classical model, the axis of rotation is transverse and runs directly through the middle of the ethmoid, similar to the way that the sphenoid's axis of rotation runs through the middle of its body. The liquid-electric model posits that the ethmoid has no axis, but rather has its movement determined by the minute motion patterns of the brain, and the inputs of its larger bony neighbors, notably the frontal, maxillae and sphenoid. Brain motion tends to rotate the ethmoid around the midsagittal plane.

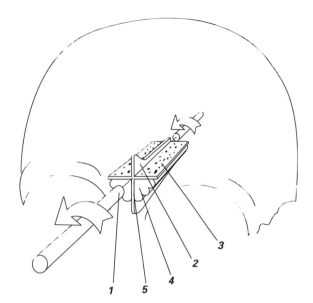

*Ethmoid motion around an A:P axis*

*1 Midsagittal axis of rotation*
*2 Crista galli*
*3 Cribriform plate*
*4 Ethmoid air cells*
*5 Perpendicular plate*

## Motion

Ethmoid motion is strongly modified by the falx cerebri. The ethmoid is like a child holding onto a large kite (the falx) with one hand (the crista galli) in a gale-force wind. The kite moves the child around, threatening his stability and possibly even lifting him off his feet in a strong gust (a traumatic blow to the cranial vault, the occiput, or the neck).

### Osteopathic Model

The classical osteopathic model (similar-motion model) has the ethmoid move in a clockwise direction during flexion, looked at from the left side of the head. At the same moment the sphenoid moves counterclockwise, the two bones acting as if geared together.

### Liquid-Electric Model

In the liquid-electric model, the ethmoid does not move as a cog, but rather dilates, rotates, flares, and contracts under the influence of its larger neighbors. Thus, the movements of the maxillae, frontal, and sphenoid distort, or squeeze, the ethmoid. The deforming it undergoes in flexion is central to the movement of the whole cranium; without the ethmoid's delicacy, its neighbors could not move so easily. The very thinness of its walls allows both easy deformation and ready reformation. The chiropractic cranial researcher DeJarnette calls the ethmoid "the stress bone of the skull," referring to its stress-absorbing capabilities.

The deformation caused by the movements of the maxillae, sphenoid, and frontal comes in an oscillatory manner, with the ethmoid rotating about a midsagittal plane. This movement is modified by slight undulating components as the sphenoid moves into torsion.

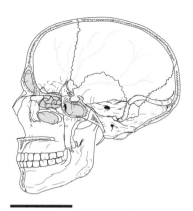

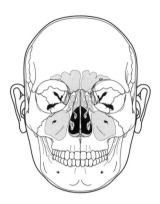

*Ethmoid air sinus, lateral (left) and anterior (right) views*

## Diagnostic Considerations

The ethmoid is a crucial mediator between the neurocranium and viscerocranium. Whatever ails the sphenoid tends to impact the ethmoid; they are linked like twins.

### Energetics

The ethmoid is part of the inner eye, and is specifically related to seeing the way ahead. If you can see that the way ahead is clear, the way ahead will be clear.

The anatomical location of the aperture of the inner eye is at glabella. The inner eye incorporates all of the ethmoid, the inferior border of the falx, and all of the sphenoid. It extends posterior to the atlanto-occipital joint and the acupuncture point Wind Palace (Governor Vessel 16).

The ethmoid "lights up like a crystal palace" during insight experiences. It loves to rotate, tending to tumble along its midsagittal axis, either to the left or right, when the individual is either not accessing or not acknowledging his ability to perceive the way ahead. In this case the area of the ethmoid becomes "cloudy," as if lost in mist.

I once took a class through a guided meditation that began with a visualization of the location and anatomy of the ethmoid and moved on to an assessment of its vitality. Then I asked the members of the class to notice their immediate response to the following instruction: "See what is right." One woman got the answer "First, go in! Then get clear! Then go out and do it!" Another had a visionary experience:

> I looked out from my pituitary, through my sphenoid air sinus, clearly saw the structure of my ethmoid, and saw through a narrow opening out into the light. It was all silver, perfect, luminous, and very peaceful.... It seems like I used to get lost in a turbulence of darkness, distraction, despair, disturbance. What I learned was that it is important to keep my heading, despite darkness, distraction, despair, disturbance.

In an individual session, I asked a client to see what was right for him in the days ahead while I touched the area over his ethmoid. He was quiet for a long time; it felt like he went way inside and disappeared in the deep structures of his head. Finally he spoke, saying "I could really see my ethmoid – it was in despair. Despair from millions of voices that all said 'No, it is impossible.'"

### Trauma and Dysfunction

Sinusitis is the most common affliction of the ethmoid. When it "tumbles" it can produce deeply disturbing psychological states in the sufferer. Perception, or the lack of it, is often involved. Think of the dissonant ethmoid as associated with the "Ds" mentioned in the student's experience: darkness, distraction, despair, disturbance.

## Interconnectedness

This is a crucial bone for the normal functioning of the cranial wave: without its deformability, normal cranial wave formations could not permeate the cranium. Further, its very deformability – caving in to pressure, absorbing impact – helps protect the sphenoid from trauma.

The ethmoid is the central bone of the air sinus network, with its own air cell network connecting the frontal air sinus to the sphenoid. The olfactory bulbs, whose fibrils pass through the cribriform plate, give us our sense of smell, which helps us connect to the world.

## Visualization

Ethmoid visualization focuses on the perception of the liquid-electric axis of rotation and the location of the crista galli. To this framework, add the ethmoid's location within the fjord of the frontal and its articulation with the lesser wings of the sphenoid, completing your visualization with the location of the vomer.

The ethmoid is a bit reminiscent of a donkey with saddlebags. The donkey, as seen in an anteroposterior viewing, is the thin perpendicular plate, with the bulbous saddlebags of the ethmoid air cells slung over each side. (The "saddlebags" have pouches in them, the supreme, superior and middle conchae.)

Visualize the cribriform plate like horizontal lowlands, pierced by the Matterhorn of the crista galli.

## TECHNIQUES

The ethmoid is reached via the frontal, sphenoid, or vomer through mechanical means, and also through directed energy techniques. It can also be accessed by way of the maxillae, which have noteworthy articulations to the vomer, ethmoid, and palatines. All ethmoid techniques influence the inner eye.

### Ethmoid Frontonasal Opposed Finger and Thumb Contact

Sit or stand to the client's left and place the "heart line" (distal palmar crease) of your left palm over the midline of the client's frontal in a simple, comforting, cupping contact. Now cross your right hand over your left, with the first and second phalangeal joints of your last three fingers curled in and resting over the back of your left hand. With the thumb and index finger take up an opposed contact on the most superior aspects of the maxillae, inferior to the frontomaxillary sutures and just posterior to the nasal bones.

Tune in to the cranial wave pattern, and initiate an accentuation of normal frontal flexion (apply posterior-directed pressure at the falx line) while simultaneously pinching the upper ramps of the maxillae medially. This will create an external rotation of the nasal bones along their modified vertical axes and decompress them from the frontal. Move into unwinding as you pick up the osseous flow. Visualize the architecture of the falx, crista galli, and perpendicular plate of ethmoid. It may be helpful to introduce some "drive" to the upper maxillae along an inferoanterior vector, to separate the superior suture of the maxillae from the frontal.

This technique allows a return to normal ethmoid position, motion, and energy by freeing the sutural interfaces with the frontal, nasal, and maxillary bones.

### Ethmoid Frontonasal Single-Thumb Contact

This technique is useful to release traumatic impaction of the nasals into the frontal.

From the basic frontal contact from the preceding technique, move your right hand into a thumbtip contact on the midline nasal suture. Apply inferior-directed pressure with enough of a posterior component so as not to slip. This will

cause the nasal bones to move into internal rotation. It may be helpful to introduce some "drive" of the nasals inferoanterior, to separate the superior suture of the nasals from the frontal.

The specialty of this technique is to create freedom of motion in the sagittal plane by releasing any compressive force impinging upon ethmoid motion that arises from the maxillae, nasals, or – in some cases – even the vomer.

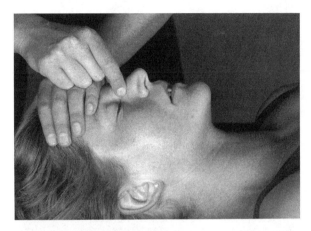

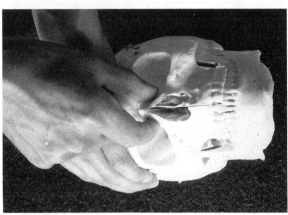

*Ethmoid Frontonasal Opposed Finger and Thumb Contact, two views*

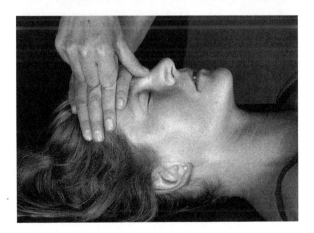

*Ethmoid Frontonasal Single-Thumb Contact*

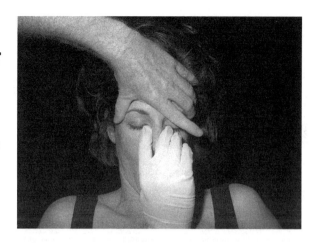

*Ethmoid and Sphenoid Oral Thumb-Based Perpendicular Plate Release, two views*

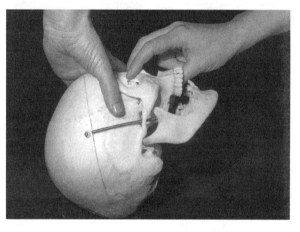

sense its effects on the ethmoid, and then unwind the ethmoid and notice the sphenoid change, and so on. Work your two hands interactively until you sense neurocranial and viscerocranial normalization. This may take the form of a prolonged still point, or a cessation of all membranous "tug-of-war" sensations, and the return of easy normal expansive rhythm.

## Ethmoid Oral Thumb-Based Contact Coupled with Occiput

This technique is one every child uses in sucking his thumb. It allows you to sense and correct ethmoid tumbling patterns (the most common ethmoid disturbances) using occipital and maxillary contacts in concert, to achieve normalization. It also helps free the maxillary air sinuses.

Sit or stand at your client's left and slip your right hand transversely under his occiput. Place your left thumb on the maxillary portion of his hard palate and place your index and middle fingers to each side of the prominence of the nasal bones. Visualize the axis of rotation of the ethmoid (transverse through the middle of the ethmoid body) and wait until you

## Ethmoid and Sphenoid Oral Thumb-Based Perpendicular Plate Release

**Far right:**
*Ethmoid Oral Thumb-based Contact with Occiput, two views*

Sit or stand at your client's right, which will allow you to use your dominant right hand for a combined oral and external contact. Place your right thumb inside the mouth on the hard palate, anterior to the palatines. Your right index and middle fingers straddle the nose, fingerpads down medial to the medial canthus of the eye. This gives you a tripod contact wherein you can separate the maxillae and zygomae laterally (by abducting your index and middle fingers from each other) and/or draw the maxillae anterior, or anterior and caudad, or even cephalad. Place your left hand into a sphenofrontal spanning contact, and use it to hold the sphenoid in either an accentuated flexion position or at the limit of extension – one of the two extremes will produce a marked freeing up of the ethmoid. This is a "floating universal joint" hold; that is, it gives you the capability to move the maxillae – and through your other hand the sphenoid – in any direction, as if you held the sphere of a universal joint, with the sphere itself floating like a tennis ball in water.

At a certain point your hands will sense what is needed and you can begin to unwind both sides interactively – that is, to unwind the sphenoid and

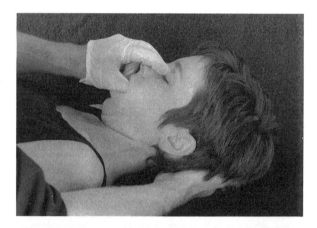

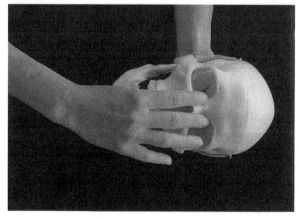

can sense its movement through thumb, index finger, and occipital hand.

Next begin to lever the ethmoid anterior and inferior by pivoting around your thumbtip. Consider the maxillary motion as hinging at the transverse palatine suture. Optimize decompression at the frontonasal, sphenofrontal (lesser wing articulation), vomer, and ethmoid sutures.

Clients can readily be taught to use this technique to move the ethmoid anterior and inferior, unwinding the falx and freeing the junction between neurocranium and viscerocranium in the process. I instruct clients with "compression head" to perform this technique on themselves while I work with posterior structure release techniques, such as opening the lambdoid suture.

## Ethmoid Oral Index-Finger Maxillary Approach

Sit or stand at the client's left, and with your right hand take up a light contact on the frontal bone. This hand's focus is on the ethmoid and its midsagittal articulation in the frontal fjord. Now slide your left index finger along the alveolar ridge of the maxilla further from you (on the client's right side, in this example) sufficiently far to get the fingernail level with, and medial to, the inside of the zygomatic arch. Next, internally rotate that finger, introducing inferior decompression to the mandible.

You are now free to experiment with index and thumb contact to the maxillae, nasals, or anterior aspects of the zygomae. What you want to achieve is a firm, meaningful contact with both sides of the maxillae in such a way that you can take the maxillary ramps off of the frontoethmoid complex and simultaneously unwind that complex with your right hand. Taking the frontosphenoid complex into an accentuated extension phase will begin to loosen the "fjord." Initiate maxillary caudad decompression at the same moment and you create a wonderful open space for the ethmoid to float free. Sense falx involvement. This is highly effective for ethmoid and maxillary sinus congestion.

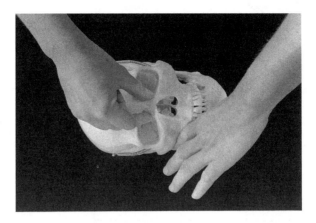

*Ethmoid Oral Index-Finger Maxillary Approach*

## Other Techniques that Can Affect the Ethmoid

- Frontal Anterior Decompression
- Fronto-Occipital Drainage
- Clear the Confusion (Unwinding the Falx)
- The CV4
- Auditory Tube Twist
- Incisive Bone Decompression and Unwinding
- Zygomae Lateral Release: Decompression
- Sphenoid Air Sinus Drainage
- Sphenoid External Coupled Contact with Zygomae
- Sutherland's Grip, taking the sphenoid into extension
- Sphenofrontal Release at Lesser Wing (Cant Hook), freeing the lesser wing from the frontal and ethmoid
- Normalizing the vomer
- Maxillary Lateral Decompression of the Median Palatine Suture
- Lumbosacral Decompression and Unwinding
- Occiput and Sacral Coupled Hold: Core Link Appraisal

# 29
# The Vomer

**Etymology**

**Vomer** Latin for plow

1 Schyndelesis with sphenoid
2 Ala of vomer
3 Plain suture articulation with median palatine suture
4 Articular surface with inferior sphenoid body and rostrum
5 Articular surface with schydelesis of sphenoid
6 Bilaminar vertical plate of vomer

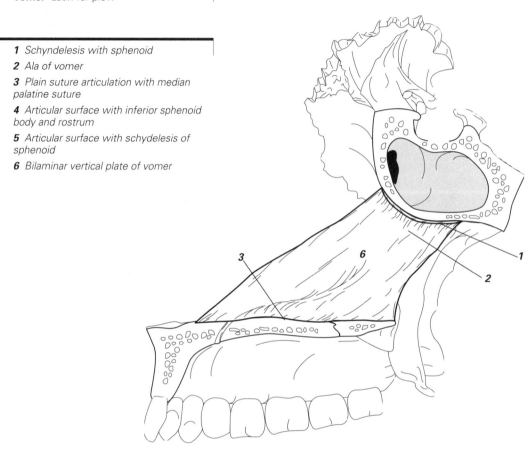

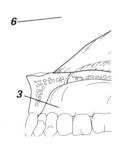

Until quite recently in history, the plow was known as the vomer. After the American Revolutionary War, for instance, Benjamin Franklin implored his liberated countrymen to move on to new times by saying: "Citizens, put down your weapons and take up your vomers."

## Embryology and Osteology

The vomer forms as two paper-thin wafers of bone sandwiching a central cartilaginous membrane, the vomerine cartilage, which extends forward to form the central cartilage of the nose. Ossification begins with one center in each wafer and is completed after puberty; this allows for frequent falls on the nose – before there is a bone to break – as the locomotor system learns the parameters and immutability of the laws of gravity.

## Anatomy

The vomer is located in the nasal cavity where it contributes the bony trellis for the mucous membrane-covered posterior and inferior portion of the nasal septum.

### Structure

The vomer is a very thin, bilaminar quadrilateral wafer of bone that spans the median gap between the maxillae and sphenoid, and maxillae and ethmoid.

## Location

The vomer forms the inferior portion of the nasal septum. It lies inferior and anterior to the sphenoid, inferior and slightly anterior to the ethmoid, and superior to the maxillae.

### Landmarks

The vomer is visible in a skull if you look posterior through the nasal orifice: it constitutes the inferior half of the nasal septum. The posterior edge is a free border, forming the medial wall of the choanae, or the posterior ovoid-shaped aperture of the nasal cavities at the nasopharynx.

## Sutures and Articulations

The vomer has two areas devoted to bony articulation and one area of cartilaginous articulation. At its superior border it articulates with the sphenoid, where its expanded tongue-shaped aspect forms a schindylesis (tongue-and-groove joint) with the sphenoid. The vomer also articulates with the

superior aspects of the palatines via small, variable, and minimal articulations at the underside of the sphenoid body, an area known as the "rostrum." The vomer articulates with the ethmoid at its anterosuperior edge by means of an irregular harmonic suture (that is, there is no interdigitation). Its inferior border articulates with four bones – both maxillae, via an irregular, notchy articulation located immediately superior to the median palatine suture, and both palatines, also on the superior aspect of the median palatine suture. The cartilaginous articulation is formed by the meeting of the anterior and inferior border of the vomer with the septal cartilage.

The vomer articulates with six bones:

- The sphenoid
- The ethmoid
- Both maxillae
- Both palatines

It also articulates with the cartilage of the nasal septum.

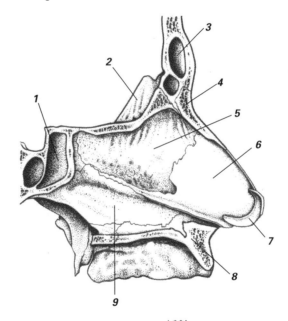

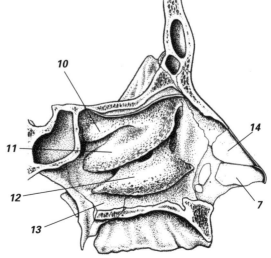

*Nasal cavity*

**Top:**
*Medial wall of right nasal cavity*

**Bottom:**
*Lateral wall of left nasal cavity*

**1** *Sphenoid sinus (double)*
**2** *Crista galli*
**3** *Frontal sinus*
**4** *Right nasal bone*
**5** *Perpendicular plate of ethomoid*
**6** *Septel cartilate*
**7** *Greater alar surface*
**8** *Right maxilla*
**9** *Vomer*
**10** *Superior concha*
**11** *Middle concha*
**12** *Inferior concha*
**13** *Left palatine bone*
**14** *Lateral nasal cartilage*

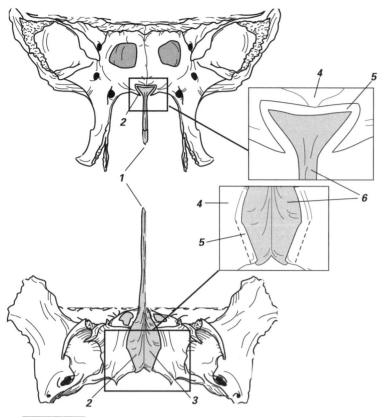

*The schynde-
lesis of
vomer articu-
lating with
sphenoid,
anterior view
(above), and
inferior view
(below)*

*1 Plain
suture articu-
lar surface of
vomer to
median pala-
tine suture
2 Schyndele-
sis of spheno-
vomerine
articulation
3 Ala of
vomer
4 Sphenoid
5 Schyn-
delesis
6 Vomer*

## Weight

A medically prepared, disarticulated vomer weighs
$\frac{1}{16}$ ounce (1.8 gram).

## Detailed Anatomy and Musculature

The vomer is a very thin, quadrilateral slice of bilaminar bone. The perpendicular plate of the ethmoid is functionally continued as the vomer.

The superior surface of the vomer has two ala, or
wings. The alae form a relatively strong triangular
spine, fluting upward like tulip petals spreading at
dawn and ending in a V-shape tongue-like configuration that slips into a V-shaped groove formed by
two delicate little lips on the underside of the rostrum of the sphenoid.[1] The apex of the V faces posterior. It is the most exquisite joint in the head.

### Musculature

The vomer has no muscle attachments.

## Physiology

The vomer is a primary speed reducer, something
it achieves partly through its schindylesis with the
sphenoid and partly through its very thinness and
malleability. Its mucous membrane helps warm
and moisten the incoming breath.

## Axis of Rotation

The vomer, in the classical model, has a transverse, horizontal axis running through the middle
of its vertical plate. In the liquid-electric model, it
is considered to have a modified vertical axis that
runs at an angle of some thirty degrees from the
floor of the nose midway through the anteroposterior depth of the vomer up to the rostrum of the
sphenoid.

## Motion

The bilaminar vomer is so delicate that it readily
deforms from the input of the much more robust
maxillae and sphenoid, and in such cases its
motion may have neither axis nor smoothness.
When the bone is "bullied" its pliancy provides for
most of its motility.

### Osteopathic Model

In the classical (similar-motion) model the vomer
moves as if it articulated with the sphenoid and
ethmoid with straight-cut gears. Looked at from
the left side of the head it moves clockwise during
flexion, exactly synchronous with the ethmoid. As
the sphenoid flexes and nose-dives, the vomer
moves into true backward-bending.

### Liquid-Electric Model

The vomer moves in a complex "wobbling wheel"
fashion in the liquid-electric model. The point of
resolution moves around the surface of an imaginary sphere about ½ inch (1.3 centimeter) in diameter located at the center of the vomer.

## Diagnostic Considerations

Considering its slim delicacy, the vomer plays a
surprisingly important role in physiological and
energetic dysfunction. Torus palatinus (see below)
demonstrates what a powerful effect it can have on
what seem to be much more robust bones.

### Energetics

The vomer is the bone that connects the throat
soul to the inner eye soul – this is where we connect what we see with what we say. One student's
experience was as follows:

*My partner was touching my vomer through the
hard palate. Hugh was guiding the class, and
mentioned that the connection between seeing
and saying was a very delicate one. In that
moment I experienced my vomer as a sheet of
light, which went all the way up to my ethmoid,
which lit up like a crystal palace ... then a hole*

*appeared above it, and I saw through that hole the real solution to everything that is happening in my life just now.*

The vomer is present time and the lead-up to perception.

It is extremely important for the functioning of the third eye. Hindu, Taoist, and Zen meditation practices all honor the Governor Vessel, the incisive bones, and the vomer by pressing the tip of the tongue to the hard palate. The tongue, like all pointed structures, is good at delivering energy, and in this case part of its energy is directed along the vomer to the sphenoid, seat of the inner eye. (Precisely what quality of energy, and where the energy goes, depend upon the meditator's use of his breath, visualization, and intent.) The Chinese master Dong Shaoming notes that when energy is properly harnessed and directed in the body "the mind is like a sword."[2] The vomer is part of the sword.

### Trauma and Dysfunction

The midline plates of the vomer and ethmoid are frequently deviated during birth, or through the countless falls of childhood, and may ossify in the deviated configuration. They seem to function best with slight deviation. The very thinness and pliancy of the vomer allow the compressions and distortions of the cranium to occur without causing the vomer to protrude into the median palatine suture or through the hard palate. When the vomer presses inferiorly onto the median palatine suture it causes a sausage-shaped deformation to the roof of the hard palate known as torus palatinus.

Torus palatinus can be treated in craniosacral work[3] by normalizing each of the bony articulations of the vomer. When treating torus palatinus your objective is to create bony space for the vomer by decompressing the maxillae from the sphenoid and normalizing sphenoid, ethmoid, and palatine position, motion, and energetic loading. It also helps to balance the reciprocal tension membrane, and to decompress the mandible to ensure that there is no ongoing impaction to the maxillary teeth. Coupled holds such as the Oral Coronal Shear Test and the Vomer Oral Thumb-Based Technique enable you to balance the vomer with its more robust neighbors. Work with the condition until the maxillae and sphenoid function smoothly without any infringement from the vomer.

The vomer may be implicated in sphenoid sinusitis by compressing the rostrum and reducing sphenoid motion. Sinusitis is a kind of crying for love, symptomatic of an individual who lacks tenderness coming in from outside.

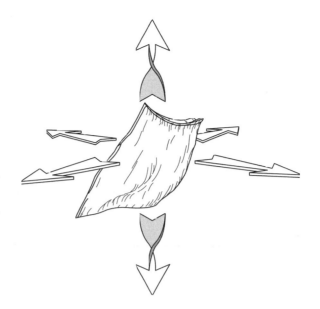

*Vomer micro-movements: possible cranial wave motions*

The vomer is covered by periosteum and mucous membrane. These layers, and eventually the bone, erode with habitual cocaine usage.

## Vomer Lesion Tests

Use the Ethmoid Oral Thumb-Based Contact Coupled with Occiput or the Ethmoid and Sphenoid Oral Thumb-Based Perpendicular Plate Release for optimum sensitivity in testing for vomer lesions. An alternative is the Vomer Oral Index-Finger Technique; however, this tends to place your body much further away from the client's head, and because of this it lacks a certain dynamic cogency that the thumb-based techniques have.

Remember to pause in "neutral" between each stage of the testing sequence.

### Synchrony

"Synchrony" here refers to the bones' action in the osteopathic model, where the sphenoid and vomer move as if geared together. Tune in until you can sense the rhythm of both bones, then assess whether they are in fact moving in synchrony. Remember that there will be some "speed reducer" effect by the time sphenoid-propagated vomer movement transmits itself through the hard palate; this is normal. Be aware that the pattern expressed may be one of opposite motion, as in the liquid-electric model.

Use interactive work to optimize the electrical, fluid, and mechanical components and allow synchrony (or opposite motion) to come back in. If that does not work, consider going to Sutherland's Grip, and beginning unwinding.

### Torsion

Maintain your contact and introduce torsion about an imaginary vertical axis through the midline of the inferior-most portion of the vomer with your oral contact. Move clockwise, then counterclockwise, and note the ease and quality of these motions and their effects on sphenoid motion, position, and electrical "feel."

Decompression will often assist normalization of torsion patterns. To achieve maxillary decompression, place one hand in an external spanning contact immediately superior to the alveolar ridge of the maxillae, just where the maxillae become slightly narrower as the tooth roots taper off. Leave a gap under the client's nostrils, and place the index and middle fingertips of your other hand above the spanning hand and onto the maxillae just beneath the nostrils. Decompress the maxillae by taking up a light but firm contact and moving them inferior when the cranial wave formations take the bones inferior. (An alternative technique to achieve a similar effect would be Incisive Bone Decompression and Unwinding.)

### Shear

Now take the hard palate lateral, thus moving the inferior border of the vomer laterally. Do the test to one side, come back to neutral, pause, then repeat to the other side. The diagnosis of a shear lesion is made according to the side that the vomer moves to most easily.

The Oral Coronal Shear Test is the best technique to correct a shear lesion. With both hands move into the side of the greatest fluidity first, until you sense release. Then gently explore the motion available on the restricted side, until it also frees up.

### Decompression

The final test is to assess whether the vomer allows free anterior glide of the maxillae – that is, whether the suture where the vomer rests upon the maxillae is flexible enough to permit motion anteriorly. Move your oral finger in a purely anterior direction, utilizing tactile adhesion rather than

actual pressure to the median palatine suture. (A fingerprint-sized piece of tissue paper between your glove and the mucous membrane enhances adhesion.)

The anterior-decompression part of Sutherland's Grip is the best technique to treat a restriction in anterior glide. Move in the direction of the greatest ease first, then gently explore and free up the restricted areas.

## Interconnectedness

The vomer is an innocent. With no muscle attachments and precious little mass it is acted upon by its powerful and dynamic neighbors. They are perpetrators and players, the vomer a pawn. But this pawn nonetheless plays an important role in maxillary torsions, which it may pass on to the sphenoid. Likewise, it may pass sphenoid patterns to the maxillae.[4]

## Visualization

To visualize the vomer, place two wafer-thin gossamers of bone together in your mind's eye. Flute their upper portion out to join the sphenoid, then add a little bulk to the underside to give it strength. Or imagine a tall crystal champagne glass, squeeze its sides together and align it in the plane that the vomer assumes inside the head. Use anatomical illustrations to help you understand the relationship with the sphenoid, ethmoid, vomerine cartilage, and maxillae.

## TECHNIQUES

## Vomer Oral Index-Finger Technique

Standing to one side of the client take up an index finger contact inside the mouth just anterior to the transverse palatine suture. Check for torus palatinus. Span the greater wings of the sphenoid with your other hand, making firm contact with glabella with the base of your index finger.

Tune in to the hard palate and vomer first. Assess motility there by energetically "going through" the hard palate until you can pick up the subtle motions of the vomer. Then "listen" to your hand on the sphenoid and discern the link between the patterns of the vomer and sphenoid. Balance the two carefully.

## Vomer Oral Thumb-Based Technique

If you are right-handed, sit or stand at your client's right side. Use both hands to raise his head up off the table surface until you can comfortably cup the occiput in your dominant hand, separating it from the table, with your dominant elbow lateral to the client's right ear. Now use your non-dominant hand to make a thumbpad contact inside the mouth on the hard palate, anterior to the palatines. The index and middle fingers of your right hand straddle the nose, opposing each other and making fingerpad contacts with the most superior aspects of the maxillae, just inferior to the frontomaxillary sutures. This gives you a tripod contact in whose center lies the vomer. (If working with your dominant hand on the face feels unnatural, change your hands over.)

Take time to tune in and then work with the unwinding patterns in both areas. You can unwind the maxillae and vomer and strongly affect the ethmoid with this technique. This is a useful technique to use toward the end of a session, since it gives you the useful capability of balancing the front half of the head with the back half. You can specialize further with it by working to normalize the relationship between the falx and the blade of the vomer, which is part of the energetic plane of the falx, and represents its inferior-most pole.

## Other Techniques That Can Affect the Vomer

- Incisive Bone Decompression and Unwinding
- All ethmoid work
- Sutherland's Grip
- Maxillary Lateral Decompression of the Median Palatine Suture
- Sphenoid Air Sinus Drainage
- Oral Coronal Shear Test
- Sphenoid External Coupled Contact with Zygomae
- Mandible Thumbs-Internal Technique, Palpation and Unwinding
- Rolfing work inside the nose

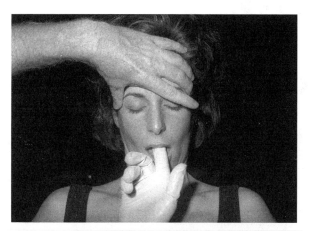

*Vomer Oral Index-Finger Technique, two views*

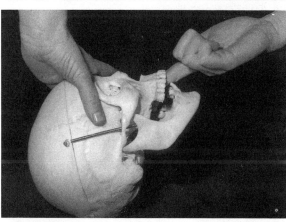

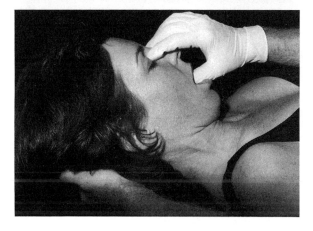

*Vomer Oral Thumb-Based Technique*

# 30
# The Zygomae

## Etymology

**Zygoma** *Greek for the cheekbone*

**1** *Lateral, or malar surface*

**2** *Temporal, or medial surface*

**3** *Orbital surface*

**4** *Temporal process, posterior-directed promintory articulating via a lightly-interdigitated suture with temporal portion of zygomatic bone*

**5** *Frontal process, articulates via dentate suture with zygomatic process of frontal bone*

**6** *Zygomaticofacial foramen, transmits zygomaticofacial branch of zygomatic nerve (part of CN V, maxillary branch of trigeminus) through zygoma to zygomatico-orbital foramen*

**7** *Zygomatico-orbital foramen*

**8** *Zugomaticotemporal foramen, transmits the zygomaticotemporal branch of the zygomatic nerve*

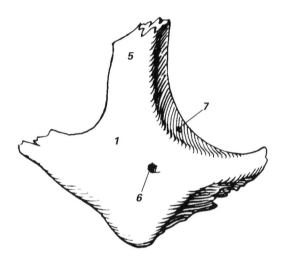

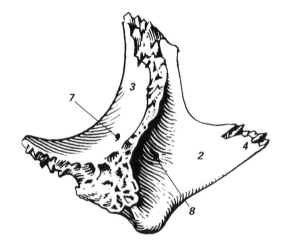

## Embryology and Osteology

The zygomae begin to ossify from three centers in a membranous matrix eight weeks after conception. These centers generally fuse together five months after conception, but occasionally remain in two parts throughout life, one superior and one inferior.

## Anatomy

The zygomae are situated at the corner of the face and make up the inferior and lateral margins of the orbit.

### *Structure*

The zygomae are short, strong, squat, four-legged, compound curvature bones of exceptionally robust diploic bone construction.

## Location

The zygomae form the lateral half of the inferior border of the orbit and three-quarters of its lateral border. They form the prominence of the cheekbones.

### *Landmarks*

Landmark the inferior angles of the zygomae by taking one line of sight lateral from the point where the nose meets the upper lip and a second line of sight inferior from the lateral eyelid. The two lines intersect at the inferior angle of the zygomaticomaxillary suture. The zygomae extend posterior as much as three finger widths from the lateral canthus of the eye. Superiorly, they reach the lateral extremity of the eyebrow. Anteriorly, they reach to a point directly inferior to the pupil of the eye.

## Sutures and Articulations

The zygomae each have four sutures. The most superficial and prominent is the articulation with the temporals, a highly variable serrated suture that is more anterior on the superior surface than on the inferior. The most robust suture is a massively corrugated, triangular cross-sectioned joint with the maxillae. This joint has twice the chord of the sagittal suture. The articulation with the frontal is interdigitated, and about the thickness of a typical sagittal suture. The most delicate suture is the meeting with the sphenoid, comprised of single-layer cortical bone that is mildly stepped or irregular.

Each zygoma articulates with four bones:

- One temporal
- The sphenoid
- The frontal
- One maxilla

## Weight

One medically-prepared, disarticulated zygoma weighs $1/18$ ounce (1.5 grams).

## Detailed Anatomy and Musculature

The zygomae have downsized, and are a diminutive relic of their former australopithecine glory. But they are still strong, diploic-boned flying buttresses. The zygoma's four sutures constitute their anatomical interest.

The drumskin-tight, double-layered fascia of temporalis adheres to the superior border of the zygomatic ridge.[1]

### *Musculature*

The muscles attaching to the zygomae consist of the:

- Masseter, superficial and profound group
- Zygomaticus minor and major
- Obicularis occuli
- Auricularis anterior
- Levator labii superioris

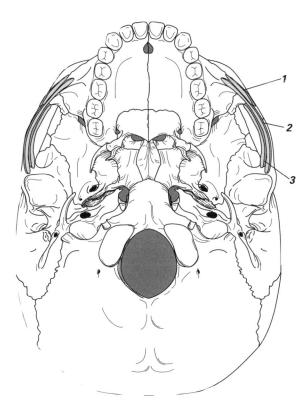

*Cranial base showing zygomatic arch with masseter muscle (shaded)*

*1 Superficial part of massseter muscle*
*2 Profound part of masseter muscle*
*3 Most profound part of masseter muscle*

## Physiology

The zygomae help protect the thin-walled temporal squama, the temporal lobes of the brain, and the pituitary. They also give cover for the underlying tendon of temporalis, the greater wings of the sphenoid, and the lateral margins of the orbit. Further, the zygomae act as speed reducers between the markedly eccentric movements of the temporals and the relative inertia of the maxillae. They are by far the most robust of the speed reducers.

## Axes of Rotation

The classical model has the zygomae with axes of rotation that run through the bones at forty-five-degree angles in the horizontal plane. This is an identical angle and plane of motion with the temporals, which helps to maintain congruity between the two bones at their articulation in the zygomatic arch.

## Motion

The motion of the zygomae is in accordance with that of the temporals, so they rotate externally in flexion, and around parallel forty-five-degree anteromedial axes. The zygomae hinge at their articulations with the maxillae and temporals. When the temporals and zygomae are working normally there is almost no movement at their suture; this helps to explain its delicacy – it has no need for an extensive surface area to dissipate excessive motion between two incompatible bones.

### Osteopathic Model

To understand the osteopathic (similar-motion) model for zygomae motion, imagine the left zygoma as a bucket handle where the handle attachments to the bucket are the zygomaticomaxillary suture anteriorly and the temporozygomatic suture posteriorly. The hinges of the bucket handle are aligned at the above-mentioned forty-five-degree anteromedial angle to the median plane of the head. If you dropped the handle just five degrees, this would be left zygoma flexion. The zygomae often present a clear, amplified reading off of the temporal bones, as well as receiving inputs from the sphenoid and (to a lesser degree) the frontal. The zygomae pass motion on to the maxillae, not vice versa.

### Liquid-Electric Model

The liquid-electric model posits a sequential, or alternating, flexion and extension cycle for the zygomae that accommodates to the "liquid" sphenoid motion. As the left greater wing of the sphenoid nose-dives and moves inferior in torsion, the left zygoma dips inferiorly, perfectly accepting the sphenoid motion.

## Diagnostic Considerations

The key to understanding the zygomae lies in their ability to modify the motion patterns, basic position, and energy of three vital bones: the sphenoid, maxillae, and temporals. They are frequently traumatized in the countless falls of childhood. Boys get in fist fights more often than girls, and get hit on the left zygoma more often than the right (most people are right-handed and swing to hit the face with the right fist, usually impacting their opponents' left sides).

Work with the zygomae in the treatment of sinusitis, before and after orthodontic work, and after all facial trauma.

### Energetics

The zygomae are the eagle's beak, war paint, Cherokee chevrons in brilliant forward-straining colors. They are pride in appearance. Every heroine in a Louis L'Amour novel has high, prominent cheekbones (and no hero has limp zygomae). In the 1992 obituary for Marlene Dietrich, the *New York Times* eulogized her for, amongst many other things, being "the dame with the gorgeous gams and the glorious cheekbones."[2]

The zygomae are the upper realm of the throat soul. They provide feelings of strength and protection when optimum. Taut zygomae may indicate an individual who has become rigid within his own being, manifesting brittleness in life.

### Trauma and Dysfunction

The zygomae form the lateral and inferior portions of the orbit and play a vital role in protecting the eyes. As bodyguards (actually "eyeguards") they are frequently impacted, target practice for a thousand different slights and abuses from postural habits of resting the head on the heel of the hand to the impacts of unhelmeted contact sports. Facial trauma is a frequent part of life. Whenever the maxillae are impacted, however minimally – which obviously includes dental and orthodontic work – check the status of the zygomae afterwards. The zygomae are worth considering in any treatment protocol, especially where trauma is involved.

The zygomae act as strong governors to the maxillae, sphenoid, and – to a lesser extent – the frontal. Normalizing the zygomae is a key component in the treatment of sinusitis, which is aggravated by any zygomatic sutural compression. The very delicacy of the temporozygomatic suture tells us that there is synchronous motion here, and that osseous pliancy takes care of most of the shock absorption required of the zygomatic arches.

## Interconnectedness

Although dominant governors of maxillae and sphenoid movement, the zygomae do not seem to exert much influence on the temporals, possibly because of the flexibility inherent in the flying buttress arch and slimline suture that connects them.

## Visualization

Studying disarticulated zygomae is the best way to learn to visualize these little bones. When visualizing a client's zygomae, it may help to imagine each of the sutures gapping and accommodating to the liquid-electric motion.

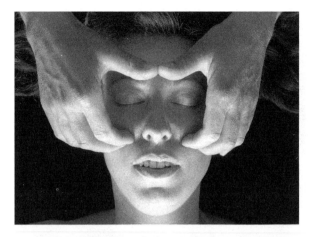

*Zygomae Three-finger Palpation*

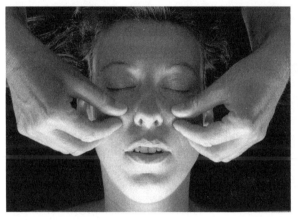

*Zygomae Lateral Decompression and Unwinding*

## TECHNIQUES

### Zygomae Three-Finger Palpation

This is an elegant, useful hold for freeing up the viscerocranium and sphenoid. Sit or kneel at the head of the table. Contact the inferior aspect of the zygomae, palpating them with a tiny, delicate, three-finger contact around their lateral angle and beneath the anteroinferior border. Remember how far anterior the zygomatic processes of the temporal bones actually come – halfway along the arch – and be sure you are anterior to this suture. (The suture is usually easy to palpate.)

### Zygomae Lateral Release: Decompression

Stay with the preceding contact, but now take out the skin slack in a lateral direction. Bring your thumbpads into contact on the anterior surface of the zygomae and maxillae (over the infraorbital foramen) and adjust your finger grip to give you added purchase to obtain the optimum contact. Once you have firm bony contact begin initiating lateral decompression.

### Zygomae "Bicycle Handlebars": Unwinding

Keeping your thumbs and other fingers in the same contact as used for the preceding decompression, you can move into unwinding, using your contact like a grip on bicycle handlebars to work with the zygomae in almost any plane. A combination of lateral, anterior, and superior traction is especially useful. Since the zygomae sit at the anterolateral borders of the skull, they can also be used rather like sensitive bucket handles to push and pull the cranial "bucket" back into shape.

*Zygomae Oral Anterior Decompression and Unwinding, two views*

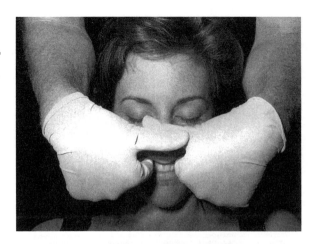

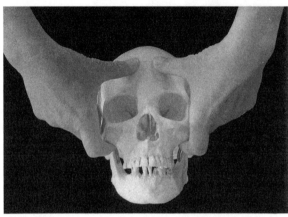

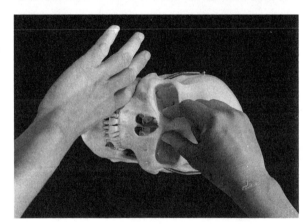

*Zygomae and Nasal Oral Index-Finger Technique*

## Zygomae Oral Anterior Decompression and Unwinding

Stand at the client's head. Place your index fingers inside the mouth, external to the upper teeth, and locate the fingertip-sized aperture immediately posterior to the zygomaticomaxillary suture. Curl your index fingers into these hollows. Wait until you can feel motility before commencing decompression or unwinding.

This technique is very good for bringing both zygomae anterior. It may help to visualize a gapping at the temporozygomatic suture on the zygomatic arch, and the sphenozygomatic suture just posterior to the orbit. This is a preliminary opening technique to working on the bones governed by the zygomae: the maxillae, palatines, sphenoid, and temporals. It is also an important ingredient in relieving sinusitis.

## Zygomae and Nasal Oral Index-Finger Technique

In medially-directed impaction, the zygomae can cause a displacement, or compression lesion, to the nasal bones. This technique, centered upon an unusual internal rotation of the index finger, works to rectify such compression. It frees the maxillae by releasing any zygomatic or nasal pressure.

Sit or stand to the client's left and place your left index finger inside the mouth, with the shaft of the finger medial and inferior to the zygomatic arch; use the inferior angle of the zygomaticomaxillary suture as landmarking for the location of your first phalangeal joint. Follow normal flexion motion by internally rotating the shaft of your index finger, taking the maxillae inferiorly. At the same time, take an index and middle finger pinching contact with your other hand, bridging the upper ramps of the maxillae. Accentuating your medially-directed pinching pressure causes external rotation of the nasal bones.

Variations consist of decompressing the nasals away from the frontal after an impaction injury, or taking the zygoma purely laterally to create more emphatic space for the maxillae.

## Zygomae Asymmetric Frontal Suture Release

This technique is designed to relieve compression mediated to the frontozygomatic suture, which will almost always have affected the sphenoid.

Stand at the client's left and rotate his head to the right. Take up a very close-contact straddle hold with your right hand on the sphenoid and glabella, so that the surface of your hand touches his temples and forehead from one greater wing of the sphenoid to the other. Then straddle both zygomae with your left index finger and thumb. Begin decompression by taking the zygomae inferiorly and into external rotation (flexion) during the flexion phase. Simultaneously, with your right hand take the sphenofrontal complex off the zygomae by introducing an extension motion coupled with superior decompression. Add slight sphenobasilar torsion or side-bending motion at the target suture if necessary.

Normalize the head with Zygomae Oral Anterior Decompression, unwinding once the frontozygomatic suture has released. If this sequence does not work, move into sensitive interactive work and then unwinding, until the sutures release and return to their normal elasticity, without using accentuations or flexion or extension.

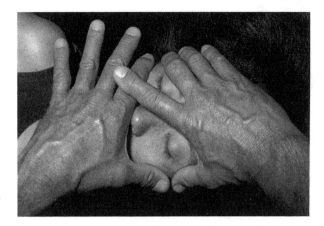

*Zygomae Asymmetric Frontal Suture Release*

## Other Techniques that Can Affect the Zygomae

- All temporal techniques
- Maxillary Lateral Decompression of the Median Palatine Suture
- Masseter release work
- Frontal Anterior Decompression
- Sphenobasilar Decompression
- Oral Coronal Shear Test
- Educating the client to desist from resting his head, via one zygoma, on the heel of a hand

# 31
# The Maxillae

**1**  *Body of maxilla, containing maxillary air sinus*

**2**  *Orbital surface of maxilla, forming part of floor of eye socket*

**3**  *Infraorbital foramen and canal, transmits infraorbital artery and nerve, part of CNV, trigeminus*

**4**  *Facial surface of maxilla*

**5**  *Anterior nasal spine, sharp anterior projection for attachment of cartilaginous nasal septum; Governor Vessel 26, "Middle of Man" located at deepest part of curve below spine*

**6**  *Conchal crest, formed by attachment of inferior concha*

**7**  *Maxillary hiatus, large aperture in medial wall of maxillary air sinus, largely covered by palatine bone posteriorly and inferior concha anteriorly*

**8**  *Maxillary air sinus, or Antrum of Highmore*

**9**  *Frontal process of maxilla, articulating with frontal bone via interdigitated suture of moderate depth*

**10**  *Ethmoid notch, diagonal ridge for articulation of middle concha*

**11**  *Zygomatic or malar process, articulates with zygoma via dentate suture*

**12**  *Palatine process, horizontal plate forming the anterior two-thirds of the hard palate*

**13**  *Median palatine suture, mildly roughened intermaxillary articulation*

**14**  *Transverse palatine suture, mildly roughened maxillopalatine articulation*

**15**  *Incisive canal, double at nasal surface, single at oral surface, transmits nasopalatine nerve, branch of pterygopalatine ganglion*

**16**  *Alveolar ridge, enlarged area of maxilla forming sockets for teeth*

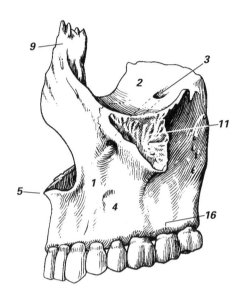

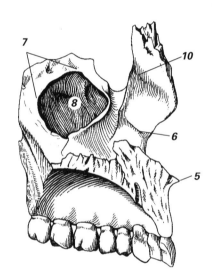

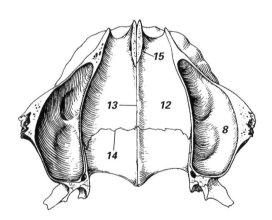

## Embryology and Osteology

The bones and muscles concerned with suckling and crying naturally have the earliest development and competence. The maxillae begin to ossify from a membranous matrix, from four ossification centers, seven weeks after conception. By the tenth week each maxilla has ossified into two portions, the incisive bone anteriorly and the maxilla proper posteriorly. The maxillary air sinus is the first air sinus to form; it begins to appear during the fourth month of fetal development.

## Anatomy

The maxillae are the second-largest bones of the viscerocranium and form the inferior and part of the lateral border of the orbit. They also form parts of the nostrils and mouth.

### Structure

The maxillae are pneumatic bones composed of robust diploic bone at the alveolar ridges, and the remainder of the bones are a mixture of much thinner diploic bone (the posterior maxillary portion of the hard palate), dense and strong single-layer cortical bone (where the maxillae articulate with the frontal), and paper-thin cortical bone that surrounds the posterior walls of the maxillary air sinus. The latter bone can be so thin because the maxillae are protected in this area by the zygomae and masseter. The air sinuses are fully two-thirds the size of the orbits, and are by far the largest air sinuses in the head.

## Location

Maxillary location is easily assessed through the upper teeth, all of which root in the maxillae. The bones extend superiorly to nasion and posteriorly to the palatines; they meet each other medially.

### Landmarks

Spatially, the maxillae seem to hide from the limelight at almost every turn. The nasal bones actually form the prominence of the nose just inferior to nasion, although the maxillae provide its ramparts. The zygomae rob the maxillae of prominence at the corners of the face. Except for the prominence of the mustache line of the upper lip, and the inferomedial half of the eye sockets, the maxillae are almost hidden bones.

## Sutures and Articulations

The maxillae are possessed of a wide variety of bone thicknesses and sutural classifications. Each maxilla presents a very robust dentate suture with the zygomae – the most recessed suture in the cranium; a serrated suture with its partner maxilla; a lightly serrated suture line with the incisive bones; a roughened and irregular harmonic suture line for the vomer; a lightly interdigitated suture with the palatines; a modified harmonic joint with the ethmoid; and a harmonic joint with the nasals. The maxillae are somewhat recessed where they articulate with the frontal by means of a dentate suture.

Each maxilla articulates with a minimum of nine bones, as well as its own teeth and the mandibular teeth opposite. The articulations are as follows:

- The partner maxilla
- The vomer
- The ethmoid
- One zygoma
- One palatine
- One interior concha
- One nasal
- The frontal
- One incisive bone (the suture often disappears by age fifty)
- Eight maxillary teeth
- The mandible, via tooth contact
- The sphenoid when the palatine bones are absent

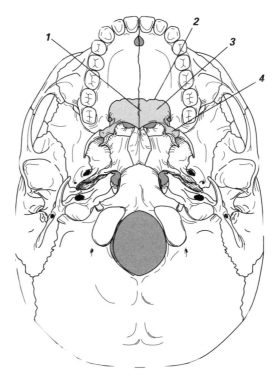

*Cranial base showing the relationship of maxillae to sphenoid and palatines*

**1** Median palatine suture
**2** Transvers palatine suture
**3** Palatine bone
**4** Pyramidal process of palatine bone

*Nasal cavity*

**Top:**
*Medial wall
of right nasal
cavity*

**Bottom:**
*Lateral wall
of left nasal
cavity*

*1 Sphenoid
sinus
(double)*
*2 Crista galli*
*3 Frontal
sinus*
*4 Right
nasal bone*
*5 Perpendic-
ular plate of
ethomoid*
*6 Septel
cartilate*
*7 Greater
alar surface*
*8 Right
maxilla*
*9 Vomer*
*10 Superior
concha*
*11 Middle
concha*
*12 Inferior
concha*
*13 Left
palatine bone*
*14 Lateral
nasal
cartilage*

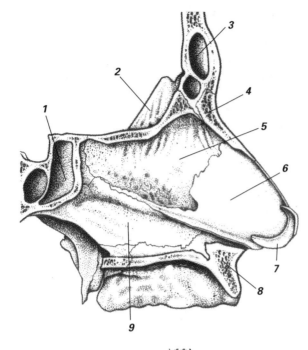

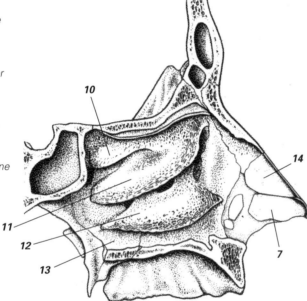

## Weight

One medically prepared, disarticulated maxilla –
including its incisive bone – weighs ¼ ounce
(7 grams).

## Detailed Anatomy and Musculature

Each maxilla has two fossae (zygomatic and sphenomaxillary), two fissures (sphenomaxillary and
pterygomaxillary), and four processes (zygomatic,
nasal, alveolar – itself containing eight sockets –
and palatine). Each contributes to three cavities,
forming the roof of the mouth, the floor and lateral
walls of the nasal cavity, and most of the floor of
the orbit.

The incisive bones are usually separate from the
maxillae until age fifty, by which point the sutures
that separate them from the maxillae often disappear. They are small, variable bones at the most
anterior part of the maxillae that house the alveoli
for the upper front two teeth on each side.

Eleven muscle groups attach to each maxilla. For
craniosacral work, the most important of these are
the medial pterygoids, masseter, and buccinator.
The very strong musculature of the tongue, which
does not attach to the maxillae, nonetheless plays
an important dynamic role, depending on how it is
used in pressing up on the hard palate when
thoughtful, playful, or stressed.

### Musculature

The muscles attaching to the maxillae consist
of the:

- Medial pterygoids (variable)
- Masseter, most anterosuperior fibers
- Buccinator
- Orbicularis oris
- Depressor anguli oris
- Levator labi superioris
- Levator labi superioris alaeque nasi
- Levator anguli oris
- Nasalis
- Depressor septi nasi
- Risorius

## Physiology

The very thinness of the walls of the air sinus
mean that the compressive forces of chewing can
be dissipated by osseous flexibility, which also
helps the maxillae avoid fracture. We swallow, on
average, eighteen hundred times per day. Each
swallow typically means a compression of the
teeth, and may add further muscular tension to
what may already be chronic temporomandibular
joint hypertonicity.[2,3,4]

All three of Sutherland's "speed reducers"[5] – the
zygomae, palatines, and vomer – articulate with
the maxillae. Motion dissipation can therefore be
understood as a vital consideration for normal
maxillary function. The maxillae are strong governors of the sphenoid.

## Axes of Rotation

The classical axes of rotation for the maxillae lie in
a vertical plane, passing through the middle of the
hard palate portion of each maxilla, lateral to the
median palatine suture and anterior to the transverse palatine suture. The axes diverge laterally
and slightly anterior as they pass inferiorly.

## Motion

The motion of the maxillae is strongly affected by facial muscle status, sphenoid and palatine motion, and the habitual position of the tongue.

### Osteopathic Model

In the classical (similar-motion) model the maxillae diverge, widening more posteriorly, in flexion. Each maxilla diverges around an axis of rotation, as defined above.

### Liquid-Electric Model

In the liquid-electric model, maxillary motion echoes that of the sphenoid. Thus, as the sphenoid moves into its liquid-electric flexion, the left greater wing nose-dives but also moves inferiorly into a slight degree of torsion while the left maxilla simultaneously moves laterally and inferiorly at its posterior margin.

## Diagnostic Considerations

The maxillae are heir to more ills than any other bone of the viscerocranium by courtesy of the proximity of their air sinuses to the roots of the upper teeth. Dental root canal decay readily passes up into the maxillary air sinus, especially when, as often happens, the root canal opens directly into the air sinus. It is a challenge in differential diagnosis to discern dental pain from air sinus inflammation pain.

### Energetics

This is the upper limit of the vishuddha, throat soul, and therefore the energetics of the maxillae relate to communication, tenacity, affection, threat display, attack and defense. This center is challenged to be a clear communicator under stress, when, optimally, your voice is clear as crystal. "You want the truth, I'll tell you the truth!"[6] – this is the throat soul, the energy of standing up and stating your rights. It is also creativity in song, poetry, and speech, as well as the opposite polarity, silence – as the ancient Taoists noted, "the source of all great action lies in stillness and in silence."

> *Those who know do not talk.*
> *Those who talk do not know.*
> *– Lao Tzu*[7]

The throat soul is conditioned with the primal imprint of receiving nurturance and unconditional love with mother's milk. It is an area associated with the upward-looking posture of devotion and ecstatic experience. (Eloquently shown in the runner's euphoria in the film *Chariots of Fire*.)

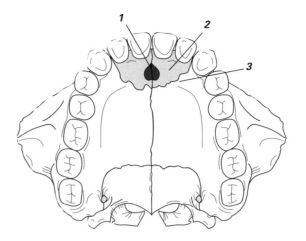

The maxillae tend to hold anger, resentment, even bitterness, as well as loyalty. Such feelings of loyalty are often misplaced. They represent gracefulness and poise in physical beauty. When possessed by feelings of superiority or disdain, we "look down our noses" at other people.

Teeth are pride, vanity, youthfulness, attractiveness, and strength. The maxillae and mandible "sink their teeth into" a loved one in a codependent relationship. In any negative state, the maxillae lose their flexibility and their cranial wave feels like it is moving through gritty molasses.

### Trauma and Dysfunction

The throat is a common site for illness and emotional distress. We become resentful if there is someone we want to speak to but are not allowed to, or cannot, tending to "bite our lip" or "bite our tongue." Minor mouth symptoms may turn around the question of speaking personal truth when afraid to do so because of the consequences; this sends the field in the area into disarray.

The maxillae are, surgically speaking, the most important bones in the viscerocranium as they are heir to more disease than any other viscerocranial bone. This is solely due to the presence of the air sinuses and the frequent eruption of root canal decay into them. The exit apertures for these cavernous sinuses are small and at the superior margins of the sinus – a good arrangement for water-dwellers because it enables them to swim with their nostrils just under the waterline while keeping the air sinuses dry. This arrangement probably dates from the extended evolutionary period of estuary and offshore living that early hominoids seem to have gone through,[8] but is a very unfortunate arrangement when it comes to effecting maxillary air sinus drainage.

For all their apparent strength, the maxillae are very easily destabilized. The widespread use of dental braces, bridges, splints, ill-fitting partial dentures,[9] and incompatible fillings plays havoc with viscerocranial mechanics.[10] The maxillae, with

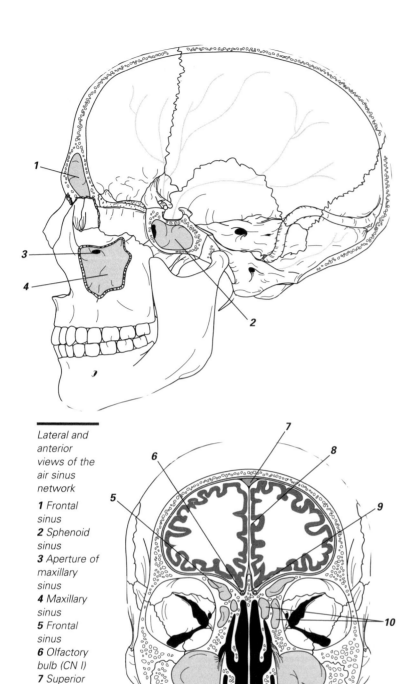

*Lateral and anterior views of the air sinus network*

**1** Frontal sinus
**2** Sphenoid sinus
**3** Aperture of maxillary sinus
**4** Maxillary sinus
**5** Frontal sinus
**6** Olfactory bulb (CN I)
**7** Superior sagittal sinus
**8** Falx cerebri
**9** Crista galli
**10** Ethmoid sinus
**11** Maxillary sinus

much less freedom of movement than the mandible, and being that much "closer to home" (i.e., closer to the sphenoid and brain) have a much harder time absorbing orthodontics that inhibit or stop cranial wave formations passing through them.[11,12]

In a perfect world all dentists would be fully trained craniosacral healers, and test their patients' cranial mechanics before and after every dental procedure.

Maxillary techniques excel at balancing the viscerocranium and treating sinusitis, "mask" or eye socket-area headaches, and frontal headaches.[13] Maxillary work, as a long shot, may help with visual problems, and after facial injury. Torus palatinus[14] can be optimized and sometimes removed with craniosacral work to the affected structures and those acting upon them. In constant-on engram conditions, and especially in masseter hypertonicity, the mandible will compress the maxillae. Sutherland's Grip is the finest technique for working with the sphenopalatine ganglion, for the treatment and interdicting of an oncoming migraine, and for releasing the palatines from a traumatically-induced injury that has compressed them.

## Maxillary Lesion Tests

For the maxillary lesion tests listed below, I would recommend the use of three contacts. The first possibility is the Ethmoid Oral Thumb-Based Contact Coupled with Occiput. You can also use the Ethmoid and Sphenoid Oral Thumb-Based Perpendicular Plate Release or Sutherland's Grip.

These tests enter areas of great privacy. Extreme sensitivity is called for, as it is remarkably easy to destabilize the sphenoid via the maxillae in clients whose heads have not recovered from trauma. While appearing robust, the maxillae are in fact as sensitive as the palatines and, in my experience, more easily destabilized than the temporals. Always pause at "neutral" between tests, to avoid overwhelming both "the mechanism" and the dreambody.

### *Synchrony*

The zygomae, vomer, and palatines act as "speed reducers" to dissipate some of the sphenoid's motion before it reaches the maxillae. Assess whether the sphenoid and maxillae appear to accommodate each other and move harmoniously, like good neighbors. If there is a need to establish synchrony, the best way to interact with the field and its structures is through unwinding. Sutherland's Grip is one of the best techniques; the Oral

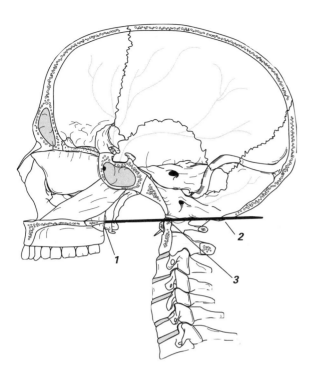

**Far left:**
*McGregor's
Line*

*1 McGregor's
Line: runs
from posterior
margin of
hard palate
2 . . . to
posterior
margin
of foramen
magnum
3 . . . and
intersects the
tip of the
dens*

the side the maxillae moves to more easily. If you
have a distinct sense that there is a difference, treat
the lesion by first going to the fluid side (that
is, the side the maxillae move to more easily).
Once the restrictions in the bone structures,
sutures, and muscles have eased off, you will find
that you can take the structures to the side they
did not originally want to go with much greater
ease. Your work is complete when they can go to
either side with equal ease.

*Decompression*

Use Sutherland's Grip for this evaluation. Test by
gently hooking the tips of the index and middle
fingers of your dominant hand around the last
molar tooth on each side and introducing a decompressive traction and intention in an anterior
plane, along McGregor's Line. There should be a
distinct sense of anterior glide, a millimeter or so
in distance. The sphenoid will not be strongly
affected unless the maxillae have been displaced
posteriorly by trauma.

If it is the case that the sphenoid is affected, the
sphenoid will suddenly swing free, usually into
extension as maxillary compression is taken off its
pterygoid processes. Maintain the decompression
until the tissues soften and appear to normalize,
then work with all the attendant structures until
the maxillae no longer impinge on sphenoid
motion, or the motion of the three speed reducers
(the palatines, zygomae, and vomer).

## Interconnectedness

The throat soul is where we connect what we see
(sphenoid) with what we say, and also with what
we feel (heart and *hara*). The maxillae are dynamic
bones that act as an interface between the viscerocranium and neurocranium, exerting a major influence on sphenoid homeostasis and the optimum
functioning of the stomatognathic system. They
are also a key player in temporomandibular joint
dysfunction and contribute a decisive component
to migraine headaches.[15]

## Visualization

It takes some time to really visualize the maxillae
as they are not prominent except for the mustache
line area of the upper lip and the lower margins of
the orbits. Visualizing the exact shape and surprising size of the maxillary air sinus is a challenge
best met through the close perusal of anatomical
paintings, drawings, and photographs, and the handling of disarticulated maxillae.

Coronal Shear Test and the Ethmoid Oral Thumb-
Based Contact Coupled with Occiput may also be
very useful.

*Torsion*

To test for maxillary torsion lesions, first focus on
your contact with the occiput or the greater wings
of the sphenoid. Wait until you feel the textures of
the cranial wave passing through the bone you are
touching, then begin to "damp" its movements –
that is, slightly reduce them. Then begin to rotate
the maxillae around an imaginary vertical axis running through the midline of the median palatine
suture. Test for left torsion (counterclockwise
motion as looked at from the vertex) and note how
far and how easily the maxillae rotate left before the
sphenoid engages. Then come back to the midline,
pause, and repeat for right torsion. Compare and
contrast the movements. A lesion is present if the
maxillae move more easily and further to one side.

Sutherland's Grip is best to treat a torsion lesion.
Move first in the direction of the greatest ease
until all tension has dissipated, then begin to
encourage, without forcing, the maxillae in the
direction that they did not want to go into at first.
This is a matter of staying exquisitely sensitive
and present to energy and movement. Use minimal
contact pressures, and stay until you sense a complete release – which usually happens all at once,
after minutes of resistance.

*Shear*

Test for a shear lesion with a pure lateral displacement of the maxillae, first to the left, then the
right. The Ethmoid Oral Thumb-Based Contact
Coupled with Occiput is usually the most sensitive technique for this test. The lesion is named for

## TECHNIQUES

### Incisive Bone Decompression and Unwinding

Sit at the client's head and oppose your index fingers and thumbs to each other on the anterior and posterior surfaces of the front incisor teeth of each side. (You may need a postage stamp-sized piece of tissue paper between your gloves and the tooth enamel to dry the saliva out, and give you the grip you need.) Move into as much wrist flexion as is comfortable for you, and endeavor to get your elbows on the table surface close to the client's head. Allow a minute or two for the saliva to dry out. Wait until you can feel the motility patterns of the incisive bones, then move into decompression – directly caudad – and unwinding.

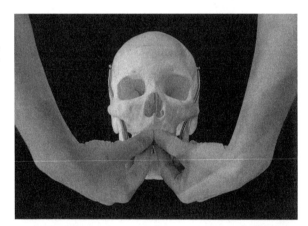

*Incisive Bone Decompression and Unwinding; for clarity the photo below shows just one hand in position.*

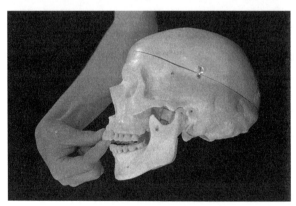

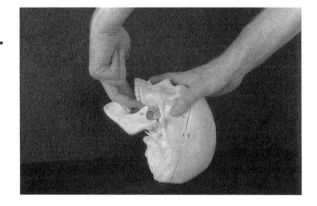

*Sutherland's Grip*

This technique is the treatment of choice for glabella-area headaches, the kind that make you pucker in at the brow. Your line of decompression passes superiorly through the vomer and ethmoid to the falx, and unwinds the falx. Once the falx is free, the headache disappears. This usually takes no more than three or four minutes.

### Sutherland's Grip

Stand to one side of the table and span the greater wings of the sphenoid with one hand, ensuring that you have contact with the base of your index finger at glabella. Take up an index and middle finger contact with the other hand, placing your fingers in a V-shape and contacting the biting surface of the upper teeth.

There are many different ways to use Sutherland's Grip. You can use it as a diagnostic tool, sensing the motility of the sphenoid and maxillae and therefore deducing the status of the palatines that lie between them (in this case your oral fingers remain flat). Or you can hook your fingers posterior to the final maxillary teeth (or the vestigial alveolar ridge if the client is toothless) and introduce an anterior decompression to the maxillae. This is the treatment that is most effective for migraine headaches.

Wait until you sense sphenoid motility before introducing anterior decompression. If the sphenoid is perfectly free, there will be little effect on it from this anterior maxillary decompression. If, however, the maxillae have impacted upon the palatines and pterygoid processes of the sphenoid, it will "kick free" in a dramatic fashion and suddenly have more movement, typically into extension. This is because the posterior impaction of the maxillae onto the pterygoids has been released, freeing the pterygoids to move in an anterior direction, which is sphenoid extension. Complete your work with very gentle but thorough unwinding until you reach a deep still point.

In cases of severe facial trauma, you may have to use considerable anterior-directed traction before the maxillae will free.

## Maxillae Internal Palpation

Sit at the head end of the table. To take up the oral contact, place both hands, palms down, above your client's face. Curl your ring and little fingers up against your palms, then flex your middle fingers to a ninety-degree angle with your palms and place one middle finger at a time on the biting surface of the upper teeth, sliding it slowly posterior until you have made contact as far posterior as possible (preferably with the final teeth). Place the index fingers on the chin, on the prominence of the mentalis muscle, flexed very slightly so that the index finger's natural tendency to want to straighten will provide a constant pressure to keep the client's mouth open. Once you have both middle fingers inside the mouth, and both index fingers on the chin, cross your thumbs over each other so that they are self-supporting.

This is a very light hold. Encourage the client to release his mandible so that there is not a continuing low level of tension in the jaw musculature. Wait for the gentle maxillary patterns to emerge into your middle fingers.

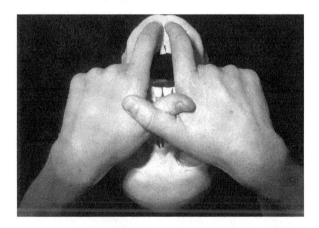

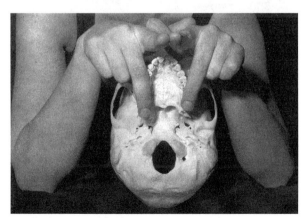

## Maxillary Lateral Decompression of the Median Palatine Suture

With the same contact on the biting surface of the maxillary teeth used in the preceding technique, introduce a lateral decompression of the median palatine suture. You may need to increase your contact pressure in a superior direction, or else slightly curl your fingers around the medial (lingual) side of the teeth in order to prevent slipping.

Nominally, it would seem that this technique would work better if performed in a hinging motion – that is, diverging posteriorly in a movement similar to classical flexion (with the posterior part of the palatine suture separating more than the anterior). However, a pure lateral decompression of the suture seems to work better in almost all cases. Your decompressive force is designed to separate the median palatine suture; find out which vector has the optimum effect.

This decompression is helpful in returning motility in "mask" (eye socket-area) headaches and cluster headaches. It is often helpful with migraines. Both the Maxillae Internal Palpation and this decompressive technique are excellent for balancing the viscerocranium, and for the enhancement of bone motility that we seek to achieve as a vital ingredient in the treatment of sinusitis. Lateral decompression may help free the sphenopalatine ganglion and the palatines themselves, and give some benefit with visual problems. It may also be useful after traumatic injury to the face.

**Far right:**
*Maxillae Internal Palpation and Lateral Decompression, two views*

## Other Techniques that Can Affect the Maxillae

- All mandible techniques
- All palatine techniques
- Sphenoid work to correct sphenobasilar lesion patterns
- Ethmoid Oral Thumb-Based Contact Coupled with Occiput
- Ethmoid Oral Index-Finger Maxillary Approach
- Zygomae Lateral Release
- Vomer balancing work
- Release of the masseter, temporalis, buccinator, and medial pterygoid muscles
- Stomatognathic system unwinding
- Corrective dentistry
- Throat soul clearing work: Arnold Mindell's Process Work, Gestalt therapy, psychotherapy (especially in cases of sexual abuse), and Voice Dialogue

# 32
# The Palatines

**Etymology**

**Palatine** from the Latin *palatum*, the palate

**1** Perpendicular plate, forms part of medial wall of maxillary air sinus

**2** Horizontal plate, forms posterior one-third of hard palate and floor of nose, and articulates via a roughened surface with opposite palatine

**3** Nasal surface, part of perpendicular plate facing nasal cavity

**4** Maxillary surface, lateral surface of perpendicular plate which forms palatine margin of pterygopalatine foramen

**5** Pyramidal process, articulates via plain suture with curved anterior face of pterygoid process of sphenoid

**6** Conchal ridge, articulates with inferior concha via plane suture

**7** Ethmoidal crest, articulates with middle concha via plane suture

**8** Orbital process, located between maxilla, ethmoid and sphenoid at rear of eye socket

**9** Sphenoid process, articulates via plane suture with underside of sphenoid body and ala of vomer

**10** Nasal crest, a bony ridge formed by median palatine suture articulation

**11** Palatine portion of median palatine suture, articulates with opposite palatine bone

**12** Posterior nasal spine, posterosuperior limit of nasal crest

**13** Greater palatine sulcus, helps form canal for greater palatine nerve and descending palatine artery

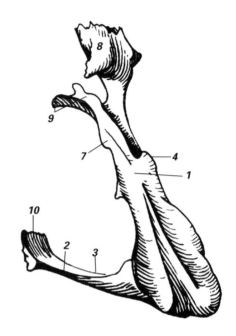

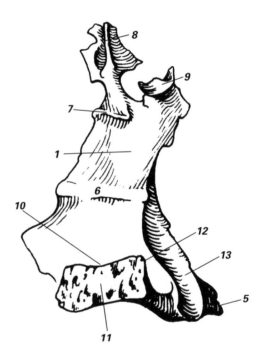

## Embryology and Osteology

Each palatine commences ossification from one center, embedded in its membranous matrix, at the seventh week after conception. The ossification centers are strategically located at the juncture of the bones' vertical and horizontal plates.

## Anatomy

The palatines are quite extraordinary. Disarticulated from the skull, their delicate, wafer-thin cortical bone construction makes them look like a leftover from a leg of NASA's lunar landing module: thin, spindly, and very interesting-looking.

### *Structure*

The palatines are composed of paper-thin cortical bone, as well as $\frac{1}{32}$ to $\frac{1}{24}$ inch (0.8 to 1 millimeter) thick diploic bone where they help form the hard palate.

## Location

The palatines make up the posterior third of the hard palate, where they can be felt and seen inside the mouth. They are interposed between the sphenoid and the maxillae and are visible in the orbits of an intact medical specimen skull as very small triangular-shaped bones posterior to the maxillary components of the orbits.

### *Landmarks*

The transverse palatine suture, the joint between the maxillae and palatines, lies at the level of the gap between the seventh and eighth teeth. This is usually visible as the place where the mucous membrane changes color and there are often little puckered-in depressions where the mucous membrane finds attachment to the sutural ligaments.

## Sutures and Articulations

The palatines are not heavy bones, but ballerinas; their interdigitations are tiny and tremulous, and limited to their articulations with the maxillae. The interface of the palatines to the pterygoid processes of the sphenoid is a flared V-shaped channel arrangement. The channel is curved like the crescent moon, with its concavity facing anteriorly to perfectly accept the convex protuberant curve of the anterior face of the pterygoid processes. The remaining palatine joints are modified plain sutures.

Each palatine articulates with six other bones:
- The other palatine
- The sphenoid
- The ethmoid
- The vomer
- One maxilla
- One inferior concha

## Weight

One medically prepared, disarticulated palatine bone weighs $\frac{1}{56}$ ounce (0.5 gram).

## Detailed Anatomy and Musculature

The palatines are exquisite, delicate, and variegated bones with an extraordinary appearance. They are composed of two plates, one vertical and one horizontal; the vertical is by far the more complex.

The palatines assist in forming three cavities: the floor and outer wall of the posterior part of the nasal orifice, whose apertures are known as the choanae; the posterior part of the roof of the mouth; and a very small part of the floor of the orbit.

The palatines have one important muscular attachment, that of the medial pterygoids. The muscle is largely attached to the medial aspect of the lateral pterygoid plates, but its most anterior and superior portion does swing around the inferior belly of the external pterygoid to attach with the palatines and maxillae. The other muscles that attach to the palatines are concerned with swallowing and gagging.

### Musculature

The muscles attaching to the palatines consist of the:

- Medial pterygoids
- Muscles of the soft palate
- Levator veli palatini
- Tensor veli palatini (which swings around anterior to the hamulus)
- Palatopharyngeus
- Uvular
- Palatoglossus

## Physiology

This is quite definitely a viscerocranial bone – all nose, mouth, and eye.

## Axis of Rotation

In the classical model, palatine movement is said to take place around a horizontal, coronal axis, similar to the axis of the sphenoid. This axis is modified by motion inputs from the maxillae, which rotate around an almost vertical axis.

## Motion

The palatines are the foremost example of speed reducers. They lessen the amount of motion between the sphenoid and maxillae via their extensive sutural surface area and malleability. Sutherland labeled them speed reducers[1] and "washers" – but what exquisitely complex washers! Delicately wedged between the sphenoid and maxillae, the palatines facilitate the free movement of both bones and accommodating the vagaries in their motion.

### Osteopathic Model

The palatines' normal motility in the classical (similar-motion) model is a slight rocking, where the anterior margin moves first inferiorly then posteriorly. As paired bones they rotate externally in flexion, following the pattern set by their big sisters, the sphenoid and maxillae. They move slightly posteriorly at their inferior and posterior margins, as the pterygoid processes retract posteriorly during flexion.

### Liquid-Electric Model

In the liquid-electric model, the movement of the palatines also follows that of the maxillae. Thus, as the sphenoid moves into its liquid-electric flexion, the left greater wing nose-dives but also moves inferiorly into a slight degree of torsion. Simultaneously, the left palatine moves laterally and inferiorly, while the right, moving in opposite motion, moves medially and superiorly.

## Diagnostic Considerations

### Energetics

When we have "had it up to here!" we have had it up to our palatines: we are about to gag, to vomit up all the feelings we "had to swallow" in a situation, or a relationship.

Treating the palatines often evokes sensitive and sad emotions; it makes many people cry.

The palatines are experienced as a gateway to the soul. One woman became anxious during a class in Zürich, when her palatines were touched. She suddenly realized that she felt terribly vulnerable, and said "If you separate these bones with this decompression, then everyone in the room will be able to look up and see my soul."

### Trauma and Dysfunction

The palatines are rarely displaced because they are so well protected. Thin-walled bones are able to deform readily, which protects them from fracturing, as well as from displacing their sutures. But a careless finger inside the mouth can easily fault them.

Treating the palatines orally can bring great relaxation in temporomandibular joint syndrome, and of emotional blockages of the oral area, thus giving you a clue as to the possible origins of "structural dysfunction" in sexual violation.

The posterior realm of the palatines is the beginning of most people's gag reflex area. The palatines are associated with anything that has made the individual gag. (The chapter on the auditory tubes gives a technique to normalize a premature gag reflex.)

In torus palatinus, the vomer forces the maxillae to protrude inferiorly through the roof of the mouth,[2] producing a sausage-shaped lump and affecting the mechanics of the cranium. While the vomer rests almost equally on the superior border of the palatines and maxillae, I have never seen it displace the palatines in torus palatinus, no doubt because of their very thinness, coupled with the mobility that their ample sutural surface area gives them. It is important to work with torus palatinus until all the neighboring structures are functioning normally (see "The Maxillae" for more details).

The palatines seem to act as the keys that lock, or unlock, the eye sockets. It is remarkable how often releasing the palatines clears up orbital problems, and can therefore be of benefit in the treatment of headaches, which so often affect the eyes.

## Interconnectedness

The palatines are important for their ability to separate the sphenoid from the maxillae. The sphenopalatine ganglion which is nestled between sphenoid and palatine bones, innervates to the mucous membranes of the entire nasal cavity, and the roof of the mouth.

## Visualization

The palatines are exquisite, delicate, and variegated bones with an extraordinary spatial appearance that rather defies description. Placed together, and viewed from directly in front in the anteroposterior plane, they describe the outline of the archetypal plump German *hausfrau*. A petite head (orbital portions), an ample bosom (upper nasal portion), an ever-increasing bulging at the hips (the choanae), and finally a skirt over full petticoats draping clear down to the ground (the hard palate) with no feet visible.

> *Palatines are hummingbird wings*
> *gently and tentatively*
> *unfurling.*
> *The third rhythm is*
> *their flying song.*

## TECHNIQUES

Some craniosacral authorities assert that it is a waste of time to treat the palatines unless you correct their more brusque neighbors first. However, each area has its own sense of autonomy and its own local and distant reflexes; each is affected in different ways by a constant-on engram. (The same applies, less emphatically, to the nasals.) Take the high road, and sense what is apposite.

The maxillae, palatines, and temporals are the most easily imbalanced bones in the cranium. Treat them all with great care. (Treat everything with great care, even when you have to work on areas that may require great force, such as the hamstrings). The palatines need to be approached with more tactile sensitivity than any other bone in the cranium, however, so it is appropriate to think of them as the ultimate on-the-body test of your skill in touch. There is no direct digital way to bring them back down if they are forced too far cephalad, so be exceedingly careful to limit and control any superiorly directed pressure (Palatine Recoveries in the techniques section gives advice on how to stage a correction in this event). Remember that the most closely guarded secret of shamanism is intent – how you visualize and plan to work with these structures changes their response to your contact. Never rush at the palatines; they may need a lot of time.

Some craniosacral authorities recommend treating one palatine at a time, and advocate doing this standing. This has never made sense to me, as it seems to invite more tension in the healer's body and, lacking a local point of stability, more wobbling and hence less accuracy. I find seated bilateral approach superior in terms of comfort and stability, and therefore in control and sensitivity.

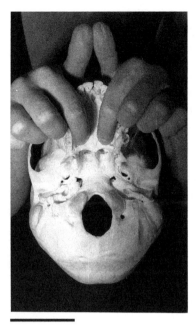
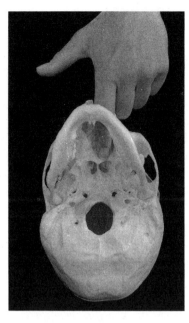

*Palatine Compression/ Decompression; for clarity, photo at right shows just one finger in the correct location.*

## Palatine Compression/Decompression

Palatine decompression involves great sensitivity. If you cannot feel palatine motility, you are not in a sensitive enough consciousness to perform this technique, in which case do not attempt it.

Use the same index-finger contact as in the evaluation above. Wait until you can feel the palatines' motility; then, as they move superior in flexion, go with them and accentuate the movement by $\frac{1}{64}$ inch (0.4 millimeter). Typically, one side will float superior into compression immediately, but the other will take a little longer, perhaps as much as a minute or two. This phenomena is explained by the alternating motion of the liquid-electric motility pattern, whose movements allow occasional "windows" when one palatine is suddenly released by not just one, but all of its neighboring bones. This alignment of forces does not happen with every cranial wave formation, and hence you may have to wait a minute or two for the optimum moment when the sutural pressure is relaxed on the palatines. Once both bones have moved superior, keep the same mild pressure, and introduce a delicate lateral force. Again, one palatine will release first, like a hummingbird's wing gently and tentatively unfurling; the other will usually follow a minute or so later.

Once both palatines have moved into lateral decompression, reverse your order of movements: bring them both medial (compression), and then inferior (decompression). The inferior motion is accomplished with the slight natural adhesion of the fingertips to the moist tissue. Then gently and slowly bring your index fingers out of the mouth with a light contact pressure along each side of the median palatine suture.

### Palatine Evaluation

Encourage the client to release his mandible during this technique so that there is not a continuing low level of tension in the jaw muscles. Sit at the client's head, and place your elbows on the table surface as close to the client's head as possible. If your forearms are too short for this, place a thick book between each elbow and the table surface. Now place your index fingers on the biting surface of the maxillary teeth and go as far posterior as the eighth tooth, then move your fingers medial until they touch. If space permits, separate your fingers very slightly, as this will enable you to feel individual palatine motion, and distinguish between the left and right side more effectively. Be sure to keep your fingers off the incisor teeth and the alveolar ridges as they are part of the maxillae.

Wait. Wait until you feel the minute motions of each palatine bone. You need more sensitivity here than for any other bone in the head. Once you can feel static position and cranial wave formations passing through each palatine, and have a sense of their energetics, you have completed your evaluation and are ready to move into palatine decompression.

## Palatine Recoveries

There are three ways to bring compressed or traumatized palatines back into a normal relationship: energetic, adhesive; and with Sutherland's Grip.

***Energetic***   This depends upon a very detailed and accurate visualization of the palatines and a fingertip or fingerpad application to the palatine contact area with an invocation, visualization, and intention to normalize – "come back down."

***Adhesive***   This will work if you use small pieces of tissue paper between your gloves and the moist mucous membranes of the palatines, providing additional adhesion. Wait for the saliva to dry out and initiate a return to the midline followed by a pure inferior movement. Keep breathing.

***Sutherland's Grip***   Span the greater wings of the sphenoid and split your index and middle fingers to put one each on the biting surface of the upper teeth. Hook behind the final teeth and decompress the entire viscerocranium anteriorly off of the neurocranium. The vectors and intention you focus and deliver to the sphenoid traction are crucial as this is what creates space for the palatines to normalize. Introduce flexion to the sphenoid as you decompress it from the sphenobasilar joint, creating the space the palatines need to move inferiorly and return to their normal seating with the maxillae.

## Other Techniques that Can Affect the Palatines

- Maxillary Lateral Decompression of the Median Palatine Suture
- Lateral Pterygoid Release
- Ethmoid Oral Thumb-Based Contact Coupled with Occiput
- All sphenoid techniques, especially moving the sphenoid into flexion
- Gagging, which, while not a "technique," involves autonomic responses including sutural releases throughout the viscerocranium and a relaxation of tension in the tentorium

# 33
# The Auditory Tubes

*Cranial base and cartilaginous auditory (Eustachian) tubes*

**1** *Articulation of cartilaginous tube with superior portion of medial pterygoid plate*

**2** *Lumen for muscular auditory tube*

**3** *Inverted J-shape of cartilaginous tube*

**4** *Musculotubal canal*

**5** *Lateral lamina*

**6** *Medial lamina*

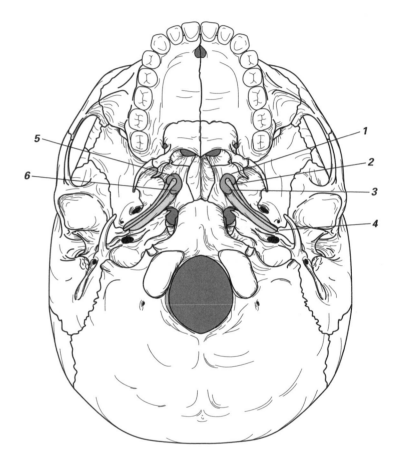

## Anatomy

The auditory (or Eustachian) tubes are exquisitely tender, limp, lightly-muscled thin tubes that run between the inner ear and the nasopharynx. they are about 1½ inches (3.9 centimeters) long. Their inner lumen, or aperture, is closed except when we swallow, gag, or are startled.

### Structure

The auditory tubes are composed of three parts: a bony tunnel through the petrous portions of the temporal bones; a J-shaped protective sheath, known as the cartilage of the auditory tube and divided into a medial and lateral lamina; and a thin-walled tube lined with mucous membrane, which is the true auditory tube, and runs through the tunnel and is protected by the cartilage.

## Location

The auditory tubes are located on the inferior aspect of the cranial base, wholly protected from the outside world. They run from the temporal bones to the medial pterygoid plates, where they open into the nasopharynx. This opening, their most vulnerable aspect, is where they are protected from foreign objects by the gag reflex.

### Landmarks

The auditory tubes can be landmarked by calculating McGregor's line (see p. 337). McGregor's Line runs from the posterior margin of the hard palate to the inferior-most part of the occiput. The auditory tubes' lowest point, where they open into the posterior wall of the nasopharynx, is approximately ¼ inch (6 millimeters) superior to the McGregor's line. A point ½ inch (1.3 centimeter) anterior from the ear canal demarks its most posterior limit.

## Detailed Anatomy and Musculature

The auditory tubes emerge from the inner ear via the lateral part of the petrous portions of the temporal bones. The auditory tube orifices in the petrous portion are located just medial to the internal carotid artery. They angle forty-five degrees anterior and medial from the petrous portion, along the inferior surfaces of the petrous portions and the greater wings of the sphenoid to attach to the superior crescent-shaped concavities in the medial pterygoid plates, just inferior to the roots of the greater wings of the sphenoid. The auditory tubes open into the nasopharynx.

The auditory tubes have two small but exceptionally vigorous muscles attaching to them.

### Musculature

The muscles attaching to the auditory tubes consist of the:

- Tensor veli palatini
- Salpingopharyngeus

## Physiology

The auditory tubes allow the eardrums to have equalized air pressure both on the ear canal and on the inner ear side, by permitting air to reach the inner ear from the nasopharynx. When your ears "pop" as you move to a higher altitude, air at higher pressure already in the inner ear evacuates via the auditory tubes to the nasopharynx.[1]

The auditory tubes naturally lie in slight extension. That is, they are very slightly twisted, or torqued, in internal rotation along their long axes. This torquing helps keep the tubes closed most of the time, which is an asset in the prevention of bacteria reaching the inner ear. When we swallow a local reflex causes the tubes to open briefly.

## Axis of Rotation

In the classical osteopathic model the axis of rotation of the auditory tubes is forty-five degrees anteromedial, identical to that of the temporal bones. In this model, auditory tube axes are temporal axes, that is, the tubes move in the same arc of movement as the temporal bones. In the liquid-electric model, both the temporal bones and the sphenoid are seen as being propagated by brain motion, which motion produces fully-floating, universal joint-type auditory tube movement.

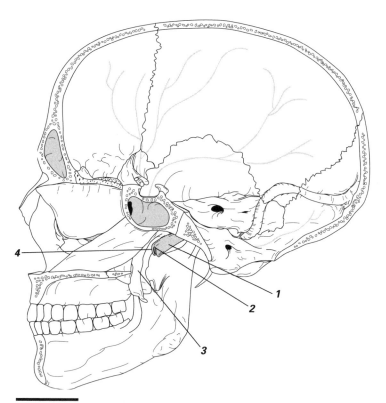

*Lateral view showing right cartilaginous auditory tube*

**1** *Medial lamina of cartilaginous auditory tube*
**2** *Lumen*
**3** *Medial pterygoid plate*
**4** *Lateral lamina*

## Motion

The auditory tubes are normally very slightly twisted, or torqued, in internal rotation (extension). Hence one aspect of craniosacral work directed at opening the auditory tubes relies on taking the temporals and sphenoid into external rotation (flexion), which will tend to open the tubes, all other things being equal.

## Diagnostic Considerations

Our chief interest in releasing auditory tube spasm or congestion is in the treatment of tinnitus, which may be caused, or exacerbated, by auditory tube closure.

If Valsalva's maneuver, and the Auditory Tube Twist, do not produce an opening of the auditory tubes, consider working with the client's diet, especially focusing on reducing and preferably eliminating all refined sugar products, dairy products,[2,3] and possibly also wheat (this last because it is one of the most common allergens, and the allergic reaction results in excessive mucus formation in the nose, nasopharynx, and auditory tubes).

### Energetics

The auditory tubes are very close to the soul – delicate, sensitive areas that we do not want anyone messing with, no matter how deft he may be. We gag to get unwanted people ("he makes me sick!") and objects away from our auditory tubes. The gag reflex protects the trachea, esophagus, and auditory tubes. Gagging also brings unpleasant associations and memories to consciousness.

The next time you are alone at night in the forest and a sudden strange sound sends shivers up the back of your neck (your "frightened cat" response – flaring out fur to look bigger), notice what your mouth does. First it instinctively opens, which has two reasons: to prepare to bite if attacked, and to hear better. This is because the auditory tubes open on these occasions, allowing sound to reach us from four different locations, rather than the usual two, which dramatically improves our ability to locate the source of the sound.

### Trauma and Dysfunction

At birth the auditory tubes are so short that the rear of the mouth is almost in the inner ear, so to speak.

As children grow and begin to move about, they begin to put things in their mouths, the better to experience them (a throwback to our time as muzzle-feeders some 100 million years ago, when this was normal behavior – indeed, one of our chief avenues of acquiring information). Thus, worms, dead flies, all kinds of bacterially or toxically loaded garbage finds its way into children's mouths, and the bacteria tracks backward along the invitingly warm, wet, and dark auditory tube, an ideal breeding ground. The bacteria reach the tympanic cavity and subsequently gain access to the developing mastoid air cell network, where bacterial multiplication results in pus formation and bony displacement and swelling within the mastoid. This is excruciatingly painful for anyone, and terrifying for a child who cannot understand what is happening, or that it will be cured soon.[4] (Breast-fed children have a significantly lower incidence of inner-ear infections and disorders than bottle-fed children do.[5])

Valsalva's maneuver is designed to open the auditory tubes and normalize pressure on each side of the ear drum. It consists of closing your nose and mouth and forcing increased air pressure back up the auditory tubes, thus opening them. With very young children who are in pain from rapid cabin pressurization in commercial airliners or during an auto ascent of a mountain pass, close the child's nose for him, seal your lips over his, and very very gently (they have tiny lungs and auditory tubes) blow their tubes open. Do this once and check if he is relieved; if not, try again for a little longer duration, and keep trying until he seems relieved and stops crying.

When the tubes become blocked in children and adults, usually as the result of a cold, it is unwise to fly. External air pressure on the eardrums drops as the aircraft cabin is pressurized, sucking them laterally, awaiting the opening of the auditory tubes to admit similarly low-pressure air. With the tubes blocked, this cannot occur and the eardrums are distended outward by the residual air pressure medial to them in the tympanic cavity; the tensor tympani muscles are overstretched, and severe pain ensues.

Pilots are prohibited from flying with blocked auditory tubes due to a history of this having contributed to the cause of fatal air disasters. The pain is so severe that it can distract the affected pilot from his duties to the extent that he may make errors of judgment, overlook an instrument warning, or forget a vital landing procedure.

## TECHNIQUES

Great care needs to be exercised when treating the auditory tubes because of their sensitive anatomy and the frequent presence of an archaic wound associated with oral sexual violation.

### Gag Reflex Normalization

People who have suffered oral sexual abuse as children often have a gag reflex that begins prematurely, before the molar teeth. With care and understanding it is possible to begin moving the point of gagging posteriorly, back to its normal demarcation line at the posterior limit of the hard palate.

The way to do this is to teach these clients to do external muscle release work on buccinator and masseter, stretching the muscle fibers either along or across their long axes, using a thumb inside the mouth and fingers external to it on the muscle bellies. Within a few weeks the gag reflex begins to migrate back to its correct place. Of course, psychotherapy can help enormously here.

### Auditory Tube Twist

*Caution This is a technique requiring a very high level of skill and must not be used on clients who have "borderline heads" – heads that destabilize easily.*

The auditory tubes naturally lie in slight extension. That is, they are very slightly twisted, or torqued, along their long axes.[6] This torquing helps keep the tubes closed most of the time, which is an asset in preventing bacteria from reaching the inner ear. Normally when we swallow the alteration of muscular and bony pressures causes the tubes to briefly move into flexion, and thus open.

This technique[7] is designed to take the natural slight torque out of the auditory tubes, which enables them to "pop" open. It is similar to the Passive-Interactive Square Ashtray hold, but in this technique your thumb shafts are aligned along the lateral surfaces of the mastoids, not their posterior ramps.

Stand at the head of the table. Explain to the client exactly what you are about to do, and instruct him to let you know the moment your

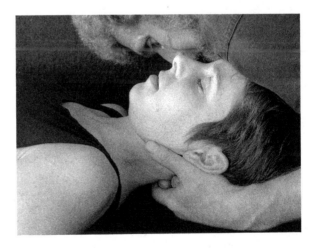

*Auditory Tube Twist*

pressure feels excessive or invasive. Overlap eight fingers under the occiput (with your dominant hand on top) – which allows more sensitivity than interlacing – and place your thumbs along the lateral surfaces of the mastoids. Initiate external rotation to the temporals with your thumb shafts by driving the mastoids medially and very slightly posteriorly (that is, accentuate normal mastoid motion in flexion).

Once you have flexion synchronous with the client's in-breath, bring the prominence of your non-dominant shoulder into light contact with the client's glabella and introduce posteriorly directed pressure simultaneous with the mastoid contacts' medial drive. Keep checking in with your client to make sure he is comfortable. Ask him if what you are doing seems effective. If it does not, adjust your pressures and angles discretely until it does feel effective to both of you. Maintain this contact, modulating your pressures and vectors until you sense and "see" the auditory tubes normalize.

End with Temporal Palming or the Oral Coronal Shear Test to normalize temporal status.

## Auditory Tubes: Direct Digital Approach

First attempt to open the auditory tubes using Valsalva's maneuver and the Auditory Tube Twist. If unsuccessful, you can try this technique. *Note that the Auditory Tubes: Direct Digital Approach is a highly skilled technique, not to be used by beginners, or those with limited anatomical knowledge.*

Explain to the client what you are about to do, and that it makes some people gag. Let him know that you will remove your finger the moment gagging begins. Make sure he is comfortable with you performing this technique on him, and understands the need for it. Stand at the client's head. Visualize the location of his tubes, and in particular the exact location of the auditory tubes' nasopharyngeal orifice. Once you have a clear image and are spatially oriented, rotate his head to his right. Align your right index finger for final approach to the nasopharyngeal orifice; track posterior along the biting surface of the upper left teeth to the final molar and locate the tip of the hamulus with your right fingertip.

At this point place the tips of your left index and middle fingers over the squamous suture that joins the temporal and parietal bone and begin a rapid (three to four taps per second) tapotement around the circumference of the suture. This serves as a neurological distraction to inhibit the gag reflex – how much it will do so is highly variable. (You have to master this tapotement equally well with both hands. In the words of Miyamoto Musashi, "Holding the long sword in both hands is not the true Way . . . . the way to train is to use both hands equally.")

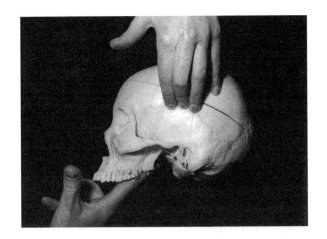

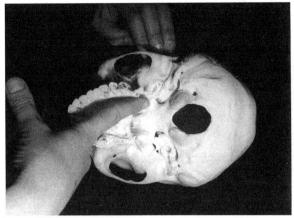

Now flex the tip of your oral finger and move it superiorly above the posterior margin of the soft palate. Stay in contact with the lateral wall of the nasopharynx, paying careful attention to location. During swallowing and gagging, the J-shaped cartilaginous part of the auditory tubes jets forward vigorously and pushes your fingertip out of the orifice. This definitively confirms that you have the correct location. Release any possible muscle spasm and mucus congestion in the tube by rapid, low-amplitude oscillations in the superior-inferior plane. This you have to learn to do while your left hand is engaged in squamous suture tapotement. You then change the head over to the other side and repeat, using your left index finger in the mouth and your right hand for temporal tapotement.

## Other Techniques that Can Affect the Auditory Tubes

- Mandible unwinding
- Temporal Auricle Decompression
- A macrobiotic diet

# 34
# The Mandible

**1** Body of mandible, horizontal portion to which ramii are attached

**2** Mental protuberance, or chin

**3** Mental spine, paired spikes of bone formed by attachment of genioglossus and geniohyoid muscles

**4** Mental foramen, transmits a branch of external carotid artery inward, and sensory portion of mandibular branch of trigeminus and mental nerve outward.

**5** Alveolar ridge, or part of body

**6** Ramus or vertical portion of mandible

**7** Angle of mandible, at junction of body and ramus, more prominent in male

**8** Articular condyle, articulates via meniscus to glenoid fossa of temporal

**9** Neck of mandible, slender portion below condyle

**10** Pterygoid fovea, or depression, anterior and inferior to condyle, where part of lateral pterygoid muscle attaches

**11** Cornoid process, formed by the attachment of temporalis muscle

**12** Mandibular notch, depression between condyle and coronoid

**13** Mandibular foramen, transmits entry of inferior alveolar nerve, largest branch of mandibular part of CNV (trigeminus), carrying both sensory and motor fibers

**14** Lingula, a thin bony lamina formed by attachment of sphenomandibular ligament

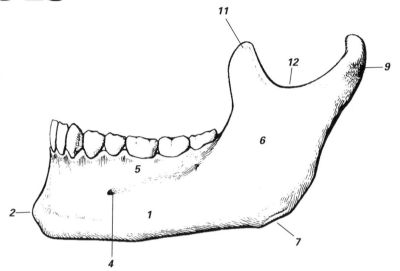

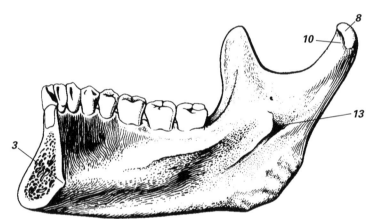

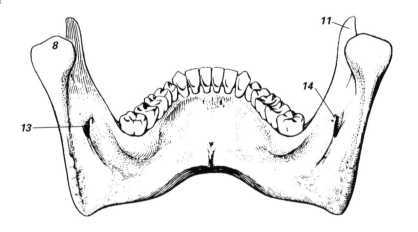

## Embryology and Osteology

Four weeks after conception the human fetus has three beautifully formed and perfectly functioning gill slits. The upper of these begins to change by the fifth week, soon to begin ossifying into the mandible. So in its genetic memory the mandible *is* a gill, and gills live to pulsate.

The alveolar ridge area and body of the mandible develop out of cartilage, the ramus from membrane. Ossification begins as early as the fifth week after conception, earlier than any other bone in the body except the clavicle. The mandible and clavicle provide the osseous anchorages and levers for two of the most vital requirements at birth, suckling and holding. At full term the mandible still consists of two halves, united by the fibrous symphysis mentis, which ossifies during the year after birth.

## Anatomy

The mandible is the largest, strongest, and by far the most mobile bone in the viscerocranium. It forms the bony framework for the inferior half of the mouth.

### Structure

The mandible is an extremely robust diploic-composition bone with multiple alveolar cavities for the teeth and a complex condylar, barrel-shaped joint surface for the temporomandibular joints.

## Location

The mandible lies at the anterior and inferior borders of the head. The temporomandibular joints are immediately anterior to the ear canals and easily palpated by placing the fingers over the area and moving the jaw into a yawn position; this makes the lateral aspects of the condyles more prominent.

### Landmarks

The chin, marked by two bony swellings on either side of the midline, is unique to *Homo sapiens sapiens*. Neanderthals had no chins; neither did *Homo erectus* or any of our more distant forebears.[1,2] The size of the prominence of the chin is highly variable; a dimple (exemplified by Kirk Douglas) may be visible over the bony midline, which is marked by the mental protuberance. The angle of the jaw is a prominent jut in slim individuals; it has a sharper, more aggressive point in the male, and a more gentle and rounded shape in the female.

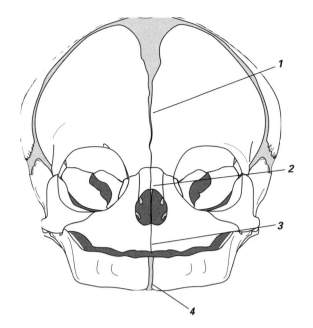

Symphisis mentis at birth
**1** Metopic suture
**2** Internasal suture
**3** Median palatine suture
**4** Symphisis mentis

## Sutures and Articulations

The mandible has one suture, at the mentis, where it articulates with the other side of the mandible. This is a symphysis at birth, which fuses by the end of the first year.

The mandible articulates with the temporal bones through two menisci; sixteen of its own teeth, and sixteen maxillary teeth via occlusal contact.

Contact between the upper and lower teeth is regarded as an important articulation of both the mandible and maxillae since the jaw is so often tense, committing the teeth to diurnal contact, and sometimes grinding.

## Weight

A medically prepared mandible weighs 1⅓ ounces (37.8 grams).

## Detailed Anatomy and Musculature

The game "Trivial Pursuit" ascribes to the mandible the distinction of being the strongest bone of the body, but this is not the case: the femur, with a breaking strain of five tons (about four thousand kilograms), is the strongest bone in the body. No doubt the game's creators meant "the strongest bone in the head" – which the mandible is, with a breaking strain in excess of five hundred pounds (two hundred kilograms).

The mandible is composed of a body, two rami, and the mental protuberance (which has two tubercles lateral to it). The protuberance of the chin

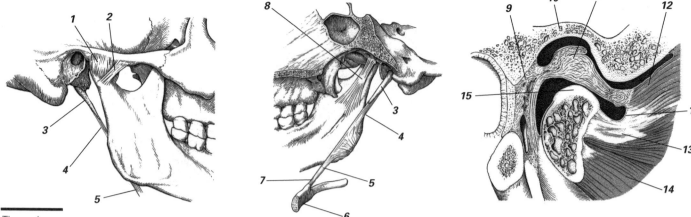

*Three views of the temporo-mandibular joint*

*1 Joint capsule*
*2 Temporo-mandibular ligament*
*3 Styloid process*
*4 Stylo-mandibular ligament*
*5 Stylohyoid ligament*
*6 Hyoid*
*7 Lesser horn of hyoid*
*8 Spheno-mandibular ligament*
*9 Retro-discal ligament*
*10 Man-dibular (or guenoid) fossa*
*11 Articular disc*
*12 Superior portion of superior belly of lateral pterygoid muscle*
*13 Tendon of lateral pterygoid muscle*
*14 Inferior belly of lateral pterygoid muscle*
*15 Articular surface of mandibular condoyle*

probably evolved as a signaling apparatus to make our threat displays more fearsome-looking. We prognate the jaw to threaten (as well as to emphasize meaning).[3] The chin also serves to protect the teeth in a fall; our quadruped relations, being that much closer to the ground, do not have anywhere to fall from, by comparison.

The body of the mandible is the horizontal portion, the ramus the vertical. The angle of the mandible is more prominent and well-developed in the male, and is the only point of sexual differentiation on a human cranium. The base of the mandible is the inferior portion of the body, the area below the alveoli. The mental protuberance swells on either side of the original site of the symphysis mentis, which makes this part of the mandible somewhat reminiscent of the symphysis pubis.

The mandible also features the mental spines, mental tubercles, and mental foramina. The last are distinct visual landmarks in the disarticulated bone. Externally, the body of the mandible has an upward-sweeping rampart known as the oblique line, climbing superiorly as it moves posteriorly to buttress the junction between the ramus and body; the oblique line is paired with a similar internal line, the mylohyoid line. Also on the internal aspect, the submandibular fossae lie inferior to the distinct ridge of the mylohyoid line; the submandibular glands nestle in these fossae. The alveolar ridge completes the anatomy of the body, and is composed of dental alveoli, the alveolar arch, interalveolar septa, and jurga.

The rami are marked by the coronoid processes anteriorly and the condyloid processes posteriorly. Their lateral faces provide attachment for the masseter, and for one-eighth of the temporalis[4] tendon externally. Internally, they accept the remaining seven-eighths of the temporalis tendon and both the medial and lateral pterygoids. The medial pterygoids mimic the (external) masseter in form and function, whereas the lateral pterygoids are

specialized as prognators of the jaw and the main muscles that propagate the masticatory process known as "trituration." The buccinator, which attaches to the mandible just superior to the oblique line and via the pterygomandibular raphe, plays the vital role (with the tongue) of locating and containing the chewed morsel of food for the teeth to work on.

Surmounting the condyloid processes are the heads of the mandible, its contribution to the temporomandibular capsule and joint. The condyloid and coronoid processes are divided by a valley-like depression called the mandibular notch. On the internal aspect the mandibular canal forms the entry point of the inferior alveolar nerve (a branch of the fifth cranial nerve), one of the sites dentists seek to approximate in anesthetizing the lower teeth.

The temporomandibular joints have been allocated a very large motor[5] and somesthetic area in the cerebral cortex and have a considerable nerve supply, both afferent and efferent. Thirty-eight percent of the neurological input to the brain comes from the face, mouth, and temporomandibular region;[6,7,8] 136 muscles above and below the mandible pivot the jaw,[9] also moving it forward as the mouth opens. The total neurological input to the brain from sensory and proprioceptor nerves during mandibular motion acts as a dominant pattern setter for the motor cortex. That is, mandibular motion sets the pattern for at least 38 percent of the motor muscles in the body, particularly in the neck, pectoral muscle area of the chest, and pelvic regions. Normalizing mandibular and temporomandibular joint function is a wise prerequisite to any attempt at normalizing the neuromuscular mechanisms of the rest of the body.[10]

The mandible has a profusion of sixteen muscle group attachments, more than any other cranial bone, and more than any bone in the body except the scapula, which has seventeen.

*Musculature*

The muscle attachments to the mandible consist of the:

- Temporalis
- Masseter
- Lateral pterygoids
- Medial pterygoids
- Buccinator
- Depressor anguli oris
- Orbicularis oris
- Depressor labii inferioris
- Hyoglossus
- Mylohyoid
- Digastric
- Platysma
- Geniohyoid
- Mentalis
- Superior pharyngeal constrictor
- Genioglossus

The masseter has the greatest contractile strength per fiber of any muscle in the body and is a major pattern-setter in mandibular movement. The lateral pterygoids are short, stout, and tenacious muscles. To release hypertonicity in them with digital pressure (see Lateral Pterygoid Release: Oral Approach, below) you need to maintain a gentle contact for thirty seconds or so, at most two minutes. The posterior fibers of temporalis are often discretely involved in temporomandibular joint conditions. They play a role in constant-on engram temporomandibular joint pain, and in muscular-contraction headaches, and can contribute to temporal bone imbalance. These fibers are the antagonists of the lateral pterygoid muscles: the lateral pterygoids protrude the jaw, the posterior fibers of temporalis retrude it.

## Physiology

A neuromuscular pattern called an engram allows the teeth to remain in the same relationship to each other no matter what position the body adopts. "Centric occlusion" occurs when we have a perfect mid-incisal line – a vertical line that passes through the gap between the superior and inferior incisors, and this alignment may help our teeth to intercuspate perfectly.

The presence of a symphysis at the mentis is regarded as evolutionarily superior (it enhances survivability throughout life) to the fused mentis we now have within a year of birth. (All fish have a mandibular symphysis throughout life.) A symphysis enables more flexibility in the tearing and chewing motions of the teeth, and it allows another variable to help ensure occlusion. Our lack of a symphysis throughout life means that it is far harder for us to obtain perfect intercuspation and centric occlusion.[11]

## Axis of Rotation

The classical axis of rotation of the mandible is a vertical line located just posterior to the mental protuberance. The mandible is said to hinge at the anterior midline, and widen at the ramii during flexion. The mandible may echo temporal motion; the amount of motion transmitted depends upon how much muscular compression the temporomandibular joints are under. The deep source of mandibular motion is located in the upper neck, or explained by Guzay's Theorem (see illustration below).

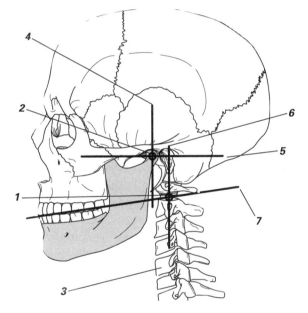

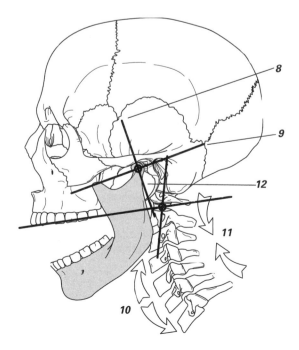

Guzay's theorum: *jaw closed (above), and jaw fully open (below)*

**1** Primary axis of mandibular motion at base of dens
**2** Secondary axis of mandibular motion at temporomandibular joint (TMJ)
**3** Cervical spine tending to slight loss of curve when biting (schematic)
**4** Vertical line through TMJ
**5** Horizontal line through TMJ
**6** Verticle line through dens
**7** Horizontal line along occlusal surface of teeth
**8** Change of verticle line during translation
**9** Change of horizontal line during translation
**10** Elongation
**11** Contraction
**12** Alterations of forces along axes 4, 5, 6, 7

## Motion

The mandible is more open to psychological input than any other bone in the head. These inputs, whether from unexpressed aggression, determination, or a fear of speaking out, cause changes in mandibular motion that range from subtle to dramatic. For instance, in states of rage the mandible is so muscularly tense that almost all movement is lost. Indeed, the person can barely separate his teeth to speak.

### Osteopathic Model

Movement of the mandible in the osteopathic (similar-motion) model is similar to all paired bones – it widens slightly in flexion. If the temporomandibular joints and upper and lower teeth are compressed, echoes of maxillary and temporal bone motion are transmitted through them to the mandible.[12] The mandible is also deeply affected by the contractile status of all sixteen muscle groups attaching to it, especially temporalis, the lateral pterygoids, and the masseter, which impart their own tonal trademarks.

### Liquid-Electric Model

In the liquid-electric model the mandible echoes the alternating, opposite-motion flexion and extension patterns of the temporal bones. The left side of the mandible therefore moves inferoposterior with left temporal flexion while the right side moves anterosuperior. If the upper neck is tense and restricted in motion, the mandible will mirror its status.[13] The mandible also receives cranial wave impulses from the sphenoid, via the pterygomandibular raphe, and the sphenomandibular ligament. Its sixteen muscle attachments provide additional impulses.

Mandibular motion is further affected by what the feet are doing. There is a deep evolutionary connection between feet, mandible, and eyes.[2] Stepping forward with the left foot, the left side of the mandible makes a micromovement into translation (that is, it moves anterior as the temporomandibular joint begins to rotate open). If you doubt this can be true, try introducing the opposite pattern as you walk, and notice how infuriatingly difficult it is.

## Diagnostic Considerations

It is hard to exaggerate the importance of the mandible in visionary craniosacral work. The proper appreciation of mandibular energetics and dynamics will make all the difference between effective craniosacral work and ineffective work. It is amazing how the rest of the body responds to an optimizing of mandibular status. For instance, neck tension and osteoarthritis, respiratory inhibition such as occurs in asthmatic states, and low-back pain may all be relieved by normalizing the mandible.

### Energetics

The mandible is the major bone of visuddha, the throat soul, which represents both expression and absorption.[14] The mandible is powerfully invested with archetypal patterns and behavioral imperatives: hominids have survived for 20 million years by baring fangs,[15,16] fighting by biting and tearing with their teeth, and eating by chewing and grinding uncooked roots, grains, and meat. For some 160,000 generations of humanity, the mandible has smiled with pleasure, chattered and trembled in mortal anxiety, and moved sideways while perusing problems. It has pouted, kissed and made up, seduced and signaled. Many Stone Age behavior patterns are still locked into our jaws and jaw muscles, and play havoc with our temporomandibular joints and temporal bones when confronted with the novel development of ongoing stress,[17] so typical of modern times.

Among the energies held in the mandible are:

***Identity*** It is the bone most associated with the individual's sense of who he is. Since the head itself is the very totem of selfhood, all cranial bones are associated with identity, but the mandible personifies it. (The hypothalamus is the part of the brain so associated.)

***Aggression*** This is where we display one of the signals of our readiness to fight – prognating the jaw. We also lift our upper eyelids and eyebrows (exposing the whites of our eyes), jut our head forward toward the target, clench our teeth, and raise our shoulders – the better to look bigger, like domestic cats fanning out their fur.

***Determination*** We set our jaws against adversity, we ponder the next move by stroking our chins wistfully. Our suppression of instinct may have begun to evolve when we first delayed the immediate urge to hunt the moment game appeared, the better to plan an effective strategy and communicate this to our fellow hunters. At this point our ancestors may have stroked their chins and thought out what to do next. Such inhibition of instinct may have set the pattern for all subsequent brain dominance patterns. The mandible is "smart determination."

**Tenacity**  We hang on with our nails and teeth; we clench our teeth; we grin and bear it.

**Sexuality**  Our relationship to our sexuality, deeply affected by childhood conditioning and the thousand wounds of love, shapes our bodies, how we hold our mandibles, and our lips. Wilhelm Reich and Alexander Lowen point out that movement is natural.[18] Sexual and sensual movement in the pelvis is natural, but often restricted because of fear, social mores, or our conditioning about sensuality and sexuality.[19] If we cannot allow natural movement in our pelvis, we transfer the need for movement to the mandible (*something* has to move) and we talk about our own, or other people's, sexuality. If we cannot move either the pelvis or mandible, we begin to armor our belly and begin to become psychotic: we feel nothing at all.[20] Some people may manifest sexual inhibition by becoming tight-lipped, or by pursing their lips as if saying "I'm not going to let out the secret that I'm a sexual being; no, not me!" The stiffness of inhibition gets caught as stiffness in the upper neck and temporomandibular joints, and acted out as anger, especially directed at other people who seem to be enjoying their sexuality.

**Sensuality**  We evert our lips to suckle, sing, celebrate by playing the saxophone after getting elected, show pleasure, kiss.

**Suppression of tender emotions**  When we are told at five "Grow up, don't cry like a baby, act like a man!" It is the mentalis muscle on the chin that quivers and oscillates, attempting to suppress emotion. The lower lip rotates out to cry, like a pout, then quickly retracts to a pencil-thin line to "keep it all in." This leaves a lasting impression on the mandible, the teeth (through clenching), and the temporomandibular joints, not to mention the heart and human sensitivity. We become soldiers early.

The English are reputed to have "stiff upper lips." In the Yorkshire region of England you are advised to "Ask no questions, tell no lies, shut your gob, an' you'll catch no flies." In Scotland the admonishment is to "hud yer tongue." Germans say that sometimes they have to "bite a sour apple" – get a difficult job finished despite the discomforts. In America you "zip your lip" to keep a

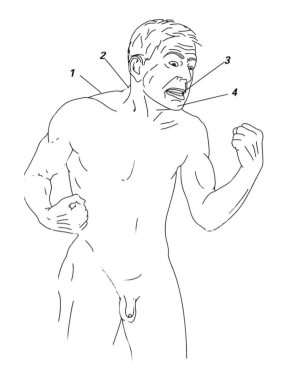

*Rage*
*1 Shoulders elevated*
*2 Neck jutting forward*
*3 Teeth exposed*
*4 Mandible protruded*

secret, become "tight-lipped" when your feelings are hurt, "keep your mouth shut" about unfavorable circumstances. The mandible is also where we "pay lip service" to something, and where we disgorge superficial energy by being "motor mouths."

There is an interesting saying in German, *auf etwas herum kauen*, which means to keep chewing on the same theme over and over again, neurotically, without finding a way out. Fritz Perls,[21] on the other hand, pointed out the positive aspect of having the ability to chew through something to its completion.

### Trauma and Dysfunction

The mandible is frequently traumatized.[22] How many scars do you have on the skin over yours? How many dental visits left a mark, physical or psychic? Who beat up on you? Who was the school bully – can you still see his face? Fist fights impact the left side of the mandible most often (as most people are right-handed and therefore punch with the right fist, which usually impacts the victim on the left side). This history of "taking it on the chin" goes some way toward explaining the mandible's strength, for we have fought for millennia. The jaw and its support structures are so strong that we can get through a stressful time carrying a lot of "battle damage." (Muhammad Ali fought the last three rounds of one of his title fights with a fractured mandible.)

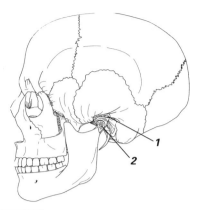 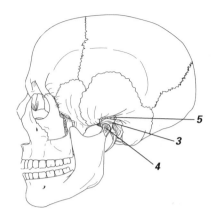 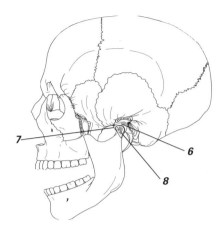

*Translation of the temporomandibular joint: note coupling of hinging and anterior movement ("translation") of condyle*
***1** Articular disc and joint capsule of temporomandibular joint, neutral*
***2** Mandibular condyle, neutral*
***3** Pulled by lateral pterygoid muscle, disc begins anterior motion*
***4** Condyle translates anteroinferior*
***5** Mandibular (or glenoid) fossa*
***6** Maximal anteroinferior motion of disc*
***7** Joint capsule*
***8** Condyle at anteroinferior limit of translation*

Nonetheless, it is emotional stress that traumatizes the mandible most. Ongoing stress locks into it, leading eventually to grinding of the teeth at night (bruxism) and the gradual degeneration of the temporomandibular joints. Anxiety, stress, and aggression alter the physiology of the jaw musculature, temporomandibular joints, and upper neck.[23,24] From my own extensive work with clients suffering from temporomandibular joint dysfunction, I know that craniosacral work is one of the most effective approaches available for it.

Go carefully when you suspect oral sexual trauma. Asking direct questions is fraught with difficulties; the questions are more likely to be met with denial and cause further internalization of the trauma. The very questions may be experienced by the client as yet another violation of his privacy. Take great care with creating a positive, supportive atmosphere.[25] Let the client know that you are there to help him. Clear yourself of any negative judgments. Rather than questioning, listen attentively to what the client says, but give equal or perhaps more attention to how the mandible actually moves as he talks (considering this movement as its own storytelling, its own poetry). Also keep an eye out for secondary physical movements or signals, especially from the pelvis and hip joints – this area is frequently the source of mandibular dysfunction.

The temporomandibular joints normally float loosely within their capsules. In anxiety, the mandible is tightly compressed into the temporal fossae, eventually leading to deterioration of the temporomandibular joint, cervical arthritis, and muscle-contraction headache. (It is wise to investigate mandibular involvement in all kinds of headache.)

The periodontal ligaments are "wavy" and can become stretched under constant compression. If a tooth is replaced or crowned too high, it will compress the opposite tooth's periodontal ligaments and upset the temporomandibular joint, which may bring on headaches or visual disturbances. The status of the temporomandibular joints can also be assessed from CAT scans, X-rays, the case history, and the mandible and temporomandibular joint testing outlined below. The most common cause of numbness of the chin is a secondary bony metastisis encroaching upon the mental foramina.

## Interconnectedness

The mandible is the most energetically loaded cranial bone. It plays a major part in sphenoid and temporal status, and may dominate maxillary function by way of the teeth. It is also a principal player in most types of headache,[26,27] and acts as a strong controller and pattern-setter for the neck, upper chest, pelvic girdle, and feet. The position and motility of the mandible is affected by all of the midline structures of the body – the hyoid, sternum, xiphoid process, linea alba, and symphysis pubis.

## Visualization

Since it is such a prominent bone, visualization of the mandible is relatively easy. See the barrel shape of the condyles, the sharp point of the coronoid processes, the strength or softness of the angle, the resolve of the chin, the set of the jaw.

## MUSCULAR RELEASE TECHNIQUES

### Masseter Release: Three Approaches

These three masseter techniques are designed to empty the muscles of tension prior to more specific work in the mouth area. The masseter has three distinct layers, separated by fascial envelopes.

### Masseter Release: Superficial Fibers

This is the most delicate of the three techniques, and aims to release the superficial fibers of the masseter. Sit or kneel at the head of the table. Curl the backs of both hands and place the middle or proximal phalangeal bones of your central three fingers in contact with the zygomatic attachments of the masseters, and the belly of the muscle inferior to the zygomatic arch. Tune in to masseter motility and the status of their energy field, and apply very delicate pressure, ⅕ to ⅓ ounce (5.6 to 9.5 grams), in an inferior and posterior direction – the direction of the fibers – and wait for unwinding to begin. Stay with the superficial fibers until you sense that all the tension has left them.

### Masseter Release: Profound Fibers

This second technique is a more robust approach, directed at the profound, or middle layer, of the masseter muscle. It uses more pressure than is customary in craniosacral work, in the order of 2 to 4 ounces (57 to 113 grams), as the situation warrants. Sit or kneel at the head of the table. Place your thenar eminences in direct contact with the masseters and your palms flat on the cheeks. Rotate your hands with wrist extension to work along the long axis of the masseter fibers, moving inferior and posterior, as in the last technique. By the time you reach the angle of the jaw, your wrists are in full extension. You may have to use massage lotion to obtain a smooth sweep.

### Masseter Release: Most Profound Fibers

This is the most direct and thoroughgoing approach, accessing the most profound layer of the masseter fibers. Sit or kneel at the head of the table. With your fingerpads, seek out the most contracted fiber bundle of the client's masseter on each side – the hot spots. Apply thumbtip contact to the one point on each side that is the most tender, hypertonic, or energetically attractive to your fingers. Align your thumbs to point almost directly in at the masseters – as directly as your thumbnails permit – and apply a deep-tissue pressure until you sense the muscle tissue relax and give way, then cease immediately.

## Lateral Pterygoid Release: Four Approaches

Some schools teach that working directly with the lateral pterygoids is unnecessary, that normalization of the viscerocranium will automatically normalize the pterygoids. This may be so, but in my experience it does not always work this way. It is wise to have many technical approaches in your tool bag, and an open, inquiring mind.

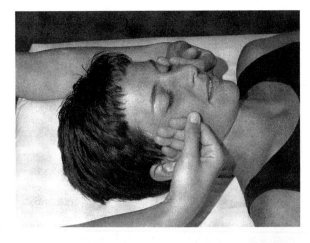

*Masseter Release: Superficial Fibers*

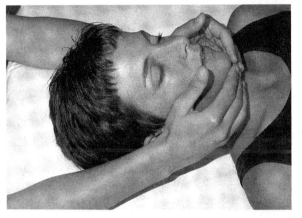

*Masseter Release: Profound Fibers*

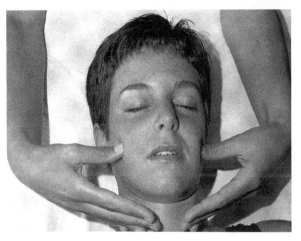

*Masseter Release: Most Profound Fibers*

### Lateral Pterygoid Release: Direct Approach

Sit or kneel at the head end of the table. Place the palms of your hand over the area immediately anterior to the temporomandibular joints. Place your index or middle finger directly over the temporomandibular joints themselves and ask the client to gently open and close his mouth. Wait until you can feel the anterior glide of the condyles easily; they become much more prominent as they move into their most anterior placement (the full yawn position), which is the position of maximum effectiveness with this technique.

Ask the client to hold his mandible as close to a full yawn position as he comfortably can, and reposition your index or middle fingers to apply medial pressure immediately anterior to the now-prominent lateral masses of the condyles. In doing this you will be applying pressure through the masseter muscles to the tendons of the lateral pterygoid muscles. Pressing too hard will diminish your sensitivity and produce sharp, wincing pain, so modulate your pressure to a tolerable level and work very slowly to release tension in the tendons.

This is a very direct approach and can produce results very quickly. However, the client cannot be expected to hold his jaw in the full yawn position for very long, and the tenderness in the muscle usually makes this unpleasant, so other approaches need to be mastered.

### Lateral Pterygoid Release: Mandible-Retrusion Approach

The most exact and capable approach to working with the mandible begins with facing the client's head while abreast of his thorax at the side of the table. Get comfortable – which may mean a chair to place your outside foot upon, one flexed knee up on the table, or your outside foot up on the table. (The adept placement of a knee or a foot provides valuable support for your own low-back and adds a dimension of valuable stability.)

Turn the client's head so that it faces your heart and align your shoulder joints with his temporomandibular joints so that your arm lengths remain approximately equal. Place one thumb at a time inside the mouth, with the palmar aspects of your thumbs on the biting surface of the lower teeth. Landmark your thumbtips as far posterior as the last molar teeth, brushing them against the upswing of the sharp edge of the ramus. (If the client has lost several of his molars, make contact with the superior-most gum line of the alveolar ridge, and also the ramus with your thumbtips.) Align your thumbs in continuous, even contact with as many of the molars and premolars as possible. Now place your index fingers external to the mouth, pointing at the top of the auricles of the client's ears – this will give you index-finger contact with the attachment of masseter. Then gently but firmly hook your middle and ring fingers posterior to the ramus of the jaw, and place your little fingers in the small recession just anterior to the angle of the jaw. You now have the jaw held in a stable, controlled, and reassuringly complete hold. I call this the Jaw Cradle. (Be careful that you are not pinching or trapping the lips, or the angles of the mouth.)

Once you are comfortable with this contact, begin to take the mandible to its most comfortable posterior limit of motion (retrusion) and begin hunting in the "feel" of the tissues for the specific locations and vectors that are hypertonic. Since the lateral pterygoids are protruders, retruding the mandible stretches the long axis of their spindles. If you introduce rotation as you retrude, you can either stretch one side at a time or focus on the hypertonic side. Maintain your posterior presence until the mandible feels quite free.

This is the most natural-feeling and pleasant way to release tension in these muscles. It is also remarkably effective in releasing muscular tension in the upper three cervical vertebrae, and in the atlanto-occipital joint.

### Lateral Pterygoid Release: Oral Approach

This is a compound technique that requires visualization of the exact origins and insertions of the lateral pterygoid muscles before you begin. It is much more effective, and considerate, than the direct digital approach, but it takes longer. Remember to check in with your own breathing, and encourage your client to breathe through his mouth, which usually encourages further stomatognathic system relaxation.

Stand at the head of the table. For the left lateral pterygoid, bring your left knee up onto the table and get in a comfortable stance. Turn the client's head about forty-five degrees to his right. Introduce the fifth finger of your right hand into his mouth and trace back to the final upper molar. Now move your finger to the inferior buttress of the zygomaticomaxillary arch, and rotate your forearm into full supination – so that your left palm now faces your left shoulder.

Now track your finger posterior again, maintaining contact with the inferior aspect of the zygomaticomaxillary suture, until you feel the sharp anterior edge of the ramus of the mandible. It may seem to partially block your path. Your task is to pass medially to the ramus but laterally to the alveolar ridge, which is now tapering out. If the ramus is blocking free access to the muscle, have the client open and close his mandible incrementally, or even rotate his mandible a little to each side, until you find the maximum aperture, or "tunnel."

The belly of the lateral pterygoid begins to be felt approximately ½ inch (1.3 centimeter) posterior to the anterior edge of the ramus. At or before this point you may feel more comfortable changing from your present fingernail-medial approach to a fingernail-lateral approach. I personally find that the fingernail-medial (palm of the operative hand facing lateral in respect to the plane of the client's

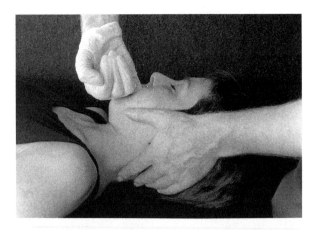

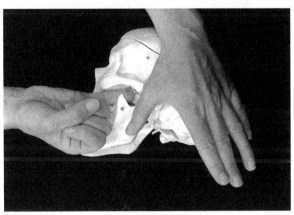

head) method maintains a more fusiform wrist, a clear energetic pathway, and offers an effective lateral pterygoid contact. The advantage of the fingernail-lateral approach is that, once in contact with the muscle, you have greater sensitivity and flexibility of response.

Be gentle and persistent; don't gouge. You can never go too deep, just too fast. You are changing the energy field of the muscle (and its engram) just by being present, waiting, listening. When the muscle has released on one side, which will take between thirty seconds and two minutes from the beginning of actual contact with it, repeat the technique on the other side.

This technique, properly done, produces a remarkable sense of relaxation and well-being. Afterward the client will feel like his mandible is a yard (meter) wide. I consider this technique indispensable for the complete evaluation and treatment of temporomandibular joint conditions.

### *Lateral Pterygoid Release: Trigger-Point Approach*

There is a fourth way to reach the lateral pterygoids – by their trigger points. The superior belly has a trigger point at the narrowest point of the zygomatic arch (easy to feel on your own or the client's head), right at the point where the fascia of the temporalis attaches to the superior margin of the arch. If this belly of the muscle is hypertonic,

the bone and fascia will feel tender right on the trigger point. The inferior belly has its trigger point immediately inferior to the narrowest point of the zygomatic arch.

Use slow, gentle, rubbing motions in a rotatory direction to ease hypertonicity, or a ⅕ ounce (5.6 gram) contact over the trigger points. Stay there with this light touch until you pick up cranial wave formations passing through the trigger-point area, or a distant cardiovascular pulse becoming apparent. Sense which way the waves move, and facilitate their passage. This will release the underlying muscle.

### Release of the Posterior Fibers of Temporalis: Two Approaches

The posterior fibers of temporalis are the postero-inferior 25 percent of the muscle, and the part most often found to be hypertonic in the constant-on engram condition of temporomandibular joint dysfunction. They are the only true antagonists of the powerful lateral pterygoid muscles. Once having achieved release of the lateral pterygoids, it is almost always appropriate, and therapeutically elegant, to release their antagonists. Work to lengthen chronically shortened muscle fibrils and the fascia of temporalis with one of the following techniques.

### *Release of the Posterior Fibers of Temporalis: Stretch across the Long Axis*

Sit or kneel at the head of the table and begin with landmarking. The posterior fibers begin at the anterior face of the auricle – at Ear Gate (Triple Warmer 21) – and extend backward to the posterior limit of the temporalis muscle which lies superior to asterian. Arrange the tips of your central three fingers so that they are located directly medial to the superior-most tip of the auricle. If you have doubts about your placement, ask the client to briefly clench his teeth: if you are in the right location, your fingertips will be pushed laterally by the contracting muscle fibers. Be sure that the tip of your index finger is posterior to a line drawn superior from the anterior-most portion of the auricle. Temporalis is located much more posteriorly and inferiorly on the cranium than instinct tells us it is. Work to reduce the tense engram holding patterns by applying medial pressure with cephalad traction (across the long axis of the posterior fibers).

Apply moderate amounts of medially-directed pressure, and then without sliding over the client's hair or skin, pull your fingertips in a superiorly

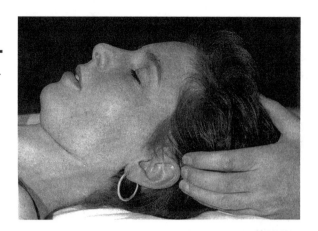

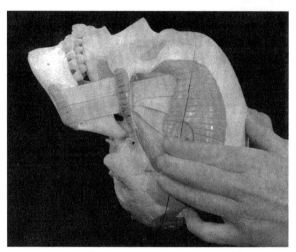

## OSSEOUS TECHNIQUES

### Mandible Thumbs – Internal Technique, Palpation and Unwinding

Begin by taking up the Jaw Cradle hold described under Lateral Pterygoid Release: Mandible Retrusion approach on p. 360.

Get comfortable and wait. Track the incoming forces and vectors from all the associated structures, and make a picture in your mind's eye of the sixteen muscle groups, the mandibular ligaments, and the temporomandibular joints. Begin to associate and identify what you feel with what you "see." Analyze the basic position of the mandible, and how far and how easily it moves in flexion compared to extension. Sense the energetic loading of the mandible: does it feel full of pent-up aggression, or full of unexpressed tender emotions? If, after five minutes, you have not naturally moved into a gentle dancing unwinding of the mandible, consider initiating one. Introducing a gentle movement into decompression may help uncover the mandible's unwinding patterns.

This technique is very effective for working with temporomandibular joint pain and dysfunction, neck stiffness and pain, and "mask" and frontal headaches.

### Mandible and Temporomandibular Joint Testing in Two Planes

This technique tests the mandible in eight directions.

Begin with simple motion testing, asking the client to open, close, triturate, prognate, and retrude his lower jaw. You can test each muscle group isometrically (against moderate resistance). To test isometrically, place your hand against the mandible in the direction you wish to test, and ask the client to push his mandible into your palm. Note the strength of his effort, while not permitting him any movement. For instance, to test for left lateral pterygoid strength, stand at the head of the table and place your right palm over the right side of his face and mandible. Ask your supine client to triturate (rotate) his mandible to his right, and note the strength with which he attempts to do this. Next, use the same principle with moderate resistance, only this time permit the client to actually move his mandible in the required direction, that is, let him "win." This will test the strength of the muscle, and also give you some information about his temporomandibular joints.

directed movement and maintain both medially-directed pressure and superior traction until you feel the muscles release. This stretches the fibers across their long axis. If simple stretching is ineffective, consider "springing" the fibers,[28] that is, stretching them and then suddenly letting them go. Repeat the springing until the feel of the muscle softens, and the temporomandibular joints move more softly.[6] This technique can be wonderfully euphoric. It often produces more parietal decompression than the standard Parietal Lift, allowing the calvarium to move further upward, creating space for the brain and energy field to expand into. It is an essential component in the holistic treatment of the temporomandibular joints.

### *Release of the Posterior Fibers of Temporalis: Pressure Across Horizontal Long Axis*

The second approach consists of using gentle but persistent releasing strokes directed along the horizontal long axis of the posterior temporalis fibers. Use the same position and landmarking to locate the muscle, employ fingertip contact over the posterior fiber group, and now work in the direction of optimum vascular drainage – from posterior to anterior.

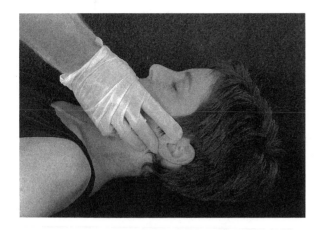

Next go through the eight-test protocol of motion testing outlined below using the healer's stance and Jaw Cradle hold already described. This protocol will give you accurate information on many different aspects of mandibular status. Of course, also take note also of the mandible's static position and its energetic song as you run through the sequence.

### Motion Testing

In each of the following movement tests we are establishing an evaluation based on three standards:

■ Ease of motion
■ Amount of motion
■ Ease and amount of motion on one side versus the other

Note how the "feel" of the mandible and its ease of motion seems to you in each direction; the restrictions or alterations in the texture of the movements are keys to deduce which structures – muscle, fascia, ligament, bone, or joint – are in need of further investigation or work. It is very useful to repeat the same motion several times until you really have the feel of it. Just once is rarely enough for comparative purposes. It is good practice, especially while learning, to allow the mandible to rest in neutral for a second or two between each test.

There are two ways to perform these tests, either robustly, as a kind of physical therapy, range-of-motion testing, or discreetly and gracefully, by sensing the cranial wave. Begin with testing discreetly, by staying within the limits of movement of the cranial wave – that is, within the involuntary motions of the mandible. If you cannot test a particular motion using discreet pressures of ⅕ ounce (5.6 grams), only then test the motion using robust pressures of ½ to 1 pound (.25 to .50 kilogram). Then go back to gracile pressures, and see if the mandible is now motile with the cranial wave.

***I: Caudad Test in the Axial Plane*** Decompress the mandible (that is, move it inferiorly) and note how it moves according to the three standards mentioned above. This stretches the temporomandibular joint capsule, the masseter, temporalis and medial pterygoid, and engages the sphenomandibular and temporomandibular ligaments at its inferior limit of motion.

***II: Posteroanterior Test in the Horizontal Plane*** Test for mandibular protrusion, or movement in the horizontal plane, in an anterior direction. This tests the joint itself, stretches the posterior fibers of temporalis, and engages the stylomandibular ligament at the mandible's anterior limit of motion.

***III & IV: Mediolateral Test in the Horizontal Plane*** Test for a pure lateral glide, first from neutral to the left side, and note the lateral glide of both temporomandibular joints. Then repeat the test for lateral glide to the right side. This tests the joint, meniscus, temporomandibular ligament on the side of the deviation, but is not particularly useful as a muscle test.

***V & VI: Rotatory Test in the Horizontal Plane*** Now take the mandible into a pure rotation to the left side, noting how it moves, then repeat the rotation to the right. Compare and contrast the two rotations. Rotation to the left stretches the left lateral pterygoid muscle, and the posterior fibers of temporalis on the right. It also tests each TMJ and retrodiscal ligament.

***VII: Anteroposterior Test in the Horizontal Plane*** Now retrude the mandible, or take it posterior. Note how this compares with the second test, which was protrusion. Retrusion stretches both lateral pterygoids, relieves tension on the retrodiscal ligament, and gives us information about the amount of "surrender" the client can allow.

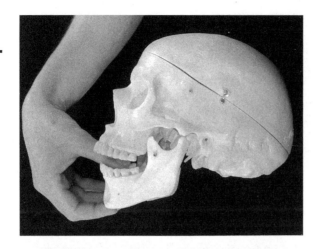

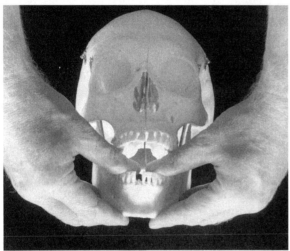

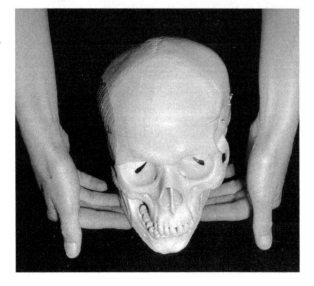

***VIII: Cephalad, Axial Plane*** Last, take the mandible into an axial compression toward the vertex. As this compresses the temporomandibular joint, you would omit it for a client known to have pain in the temporomandibular joints. This tests the meniscus of the temporomandibular joint, the mitility of the temporal bones, the status of the Tentorium Leresri, and the pliancy of the squamous suture. It does not directly test any muscles.

***Completion*** End with free-form testing, rather like testing a universal joint. This leads naturally into unwinding, which is the optimum treatment mode for the mandible and all that ails it.

## Mandible Unwinding from the Vertex

Standing to one side to unwind the mandible, as in the preceding techniques which use the Jaw Cradle, gives you the best admixture of sensitivity and firm contact, but it becomes awkward when the mandible begins to move into unwinding on the side away from you. In this situation, consider moving to the head of the table, superior to the client's vertex. Reposition your thumbs on the biting surface of the mandibular teeth and curl your other fingers in under the body of the mandible. This position, while lacking in specificity, is easier to maintain for long periods than the hold used in the preceding techniques.

## Mandible Compression

Do not use this technique in clients with temporomandibular joint pain.

Sit at the head of the table and take up a gentle, listening contact with the inferior border of the mandibular body. Once you can feel cranial wave formations passing through it, initiate mandibular compression by placing all eight fingers under the body of the mandible, and putting your thumbs (not shown in photo) over the mental foramina to create some lateral stability. Open his mouth to ensure that his lower teeth do not touch his upper teeth. Your objective is to compress the mandible into the temporal bones via the temporomandibular joints, and not to create maxillary compression. Track the progression of your compressive intent and force through the temporomandibular joints and their meniscus, through temporal bone motions, tentorial tension, parietal decompression, and finally falx resistance. Once you sense all of these tissues release under your compression, change your intention and direction and take the structures ever so slowly back down through decompression, inviting each structure to release as you do so.

End by checking the mandible to ensure that no residual compression is left in its structure. Place your hands in the standard mandibular testing contact (Jaw Cradle) – thumbs inside the mouth on the biting surface of the lower teeth, align your index fingers along the inferior aspect of the zygomatic arches, your middle and fourth fingers behind the ramus of the mandible, and your little fingers just anterior to the angle of the mandible. Introduce specific mandibular decompression, then test for freedom of motion in all directions, and finally become interactive, employing "steering-wheel" or unwinding work to fully free the mandible.

## Ten Reasons to Unwind the Mandible

Consider using this itemization to broaden your understanding of the scope of a relatively simple technique, like the Mandible Thumbs-Internal Technique, which can be used for the following:

■ To release the atlanto-occipital joint and free the back of the neck, especially the upper three cervical vertebrae.

■ To release mandibular compression mediated to the sphenoid through the maxillae, and affecting the palatines, vomer, and ethmoid (releasing mandibular compression will also help free up the temporal bones, and as a result help normalize the tentorium).

■ To free the throat soul (expression) and thus free the voice to speak out clearly, without impediment.

■ To release "archaic wounds" of oral sexual abuse, incest, and/or intolerable physical pain affecting the area (when pain is too great to stay with and process at the time, it gets parceled away in "another room"[7] for future uncaching and digesting).

■ To induce euphoric states of whole-body relaxation via the interface of the mandible's motor nerves with half of the body's motor nerves in the motor cortex (specifically, unwinding the jaw releases the face, back of neck, pectorals, and pelvic girdle).

■ To work with all common types of headache – muscle contraction, eye and sinus, migraine, menstrual migraine, and cluster headache.

■ To begin the normalization of the stomatognathic system, including helping to normalize the hyoid.

■ To release sacral and pelvic energies, whether locomotor, sexual, or spiritual (this is effected by taking advantage of the neurological and energetic mirroring between mouth and perineum and symphysis mentis and symphysis pubis).

■ To work with aggression, determination, the suppression of tender emotions, and identity.

■ To help rectify imbalances of the musculoskeletal system as far away as the feet through the ancient survival reflexes that connect jaw to foot.

## Twelve Reasons to Release the Lateral Pterygoids

This is an itemization of twelve reasons to work with the lateral pterygoid muscles. See Chapter 18, The Stomatognathic System, for further details.

■ To release the sphenoid from a chronic flexion lesion, which may relieve "flexion head" symptoms such as frontal headache, low-back pain, and sinusitis. (Hypertonicity of both lateral pterygoids in the absence of mandible prognation will force the sphenoid into flexion).

■ To release chronic contraction on the mandible, its temporomandibular joint menisci, and its joint capsule, and to make the translation of temporomandibular joint rotation smoothly congruous with prognation.

■ To equalize tension with the lateral pterygoids' antagonist, the posterior fibers of temporalis, especially in the treatment of muscle contraction headache.

■ To help release compression on the sphenobasilar joint and sphenotemporal sutures. (This is especially useful in the more serious sphenobasilar lesion patterns like vertical strain, lateral strain, and "compression head.")

■ To work with physical and emotional trauma – archaic wounds – particularly to release memories and tissue contractions resulting from dental trauma, or oral sexual violation.

■ To bring breadth back to the jaw. (The main reported experience from clients after their lateral pterygoids are released is that the jaw feels a yard (meter) wide.)

■ To work toward opening the throat soul in cases of asthma, individuals who are incommunicative or withdrawn, and in autism and psychosis.

■ To treat tinnitus, since pterygoid spasm can lead to pressure on the auditory tubes via sphenoid torsion, vertical strain, or sphenoid low lesion patterns. (Increased pressure exerted by the mandibular condyles into the fossae of the temporomandibular joints can force a slight approximation of the internal carotid artery to the auditory tube, thus leading to the "roaring" sounds that emanate from the internal carotids, which is the hallmark of some types of tinnitus.)

■ As part of the treatment protocol in whiplash injury, for loss of short-term memory, vertigo, and post-whiplash malaise. (Work with the lateral pterygoids will help normalize the temporals by reducing traction exerted on them by the retrodiscal ligament.)

■ To treat bruxism (grinding of the teeth), and interrupt the constant-on engram that can lead to frontal headache and temporomandibular joint deterioration.

■ To optimize visual clarity through sphenoid and temporal (for the lateral geniculate ganglion) release.

■ To obtain the full benefits of the mandibular relaxation response, which consists of muscular release in the back of the neck, pectoral muscle area of the upper chest, and the entire low-back and pelvis. (Specific lateral pterygoid muscle work may reflexively trigger a release of perineal, sacral, and hip rotator hypertonicity and assist in allowing the pectoral muscle area to normalize after a stressful period.)

## Temporomandibular Joint Considerations

This list is designed to cover most of the causes of temporomandibular joint pain and dysfunction. Consider using this as a checklist, or questionnaire, before working with a new client suffering from temporomandibular joint dysfunction.

It is very important to recognize that you may be altering the client's dental mechanics when you work with his temporomandibular joints. The correct procedure here is to contact his dentist and cooperate with him in achieving optimum function. The dentist and his assistants may have spent many, many hours getting the client's bite, intercuspation, and jaw mobility up to their own standards of excellence. We need to respect their work and move very carefully in our interactions with the stomatognathic system so as not to create unwelcome changes.

Enlightened dentists all over the world now work in close cooperation with craniosacral therapists of all persuasions: cranial osteopaths, chiropractors using sacro-occipital technique, and physical therapists or massage therapists specially trained in this work. Precisely because working to optimize the flow of cranial waves through the temporomandibular joints and associated areas of the biting-chewing-swallowing mechanism operates at such a different "wavelength" from conventional orthodontic work, it can create profound changes not anticipated, or allowed for, in the dental work. This needs to be fully understood.

Breast-feeding is the optimal form of early pattern-setting for the jaws and temporomandibular joints, with the mother holding the baby reassuringly close to her and her heartbeat, giving him up to ten minutes on each breast. Changing the baby over to the other breast gives a complete reversal of position, a change of nonequal muscle pulls, mandible rotation, and lip and tongue activity. In bottle-feeding, the baby is generally not changed over at all, and simply held on the mother's left side with the result that a very one-sided neuromuscular pattern may be imprinted at the formative stage, and at the blueprint level, of the stomatognathic system. The bottle is also held at a different angle than the nipple. There are many reasons for a woman to choose not to breast-feed, and in these cases it will help the development of the infant's mouth if she remembers to change sides in bottle-feeding and to take care with the angle at which she holds the bottle.

### *Breast-Feeding*

Ask the client:

■ Were you breast-fed or bottle-fed?
■ Do you have any idea how long it was before you were weaned?
■ Do you remember if you sucked your thumb?
■ How old were you when you stopped sucking your thumb?

### *Dental Braces*

Ask the client:

■ When did you have your braces fitted?
■ Why were they fitted?
■ How long did you wear them?
■ How did (does) it feel to wake up in the morning with braces on?
■ Were (are) you glad you had (have) the braces?

### *Emotional Status*

Ask the client whichever of the questions below you feel are appropriate and are comfortable asking. (The psychological states that we are asking about, or their opposite – such as the person who hates his work – are reflected in the mandible and functioning of the temporomandibular joint.)

■ Do you consider yourself a happy person?
■ Do you enjoy your work?
■ Do you have a primary relationship? How is it?

■ How would you describe your family relationships?

■ Would you say you are ambitious or easy-going?

■ How is your financial overhead? Is your rent/mortgage easily manageable for you?

■ How well do you manage to express yourself in a confrontation?

■ Do you ever "clam up" or "swallow your truth?"

■ Do you mull over your words for hours or days before speaking?

Consider the appropriateness of asking these next two questions to discover whether the individual has been forced to have oral sex, which is a "secret" cause of extreme temporomandibular joint contraction and compression:

■ Are you aware of any oral sexual abuse in your early life?

■ Have you suffered from oral sexual violation as an adult?

## Psychological Habits

How would you, the healer, describe the client's attitude to life?

■ Does he have a "stiff upper lip"?

■ What is catching in his throat?

■ Does he only give lip-service to his ideals?

■ Does he "hang on by the skin of his teeth"?

■ Is he "fed up to his back teeth"?

■ Does he "sink his teeth into" his partner?

■ Does he have the ability to chew through a project until its completion?

■ Does he "grin and bear it" and "put on a happy face"?

■ Can he express love?

■ Can he let love in?

■ Is he able to express nuances of feelings? (The typical American male is reputed to have just two modes of expression with his mate: anger or silence.)

## Other Dental History

Ask the client:

■ Do you have all of your wisdom teeth?

■ Have you had any teeth extracted? When, and was it painful?

■ Have you had root canal work/bridges/crowns/dentures/partial dentures?

■ Are you afraid of dentists?

## Trauma to the Face and Mouth

Ask the client:

■ Have you been in military service?

■ Have you had any automobile, motorcycle, skiing, surfing, or horseback-riding accidents to your head?

■ Have you had any sports injuries – baseball bats, hockey sticks, cricket balls – to your head?

■ Have you practiced any "full contact" sports like karate, tai kwon do, or boxing?

■ Have you had any operations or serious illnesses to the mouth and neck area?

■ Do you tend to get sinusitis? Have you ever been operated on for it?

■ Did you ever take any medication that stiffened your jaw?

## Diet and Oral Habits

Ask the client:

■ Do you adhere to a vegetarian, macrobiotic, or any particular diet? (Some macrobiotic adherents chew each bite of food one hundred times.)

■ How would you describe your diet?

■ Are you careful in selecting what you eat?

■ Do you eat any fruit or vegetables on a daily basis?

■ Do you chew gum or tobacco?

■ Do you smoke cigarettes, cigars, or a pipe?

■ About how many cups of coffee do you drink per day?

■ Do you play a wind instrument?

## Seat Belts

Ask the client:

■ Do you wear a seat belt when you drive? All of the time?

■ Is it a lap and diagonal seat belt or a racing harness?

■ If you use a diagonal belt, how close does it pass to your sternocleidomastoid?

■ How much tension is the belt under?

■ Does the belt tension distress you?

## Work

Ask the client:

■ Do you use a telephone at work?

■ How much time do you spend on the phone?

■ Do you work at a desk?

■ "You are a workaholic" – How would you answer this accusation?

■ Do you tend to support your jaw with cupped hands while studying?

■ Do you grit your teeth to get through an unpleasant project?

### Telephone Usage

Ask the client:

- How do you hold the telephone: (1) with a conventional receiver? (2) compressed between your shoulder (raised and tense) and your jaw (compressed and displaced)? (3) with a headset (the optimum arrangement)?
- Do you find almost all talking on the phone stressful (true for many older people)?

### Hobbies

Ask the client:

- Do you have any hobbies that stress your temporomandibular joints?
- Do you play the violin (and therefore hold it on one side, compressing and rotating your mandible)?
- Do you use a rifle (compressed under the jaw and jolting the structures of the jaw and cranium with each shot)?

### Exercise

Ask the client:

- Do you take any form of exercise? What type, how much, and how often?
- What exercise did you used to do?
- Can you feel your teeth gap when you walk?

### Posture

- Please show me how you read a book.
- What postures do you use while studying?
- How do you sit when watching TV?
- How do you carry a heavy bag or suitcase?
- Do you by habit carry your bag from only one shoulder? (This is very distressing to the physiology of the cranial base. Holding the bag in the hand is better; a daypack or fanny pack is best.)

### Sexuality

If it seems appropriate, and you are a licensed health care practitioner in a related field, ask the client the following. Note anything he may say (mandible movement) and note also what he may do, the secondary signals, especially from the pelvis and hip joints (source movement). The secondary signals express what the dreambody feels. Particularly note the postures the client adopts, and look for temporomandibular joint compression and masseter prominence.

- How would you feel about answering a few questions concerning sex?
- Would you describe your sexual relationships as satisfactory?
- Is sex pleasurable, or uneasy for you?
- Would you say that sometimes sex makes you grit your teeth?
- Is oral sex distasteful for you?
- Has it ever been forced on you?

### Ask yourself:

- Is he tight-lipped?
- Does he purse his lips?
- Is he stiff-necked?
- How does he move his body?

### Sleep

Ask the client:

- Do you suffer from recurrent nightmares?
- Have you ever been diagnosed as suffering from post-traumatic stress disorder? (This is a condition seen in those who have survived exceptionally harrowing events, such as Vietnam veterans who have recurrent nightmares, and have difficulty reintegrating with society.)
- Do you grind your teeth at night (bruxism)?
- Are your dental crowns affected by bruxism?
- Have you ever worn dental splints to avoid further deterioration?
- Have you tried meditation, psychological counseling, or biofeedback to cure your bruxism?

*Constant-On Engram*

Observe the following of the client:

- When he speaks, does he hardly open his mouth?
- Does he complain of frontal headaches, sinusitis, and temporomandibular joint pain?
- Does he obviously live a very stressful lifestyle, but deny it?
- Does he drink coffee and alcohol immoderately, smoke, and then take recreational drugs to slow down again?
- Does he seem to have hyperthyroidism, or be verging on it? (Hyperthyroidism is characterized by night sweats, sweaty feet and palms, jumpy and excitable demeanor, heart palpitations or extra systoles, and paranoia; in this case the client should be referred for medical assessment.)

Ask the client:

- Do you stimulate yourself (caffeine) when tired, or do you rest when tired?
- Do you work more than sixty hours a week?
- How many jobs do you hold down?
- How many people do you take care of?
- How many people financially depend on you?
- When did you take your last vacation? (a revealing question – watch the secondary signals closely).

## Other Techniques that Can Affect the Mandible

- All sphenoid work via the pterygoids, muscles, and the sphenomandibular ligaments
- Sphenoid External Coupled Contact with Mandible
- Frontal-Zygomae-Mandible Triple Spread
- The CV4
- Temporal Auricle Decompression, Temporal Palming, and Square Ashtray
- Hyoid unwinding
- Neck unwinding, and osteopathic and chiropractic adjustments
- Muscular and energetic release work to the sternum, xiphoid process, linea alba, rectus abdominus, and symphysis pubis
- Psychotherapy, especially Voice Dialogue: talking out deeply troubling issues that have become pent-up in the throat soul and the mandible
- Acupuncture
- Deep emotional release, Arnold Mindell's process work, Bio-energetics, biofeedback, and regression therapies

# SPECIAL
# APPLICATIONS

# 35
# Craniosacral Work with Infants

At birth a child *is* all there:[1] all of his emotional, instinctive, and perceptive apparatus is in place; underdeveloped maybe, certainly limited in grown-up verbal skills, but sensorially intact. The psyche of the child is as soft-shelled as his skull. Everything impinges on him, and it is well to remember this in treating children.

When you work with children, tell them, both verbally and attitudinally, "I'm going to help you." From birth their intuitive heart sensors are open and receptive, and they will either warm to you or withdraw from you depending on the quality of your field. Treat them with exactly the same respect and care you would an adult.

*Rebecca, fourteen months old, had known Thomas since she was born. She had always been fond of him. They giggled a lot together. Besides, Thomas was her daddy's best friend. A busy doctor, Thomas had a patient die that day. It was a great loss. To make matters worse, a nurse had made a crucial mistake at the last minute, and Thomas, his sadness mixed with anger, took her aside afterwards to explain her error to her, hoping to show her a useful way to avoid repeating it in the future. The nurse balked, refused to acknowledge that she had made a mistake, and started yelling at Thomas, reflecting his anger back at him. They parted on cool terms. It was a bad day for everyone concerned. Tired, sad, angry, overwrought, Thomas looked at his watch and realized he was an hour late for his appointment to visit Rebecca's dad's house for supper. When he got there and walked through the door with the shadow of death behind him, Rebecca took one look at him and*

*without a second's hesitation let out a blood-curdling scream. Thomas had not had time to say a single word. Turning her back on him in one swift move, she refused to look at Thomas, or let him touch her, for the next twenty minutes.*

## Twigs

"As the twig is bent, so doth the tree incline."[2] Sutherland used this quotation to illustrate his belief that minor uncorrected cranial defects in the newborn (twigs) led to gross physiological deformation in the adults (trees).

Long before birth the fetus can sense its environment perfectly well acoustically;[3] in fact, some sounds are actually louder to fetal ears than they would be in the outside world because water – the amniotic fluid that the fetus floats in – conducts sound better than air, and since the ears evolved in water[4] they cope with it superbly. This may even mean that some babies are born with hearing damage if their mothers had occupations that exposed them to high noise levels. There seems little doubt that the baby is already bonded at birth with not only the mother's body, but also his parents' voices.[5]

A newborn baby has no sutural interlocking or interdigitation between adjacent cranial bones. The bony plates of the cranial vault are free to float like icebergs in an elastic sea of membranous dura. "The mechanism" of fontanels, pliant cartilage, tender membrane, open sutures, cerebrospinal fluid, and falx and tentorium has evolved so that what is, evolutionarily, a huge head can pass through a small birth canal intact.[6,7,8] This is achieved by progressive and controlled cranial implosion.

If these molding mechanics were not over-whelmed by an abnormally long duration of compression[9] in the birth canal, or by drugs, vacuum extraction, forceps, or fear, the newborn's head will be "right" within three days.[10] It will have come through birth within its stress limits, and it has its own mechanisms for correcting itself. The reciprocal tension membrane carries its own tissue memory blueprint, which shepherds individual cranial bones, and groupings of bones, back into the optimum position they had in utero. The inherent tension and elasticity of the reciprocal tension membrane ensure this.[11] Crying and suckling reflexes help mold the newborn cranium; so does each breath. The cranial wave and natural rhythms of cranial expansion and contraction also help restore normal cranial physiology.

A prolonged birth may over-reach the capabilities of the tissues, resulting in a distorted bony cranium that does not normalize within three days,[12,13] or three months.[14] Visible deformity and lost articular motion incurs mechanical and neurological penalties, though perhaps long-delayed. These can relentlessly pursue the individual from cradle to grave.

## Why Parents Seek Craniosacral Work for Their Children

Parents usually call a craniosacral practitioner because their child's head does not "look right." The second most common presenting complaint is an absence of the suckling reflex, which may be connected to excessive slobbering, and difficulty in swallowing. Parents also become concerned with extreme restlessness and crying, which is perfectly understandable. Another common worry is suspicion of a developmental delay. The infant should:[15,16,17]

■ Roll from back to abdomen unassisted by five to six months of age
■ Be holding his head up controllably at six months
■ Be sitting erect at six to seven months
■ Be crawling by ten months (cross-crawl) and standing soon after
■ Be walking at one year
■ Be attempting verbal communication at about eighteen months

(This is an interesting replay of our evolutionary sequence: 500 million years of evolution replayed fast-forward in 18 months. Rolling is an oceanic, sea-serpent movement, from which the infant moves to the four-legged cross-crawl that mimics quadrupeds, to the desire to climb – dating from our arboreal time – through the emergence of strident bipedalism, and finally communication through speech.)

## Assessment

In treating an infant, start just as you would with an adult, in respect and wonder. Wipe away any condescension: this may be a small being, but not an inferior one. This is a hypersensitive conscious medium that responds instantly and continuously to the smallest shifts in your heartfulness and intention, as well as to variations in the quality and force of your own field. If you are having a bad day, and are harried, you may be upsetting the infant's equanimity. On a bad day, you may have difficulty tracking him and sensing his cranial wave, but if he is not obsessed with himself, he will be tracking you unerringly.

Start by sitting quietly with the infant. Take off your street armor and discard "gaining mind" and any sense of chronological impatience. The infant is in a different relationship to time; a minute to him is ten to an adult. Move into your glamour and soften and fine-tune your sensitivity to its greatest availability. Tune in to his soul state, talk to him and sense his richness, potential, and gifts. Then perceive what ails him, and how this is manifesting. Once you can sense what the trouble is, move to an assessment of what can be done about it. Then start your work.

Remember to step back frequently to adjust to what is actually present.[18] An infant will respond to your intention and physical input five to ten times faster than an adult.

## Treatment

Children rarely sit or lie still for craniosacral work. There are three strategies to consider that will at least minimize their craving for motion. The first, with an infant, is to have the mother breast-feed him, which takes up to ten minutes on each breast. Stand over the mother's shoulder and work from there, as the infant suckles. You will have to base your treatment upon bone position and energetics as it is extremely hard to sense the cranial wave in the midst of voracious feeding activity.

The second option is to work while the child sleeps, or before he gets overly tired in the evening: dusk is the best time for this. The third option is singing: if a parent or sibling can sing a lullaby while engaging the infant in eye contact, you may have sufficient time to complete your work.

### Examination Protocol for the Distressed Infant

Start your physical examination at the feet, perhaps, or the heart, as going straight to the head is more frightening for the infant. (This is true with children as long as the sutures and fontanels are open.) Hold the feet and wait until you can register a complete breath there. If there is no detectable cranial wave at the feet, move up to the hip sockets and check their mobility. Test full hip-joint circumduction, remembering that at birth all of the joints are composed of cartilage. Full hip-joint circumduction, repeated several times over a period of minutes on one hip at a time, usually "jump starts" the cranial wave in infants who lack it.

If the pelvic girdle still has no cranial wave after circumducting the hip joints, move into lumbosacral decompression and spinal unwinding. With a newborn baby you can use a core-link hold, cradling the pelvis in one palm and the cranium in the other. You can do this over your table, or with the child suspended above your lap, which is more reassuring for him. Infants instinctively like this contact, and it gives you the freedom to unwind the spinal column, the atlanto-occipital area, and both the cranial base and the cranial vault.

After hip circumduction and core-link unwinding, move next to a contact with one or both femoral trochanters, with the other hand deployed on the sacrum. Begin to pump the tiny sacrum by very gently taking it into flexion and extension alternately, emphasizing flexion to induce a flexion cranial wave, while externally rotating the femurs at the same time.

Check eye movement, and bear in mind how vital the sphenoid is to eyesight and the external eye muscles.[17] If the breath moves properly, the eyes will roll easily and the buttocks will seem to be floating as you do a supine sacral treatment.

The infant's body is so malleable and interrelated that even the normalization of a fibular subluxation can release a frontal overlap. Think of the connective tissue as a giant sheet of plastic wrap enveloping the whole body. It's all connected. Press at one point and stress will mount, or recede, at another.

### Unwinding

Unwinding is the technique of choice in working with children; it is natural, effortless, and they immediately know what you are doing. After all, it was not so long ago that they floated in their own secret inner sea and swam their own unwinding patterns, with the occasional exuberant kick at the mother's abdominal wall thrown in for good measure.

### Archaic Wounds

Archaic wounds come in early.[19,20] Remember that children's relationship to time is quite different to that of adults until late puberty. They experience a traumatic event as taking up an inordinate amount of time in their memory. A bad thirty minutes at the dentist is remembered in a child's dreambody as the equivalent of two weeks to an adult – it has an enormity of shock to it that is hard for adults to grasp, unless we can remember what it was like ourselves. So when you move into discussing a trauma with children old enough to tell you about it,[21,22] bear in mind their relationship to "time domains." Children remember[23,24] in emotional time, not in chronological or sequential time. They greatly expand that which was – or is – emotionally painful.

### Treatment Options

Treatment possibilities for work with infants and children are listed below. Corrective contacts may be taken up anywhere except on the fontanels.

■ Contact with the occipital bowl and orbital ridges, like a Frontal Cup and Straddle contact, is good for normalizing brain motility.
■ Use a very delicate Temporal Palming contact to correct rotational lesions of the atlantoaxial joints.
■ Employ deep lymphatic drainage to the parotid gland, the area immediately posterior to the angle of the jaw, and the anterior triangle of neck areas. This is especially useful to free the atlanto-occipital area of congestion, and it usually helps relieve mastoid congestion or inflammation.

■ Use a quad spread or lateral structures technique such as Temporal Palming for skull molding. Use a direct, gentle, and progressive approach to get results. Be careful not to frighten the child.

■ Use Temporal Auricle Decompression or a tiny One-Handed CV4 to mediate correction to the temporals.

■ Use any of the sacral or iliac techniques to normalize the hips, sacroiliac joints, or pelvis.

### Epilepsy

The basic energetic dissonance in epilepsy is that one hemisphere is "excited" and absorbing most of the cortical electrical activity. When the imbalance becomes overwhelming, there is a sudden and overpowering shunt of electrical energy[25] across the corpus callosum into the dormant hemisphere, which results in body convulsions similar to those induced in electroconvulsive therapy.

To work with epilepsy, use spanning contacts, directed energy, and an inner intention of great calm. Your focus is to diffuse the field and encourage both hemispheres to work together. Consider using the following techniques:

■ Clear the Confusion
■ Directed Energy to the Mammillary Bodies
■ Sphenoid Air Sinus Drainage
■ Middle of Man
■ Frontal Cup and Straddle, with neck unwinding
■ A coupled contact where one hand is at, or anterior to, the vertex and the other covering Wind Palace (Governor Vessel 16, located at the atlanto-occipital joint) on the neck; sending energy through the falx

## Summary

Although infants will not be able to tell you in words when something you are doing upsets them, they will certainly tell you by wriggling, screaming, biting, or trying to disengage your hands from their "home." When what you do is "right," they let you know with euphoric burblings, bubble-blowing, and ecstatic still points. They wriggle their little toes happily when a compressed suture opens up.

Sense what the infant needs, how much he can handle, and when the reciprocal tension membrane has enough elastic memory to spring "the mechanism" out again. Stop when you are ahead; have the child brought back another day, rather than overloading his "mechanism."

# 36
# *Bad Backs*

## Evolution

In the past 3 million years we have doubled in body size.[1,2] In the 30 years to 1991, European and North American youth added 5 inches (12.7 centimeters) to the preceding standard of average height at age twenty-one.[3,4] The bigger and taller we become, the more the leverage and pressure on the low back increases, especially when we bend over to lift a weight. Little wiry fellows get on much better with their backs.

Neurologically, the back is the most insensitive area of the body: we are only able to locate a pin prick with an accuracy of within 3 or 4 inches (7.6 to 10.7 centimeters), while sensitivity on the face is within a fraction of an inch (1 or 2 millimeters). Like the gills we have in embryo,[5] or the deep-diving reflex on our foreheads, the vulnerability and insensitivity of our backs comes from evolutionary choice. It may represent the last remnant of some ancient back armor,[6] a discreet version of the enormous projecting plates of the dinosaurs, or simply the way our nervous system has parceled out a finite amount of sensitivity.

Bending the back forward to work or lift seems effortless at first, because we are so dimly aware of the muscle work going on. In our legs, we feel strain immediately and know to stop using them, to straighten up and rest.[7] We often don't feel the pain in our back muscles, except dimly, until it is too late and the continued lifting and forward-bending has resulted in the underlying disc becoming first stretched then injured. The bipedal posture, adopted some 5 million years ago,[8] makes more demands on the intervertebral discs than knuckle-walking did. It is arguable that our spines have not had a chance to adapt.

Our backs are indeed insensitive, taken for granted, and vulnerable. Sitting in chairs aggravates the back, with further exacerbating factors coming from poor diet, poor posture, stress, driving, working in offices, and lack of outdoor exercise. Human beings, after all, were not exposed to this admixture of factors until the advent of the industrial revolution, just 300 years ago.

But the deepest causes of the disc fractures and nuclear protrusions that are the immediate sources of most back pain are psychological and spiritual. Serious back pain is foreshadowed in the individual by a profound sense of a loss of support from those closest to him, a loss of social status and self-esteem (especially in men), or a loss of direction in life. The carelessness of depression or heartbreak makes us more accident-prone, and more liable to hurt our backs.[9] Impatience, fatigue, and negligence brought on by overwork make Friday afternoons the peak time for the occurrence of sudden and debilitating back pain. The back is also where we tend to stuff away our shadows, and that hurts us too. In body language, when we "turn our backs" on something, we ignore it. We certainly ignore our backs themselves, until they get our attention.[10] Thus, back pain can mirror aspects of our shadow (that is, our unconscious) that we have attempted to "put behind us" or "place out of sight." Thus, while there are many causes of back pain, the most important are often the closest to the soul and to what D. H. Lawrence termed "life's mistake."[11]

Statistics make it clear that low-back pain is a major cause of distress in the Western world.[12] By the age of thirty, approximately 90 percent of Western humanity has experienced at least one acutely painful and debilitating episode of low-back pain.[13] In the United Kingdom there are 5,000 disc operations a year.[14] In the United States, 60 million people suffer from back pain, with one person in five experiencing back pain during any given two-week period. More than 100,000 laminectomies are performed each year in the United States.[15] Forty-five million working days are lost each year because of back pain, and $2.4 billion (1988 dollars) is spent on temporary measures like pain killers and muscle relaxants.

In 90 percent of their investigations into patients' low-back pain, medical doctors find no cause, no matter how many tests (e.g., MRIs, X-rays, blood tests, and CAT scans) they order. Metastases, or secondary eruptions from a cancer elsewhere in the body, are the most common disease (note: *disease,* not injury) affecting the spine, but they account for less than 1 percent of low-back pain.[16]

Craniosacral work offers highly effective ways of working with both the causes and symptoms of most kinds of spinal pain. It also offers education, understanding, and self-help tools to the often bemused and usually needy client.

## Anatomy and Physiology

Intervertebral discs permit the strength of bone to be married to the sinuosity of skin; they are what allow snakes to slither and swim. Quadruped discs, like those of the great apes, have evolved to allow freedom of movement and shock absorption for an almost horizontal spine. Apes sit, but they don't sit confined by chairs. All-fours mobility means that the lumbar spine naturally stays in lordosis (slight backward-bending), which keeps the disc essentially invulnerable. Watch a gorilla's free, swaying walk and you see nature's answer to the prevention of disc injury: perfect lumbar posture and stable flexibility.[17]

### The Discs

The intervertebral discs are composed of a central jelly-like nucleus encapsulated by concentric rings of tough and flexible cartilage called the annulus fibrosis, a harder version of the cartilage that composes our ears. Cut across its horizontal axis, the disc looks like an onion cut the same way, with the exception that a human disc has a nucleus (the nucleus polpusus, or "pulpy nucleus") at its core. The nucleus is encapsulated so effectively that when a person lies on his back it still has a resting pressure of forty pounds per square inch[18] (about 2 Bar), which is more pressure than supports the average car tire.

Discs have no blood supply. They keep their tonus through movement and the continual absorption and elimination of a fluid likened to

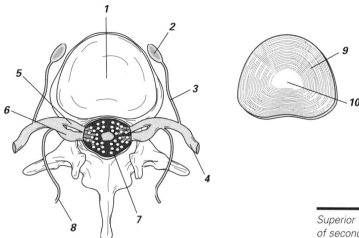

synovial fluid. At the age of eighteen the annulus is 72 percent water, the nucleus 81 percent. At the age of thirty-five the water content decreases to 65 percent and 78 percent,[19] respectively. As long ago as 1724, R. Wasse[20] calculated that we lost slightly more than 1 inch (2.6 centimeters) in height each day due to standing and sitting. We regain the lost fluid, and height, whenever we lay down for an extended period.

### The Spinal Cord

The spinal cord lies immediately posterior to the discs, separated by 1/8 inch (3 millimeters) of spinal ligaments, fat, dura, arachnoid tissue, and cerebrospinal fluid within the subarachnoid space.[21,22] The spinal cord is an elongation of the brain, and of course an extraordinarily vital structure. If the cord is chemically irritated, physically vibrated, or even slightly compressed, some degree of pain, numbness, or loss of function occurs. If the cord is emphatically compressed or sustains heavy internal bleeding, paralysis occurs below the level of the injury.

Because the spinal cord is so vital, it has additional protection in the form of the spinous and transverse processes, stout bony projections that help shield it from external injury. (It is also protected by large groups of dense and deep back muscles.) While the bony arches do form an effective armor plating, they restrict the cord to a tightly defined space. With the slight (5 percent) elasticity of the spinal dura and the malleability of the fat surrounding the dura mater, the cord has some room to move, but nowhere it can escape to. Its freedom is also limited by the distal attachments of its spinal nerves.

## Dysfunction

### Axial Compression

When we stand, the discs begin supporting the weight of the body above them, which is referred to as "axial compression." If an individual weighs 150 pounds (67.5 kilograms), the axial compression to the fifth lumbar disc causes the pressure on it to rise to more than 150 pounds per square inch (10.2 Bar), considerable pressure for an organic structure to cope with. A. Nachemson found that if the pressure on a disc was taken as a nominal 100 when a person stood upright, it dropped to 70 when he lay supine. Standing pressure increased to 150 when he stood bent slightly forward, and to 210 when bent well forward. Lifting a weight while bent forward resulted in a pressure exceeding 400. When seated, pressure was 150 if seated straight, 180 if bent forward, and 270 if bent far forward.[18,23] Sitting, bending forward, and especially forward-bending accompanied by the lifting of weight all cause the nucleus of the disc to begin to push, or "squish," toward the rear of the disc, creating a bulge in the annulus fibrosis. If this posture is habitual enough, the posterior rings of the annulus begin to stretch, and therefore weaken. When this person then lifts 20 pounds (9 kilograms) at arm's length and then bends forward, axial compression propagates the disc posteriorly in the same way, and the already weakened disc begins to bulge further.

### Bulging Discs

With bulging discs, the client will typically experience back pain at the level of the bulge, accompanied by some degree of pain or numbness if the bulge presses on a nerve root, felt along some or all of the distribution of the affected spinal nerve (it usually radiates down a leg). The client will also experience muscle "self-splinting" – an instinctive body reaction whereby muscles stiffen over an area or a joint in an effort to reduce the chance of any further damage from underlying injury (whether a ruptured disc or a broken bone).

In the low back, this self-splinting chiefly affects the iliopsoas[24] and sacrospinalis muscles.[25] Self-splinting is an immediate effect, not a cause, of back trouble. The client may be unsure of the causative incident, and there may be no single precipitating cause. Bulging is more the result of prolonged sitting, and long-term laxity in posture combined with a lack of exercise. Common sense tells us that it may be exacerbated by obesity, but statistics seem, at first glance, to dispute this.[26] On closer examination, the orthodox concept – that most obesity occurs at or below the level of the

affected disc, and therefore does not increase the pressure upon it and predispose it to distress – is suspect. Locomotion is markedly affected by lower abdominal, thigh, and buttock obesity.[27] The resulting postural and locomotor changes are bound to adversely affect fluid lumbar integrity[28] and the passage of delicate cranial wave formations. The way that low-back pain responds to the correct use of the self, as demonstrated by Feldenkrais Work[29,30] and Continuum,[31] seems to confirm this hypothesis.

If the spinal nerve irritation from a bulging disc in the lumbar spine is minimal, but the bulge presses on the posterior longitudinal ligament or the spinal dura, referred pain is felt in the overlying muscle tissue, and/or the sciatic nerve when the client raises his leg (the Lassegue test). Pain in the lumbar area may also be brought on if the client raises his neck when lying supine. Neurological insensitivity in the low back area means this muscular pain takes up to twenty-four hours to manifest.

### Fractured Discs

Disc fractures have the same causes as disc bulging, but are more serious. The outer rings of the annulus fibrosis do not simply bulge, they fracture (or "tear") and create pain if they push into a pain-sensitive structure such as a nerve root, the posterior longitudinal ligament, or the acutely pain-sensitive spinal dura.[32] Again the pain is referred along the spinal nerve or into the muscles of the low back, and is felt in the sciatic nerve when the client raises his leg, or neck, when lying supine. All the client may have noted at the time he was forward-bending and lifting was a slight popping sound in his back, which he then forgot about as there was no immediate pain. Thus, the client may at first be unsure of the causative incident, but if you ask him to review the past twenty-four hours he can invariably recollect the cause.

### Ruptured Discs

If pressure on the stretched annulus continues beyond the stage of bulging or fracture of a few of the outer rings, the annular rings may tear completely and the nucleus will then rupture posteriorly. As in bulging or fracturing, depending on the site and extent of the rupture it will apply pressure to nerve root, ligament, or spinal dura. If the rupture is central and extensive, it will apply pressure to both sciatic nerves. In rupture there is immediate, immobilizing pain, experienced as being "like a knife in the back." It may be accompanied by acutely painful involuntary "rolling" or "squirming" sensations in the low back musculature. The sufferer doubles up on the floor, in severe pain and, when he can manage to get there, takes to his bed.

If a spinal nerve or the spinal dura is pressed by a ruptured nucleus, changing the position of the spine may move the nerve or dura enough to reduce the pain. Muscle self-splinting usually produces an "analgesic posture," where the client leans over to one side, a position that reduces pressure on the rupture and therefore diminishes its impingement on the nerve root or spinal dura.

Some 42 percent of all disc lesions occur at the fourth lumbar joint.[33] If the disc bulging or rupture occurs at the disc between the fourth and fifth lumbar vertebrae, the fourth lumbar nerve may be affected, possibly leading to pain in the inner quadrant of the buttock, the posterolateral aspect of the thigh and calf, the medial border of the foot, and the medial aspect of the big toe, which may tingle. (There may also be pain on the dorsal surface of the foot.) The client senses that the pain originates in the mid-lumbar area or the iliac crest and will point there if asked to locate its origin. Fourth lumbar joint lesions may also compress the fifth lumbar nerve (see below).

About 37 percent of disc lesions occur at the fifth lumbar joint (i.e., the lumbosacral joint).[33] If the disc protrusion occurs between the fifth lumbar vertebra and the first sacral segment, there is likely compression of the fifth lumbar nerve, leading to the typical analgesic posture and sciatic nerve pain distribution that osteopaths see every day, extending down the posterior thigh, knee, and calf to the lateral border of the foot and outer three toes. It sometimes affects the lateral half of the big toe. Compression of this nerve often leads to referred pain to the superolateral buttock area of the compressed side, but this may also be due to muscular hypertonicity in the gluteus medius, piriformis, and coccygeus groups, itself either causative of a sacral imbalance that may have predisposed the lumbar disc to rupture, or caused by fatigue from prolonged holding of the analgesic posture. This posture is usually, but not always, a lateral flexion (side-bending) away from the injured side. The ability for supine straight-leg raising is diminished.

In severe cases of compression of the first sacral nerve, sciatic pain will radiate from the upper buttock to the toes, leading to pain, numbness, and loss of muscle power. When the rupture is central and sufficiently extensive that it presses on the sciatic nerves on both sides, surgery seems to be the only effective remedy.

***Pathology*** There is a basic rule of thumb in tissue pathology: once a tissue is severely injured it heals by downgrading into a simpler, less specialized form. Skin, for instance, heals by forming scar tissue. Scar tissue is inferior to the original skin in that it usually lacks sweat glands, hair follicles, some pigmentation, and elasticity.

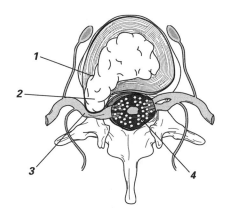

Some medical authorities say that the disc, once fractured enough to allow a rupture, does not heal.[34] Other medical evidence, based upon the six-month "spontaneous cure" rate, supports the possibility of some limited healing.[35] The protrusion may diminish in size if it is located external to the posterior longitudinal ligament.[36] Some healing of the disc fracture does *seem* to occur, but the improvement the client experiences may have more to do with a reduction of self-splinting, and of spinal nerve inflammation, than with the knitting together of the disc fracture. In the future, the fracture may open up with less provocation than an uninjured disc would need to tear. For instance, if the client lifts a weight with a careless posture, sleeps in a soft bed, or spends the night in an airline seat, his back may let him know within hours that it is over-stressed. Because of the presence of the unhealed fracture, some degree of local self-splinting may be ongoing. Undamaged disc(s) adjacent to the wounded area tend to accommodate more motion, which may stress them, and predispose to further injury.

***Referred Pain and Self-Splinting*** The old medical perception was that low back ache was due to spasm in, or overwork of, the low back muscles. This is but one part of the picture – it is rarely true that only the muscles are involved. While the muscles are affected, their misuse or overuse has allowed a bony displacement or a loss of natural cranial wave movement, which is the primary cause of the muscle pain.[37] Mistakenly assuming the muscles were the causative factor, treatment was directed at easing the painful spasm, which was thought to be an isolated problem with no connection to a disc or a facet joint, let alone the spirit. Heat, massage, and corrective physiotherapy were (and still are) applied, and millions of dollars wasted each year in this comforting but otherwise useless ritual.[38,39] While "self-splinting" in disc rupture is responsible for the analgesic posture as depicted on page 381, it is of critical importance to realize that if the underlying disc rupture remains, it may be unwise to remove self-splinting through the use of muscle relaxants.

The fact that low-back pain disappears *immediately* when corrective manipulation or craniosacral work is given both illustrates and proves the relationship of muscular back pain to disc injury. Neither heat nor massage can accomplish this, because they do nothing to remove the underlying cause of the malaise. The blueprint level, the place that things come from, has not been touched, let alone listened to, or redressed.

## The Causes of Back Pain

### Trinities

There is a saying in the aircraft industry that there are always at least three causes of an aircraft accident. If a plane is flying at night at 33,000 feet (10,000 meters) within easy gliding distance of an airport, there is no cause for alarm if all of its engines suddenly fail; this is just one cause. But if because of an altimeter failure the same plane is flying much lower, say at 10,000 feet (3,000 meters) you have a second cause, making things more serious. If a third factor is added in, say that the navigation system also fails, making it impossible for the pilot to find an airport or flat landing spot, you have the strong likelihood of disaster.

In clients with bad backs, watch out for threes: hurry, fatigue, and anger; obesity, stiffness, and lack of emotional support; or driving, heavy lifting, and a poor diet. Learn to perceive such trinities when you ask a client what happened to cause his back pain, and keep inquiring until you get the whole picture – if you miss one element of the causative trinity, your treatment will not be as effective, and may even be futile. I sense that I have the real thing when I can make a cognitive picture of what happened. If one cause is missing, something does not *feel* right. Be sure you find the human element – it is often withheld (after all, no one wants to admit to having done something stupid).

### Forward-Bending and Rotation

Severe disc injury usually occurs when lifting something heavy is combined with both forward-bending and rotation. As noted earlier, forward-bending in order to lift a weight more than triples the pressure on lower lumbar discs. A healthy disc can handle a superimposed axial compression of 1,000 pounds (454 kilograms) without damage[40] – almost twice the world-record weightlift.[41] But an already weakened disc may rupture with as little

as 50 pounds per square inch (3.2 Bar) of axial compression. When we bend forward the discs are suddenly vulnerable. With forward-bending, rotation, and lifting, the annular rings of the disc tear, having already been stretched and weakened by slouching, and the nucleus bulges away from the point of maximum axial compression, in a posterolateral direction. (The tear is rarely in a purely posterior direction, because of spinal rotation and because the posterior longitudinal ligament is ⅛ inch [3 millimeters] thick there, whereas it is much thinner – about ¹⁄₃₂ inch [0.8 millimeter] – at its lateral extremities.) If pressure on the nucleus is high enough, and the torsion and forward-bending posture tortuous enough, the nucleus ruptures through the tear in the annulus like juice from a crushed orange, impinging onto a nerve root, or the spinal dura (occasionally both).[42] The vulnerable spinal nerve gets propelled into the posterior wall of the intervertebral foramen and may impinge on the facet joints, the anterior part of the capsular ligament, and the lateral border of ligamentum flavum. There is no doubt to the sufferer what movement caused it; the pain often transfixes him in mid-movement.

*Jean injured her back while toilet-training her two-year-old son Arthur. It was a narrow bathroom in an old London house, and to pick him up she leaned forward, then rotated to reach the door handle. Arthur's weight held at a slight distance coupled with forward-bending and rotation proved too much for her fifth lumbar disc. She collapsed on the floor from sudden, excruciating pain. (Had she backed out of the room, separating forward-bending from rotation, everything would likely have been fine.)*[43]

### Peak Occurrence

More people hurt their backs on Friday afternoon than at any other time. (For similar reasons, the last ski run of the day is statistically the most dangerous.) We are in such a hurry to get things finished before the weekend that we do not take proper care. We are usually tired too, and often in ill humor. Left alone to finish the job (no support) and with just one more heavy thing to move, we say to ourselves "oh well, let's get it over with," and because we are tired and irritable we do it in a sloppy, careless way. Any time that we put hurry, fatigue, and anger together we have a volatile trinity. Using intelligence, taking a leisurely tea break to consider how to move something deftly, or admitting defeat are all far better than suffering months of disability from a disc injury. Coughing or sneezing while bent over can also overstress a disc; better to stand up straight before the explosion!

### Psychological Components

The most common situation causing back pain in men is pregnancy – their wives' – particularly during the third trimester. At this time a man usually feels a lack of sympathy, support, and appreciation, yet cannot express these feelings easily, as he sees all that his wife is going through herself.[44] But his world is also turned upside down, and his wife may be so preoccupied with her pregnancy that she forgets that he needs support as well. The more sensitive reasons that led to their relationship may be forgotten, as the couple prepares for the upcoming birth. The frequency of male back pain at this time was confirmed by a British study that showed that men get back pain more often during the third trimester of their partner's pregnancy than at any other time. The peak age of occurrence was twenty-eight.[45]

The phenomenon of a perceived lack of support from a loved one is a consistent factor in back pain,[46] but generally the spouse equivalent in question hates to hear about it. Be careful not to take sides. See the whole picture.

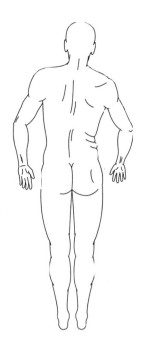

*One client showed me his X-rays, which displayed severely compressed and deformed lumbar vertebrae. Compressed as if by lifelong weight. "Who has he been carrying all this time," I wondered? "What stresses in life have worn him away in his place of support?"*

*I touched on the matter, briefly. Did he feel supported in life? Tears welled up. He shook his head mutely. On instinct I asked him if he felt that his mother had supported him. "Never!" Did he feel supported by his wife? He bit his lower lip, but this was followed by a quick flash of optimism – "Maybe she'll support me now that it is proven I'm so sick!"*

*I saw the woman in question, in his company, some time later. He said to her, "Hugh says I need some support from you in my life, that I lack support...." She tossed her head and replied disdainfully, "Oh, yes, still looking for your mother." He had been looking for his mother in her. But she wanted a lover and a husband, not a son. The impasse settled in his spine.*

### Chairs

Sitting in any kind of chair is hard for the back. For Western bodies, unaccustomed to sitting on the floor, there is no easy alternative. President Kennedy had a tall desk installed in the Oval Office so that he could work standing up, which eased his chronic back pain. It may take years of

yoga and stretching exercises to reach the point that you can sit, kneel, or squat easily and for long periods on the floor, but all of these postures are ultimately better for the back than sitting in a chair. (It may also help men avoid the kind of prolonged prostate congestion that may be one predisposing factor among many in prostate cancer. This may be one reason that the Chinese incidence of prostate cancer is one-fiftieth the American rate.[47]) Chairs take away the natural flexibility and load-sharing contributions of the legs and keep the pelvis relatively immobile. Thus, claims for "orthopedically designed" seats have to be seen in light of the fact that siting in a chair, in and of itself, is bad for the back. (It doesn't mater how well the prison is designed, it is still a prison.) One study showed that 12.6 percent of worker's back pain was caused by prolonged sitting; when sitting was interposed with standing, only 1.5 percent of the workers developed back pain.[48]

Car seats, no matter how well designed, are also small prisons.[49] Bicycles and motorcycles are much healthier for the spine, if not also the soul, as they are usually designed so that the heels are directly below the buttocks, which allows a free and naturally effective slight forward curvature of the lumbar spine. Truck and bus drivers, who drive in a more upright position, have a better basic position than do car drivers. Economy-class aircraft seats offer few blessings, except that you can leave them to move about the cabin frequently, which makes a dramatic difference, as the statistics above demonstrate.

### Beds

Soft beds exacerbate and may even be one cause of back pain. I consider a futon, the Japanese cotton fold-up mattress, superior to all but the best orthopedic "wonder bed." Because a futon is much firmer than almost all conventional spring mattresses, it takes some getting used to, and a small percentage of people with injured backs simply cannot acclimatize to them at all. In this case, using a spring mattress with a board underneath is to be preferred. The disadvantage of staying in bed during a back pain episode is that it leads to a loss of muscle tone throughout the body, rendering the spine less stable upon the return to the upright posture.

During a back crisis, it is better for the client to sleep on the floor in a sleeping bag – if he can manage it – rather than any bed except a thin futon. The only time not to utilize the floor is when it is cold and damp, or if the client is so slim and bony that he cannot get remotely comfortable. Placing boards under a springy mattress is better than nothing, but still pretty futile.

I remember my father, an osteopath in Scotland, working with a policeman. The man had been called to a pub to quell a disturbance, and had been beaten up by three men for his trouble. A disc ruptured, leaving him on the floor, bent double. Unable to work, he took to sleeping on the floor on my father's advice, and found that it gave him tremendous relief. A new problem arose when, a month later, he realized that he enjoyed it so much he did not want to rejoin his wife in bed.

### Surprise

One of America's star gymnasts was in college shortly before the 1988 Olympics. Upon enrollment, he and his coach had gone through the lists of available classes and credits and chosen those that would fulfill his educational goals yet not create any undue risk to his gymnastic development. No football, no metalworking ... but theater sounded fine.

One day during theater class the gymnast was helping paint the set for the forthcoming production of King Lear. In walking to the middle of the stage to pick up a two-gallon (eight-liter) can of paint, he bent down and rotated slightly so that he could heft it without breaking stride, but collapsed mid-step in agonizing pain. Unexpectedly, the can was empty, and his unresisted jerk caught his spine unprepared. He missed the Olympics.

### Speed

Arm, back and leg muscles seem to work at different speeds. Most nerves conduct impulses at 200 feet per second, but some sensory fibers associated with touch conduct at only 3 feet per second.[50] (Heart muscle spreads its wave of contraction at 70 feet per second.) Leg muscles seem to trigger into action that crucial little bit faster than back muscles do. Lifting slowly can make the crucial difference between elegance and injury. It seems to allow us the integration and coordination time to keep the back and its discs protected.

### Sexuality

Sexuality and the will to live are the two strongest forces within us. Natural sexuality has the power of a force of nature, like a tidal wave or volcano. If bottled up, the dreambody suffers, particularly in the low back and pelvic areas. (The low back houses the sacral soul center.)

How we relate to our sexuality is largely dictated by our conditioning. Most societies and many major religions (except paganism, Taoism, and tantric yoga) begin to impose comprehensive strictures on sexual behavior shortly after birth. Sex is condemned and so becomes secret, dirty, something to be done only in the dark of night.[51,52]

Sexual repression has not always been the case. Sometimes cultural condemnation becomes so pervasive that the only way individuals can have open and free sexual pleasure is through using alcohol or recreational drugs.

The low back, fun-loving and delighting in sinuous snake-like undulations, has a very hard time with Calvinistic messages. When a sexual being – and we are all sexual beings – is not sexually met, energy accumulates, or "backs up," in the buttocks, perineum, and lumbar spine.[53] The hands, desperate for tender touch, may develop arthritis in its absence. If sexual energy is bottled up, the sacrum becomes confused and rock-like, losing its cranial wave. A lack of euphoric sexual outlet condemns the back first to stiffness, later to rigidity. Soon this rigidity permeates the whole body,[54] as any sensual movement becomes somehow threatening, subliminally associated with sexuality. As this rigidity makes any vibratory movement taboo, the vertebrae and their discs, confined to a straightjacket, lose their cranial wave and begin a slow process of deterioration.[55] The discs, lacking open motion, become brittle, absorb shock less effectively, and fracture easily. The more sexuality is bottled up, the more angry – or depressed – an individual becomes.

In contrast, sexuality occurring within a deeply loving and supportive field becomes a spiritual experience.[56] The spiritual heart opens to the genitals and fuses with them, the genitals becoming its south pole. Tears of sexual ecstasy express the energy of the heart rising to the level of the inner eye. Tantric practice uses this energy to extend the field all the way to the Bindu ancillary soul center just posterior to the vertex, which is the north pole of the heart.[57]

### Diet

Even a short period of undernourishment, an imbalanced diet, or a diet of junk food is, in my experience, invariably implicated in low-back pain.[58] Do check for this, and encourage the client to improve his diet. Reducing or eliminating dairy products and sugar helps. Caffeine inhibits deep neurological rest, and healing generally does not start until relaxation reaches the level typically attained on the third day of a well-earned holiday – a deep, thorough letting go. If dietary changes are carried out, the back frequently responds positively within days. During an episode of back pain, as at other times, it is very important that the sufferer eat lightly but well, consume adequate first-class protein (one that contains all the essential amino acids), and drink plenty of water (to hydrate the disc). All of this will help recovery.

A person's attitude to food is synonymous to his attitude to love, and love, or its absence, is a central factor in low-back pain (as instanced in the client with the compressed and deformed lumbar discs, mentioned above). Taking care of ourselves by devoting more attention to diet means that we are beginning to love ourselves again. M.F.K. Fisher, called "America's greatest writer" by W. H. Auden in 1963, had this to say in 1943:

*People ask me: Why do you write about food, and eating and drinking? Why don't you write about the struggle for power and security, and about love, the way others do. They ask it accusingly, as if I were somehow gross, unfaithful to the honor of my craft.*

*The easiest answer is to say that, like most humans, I am hungry. But there is more to it than that. It seems to me that our basic needs, for food and security and love are so mixed and mingled and entwined that we cannot straightly think of the one without the others. So it happens that when I write of hunger, I am really writing about love and the hunger for it, and warmth and the love of it and the hunger for it.*[59]

## Healing

### Walking

Walking over rough country can totally normalize a bulging disc, a facet displacement, or a vertebra that has locked down in a rotated position.[60] What happens is that the "universal joint" movement of walking over uneven ground, especially for two uninterrupted hours or more, teases first the self-splinting muscles and then the displaced vertebra into loosening up. As the tissues loosen, the cranial wave returns, and the dreambody delights. At some point, the needed correction to both disc and spirit takes place on its own, nature's way.

Before suggesting this to a client, you must, as a responsible healer, consider his level of fitness. If he has not taken a two-hour walk for several years, this course of action would create more problems than it cures. You also must consider the degree of disc injury: when there is sciatica extending below the knee, do not encourage walking for more than ten or fifteen minutes at a time, if that. Where there are more pronounced signs of nuclear rupture, any walking will aggravate the situation.

### Siestas

My niece, at age four, called a siesta a "fiesta." I like the idea. Siestas are little treats for the back and the spirit. Little self-healings. Winston Churchill noted that "You must sleep sometime between lunch and dinner.... Take off your clothes and get into bed."[61,62] While everyone else was stirring in their milk during coffee breaks at National Security Council meetings, John F. Kennedy used to catnap, especially when there were tough choices that had to be made. He would wake up refreshed[63] after ten minutes, knowing exactly the right course of action to take.

A siesta is a definite asset for the spine,[64] especially if you can lie down. We are about an inch (2.6 centimeters) taller on awakening in the morning because the discs (especially the nuclei) absorb necessary fluid when weight is off them. (Astronauts gain 2 to 3 inches [5 to 7.6 centimeters] in space for the same reason.[65]) This is vital for disc health. Some absorption of fluid occurs during a siesta, and the psyche clears its desk. These improvements may be enough to make the critical difference in people with marginal low-back pain.

### The Nurturing of the Great Mother

In her inspiring book *The Solace of Open Spaces*, Gretel Erlich[66] meditates on the healing that open wilderness gives the soul. It is a baptism in the universal source. Despite Americans' enthusiasm for gyms, I have never been able to convince myself that such exercise does any real good, as there is no nurturing of the soul. My preference is for an hour a day outside. Walking in open spaces cures the spirit of its source of back pain. Aloneness can allow a great nurturing, a return to inner alignment to the spine.[67] Company can also help: if you can walk for an hour in the countryside and "talk out" your feelings with a good friend, you cannot remain in an anxiety state.[68]

### Soul Insights

In one of my classes, a chiropractor told the story of a client with low-back pain. The man was well-built, in his late thirties. She took X-rays and performed the necessary tests; nothing seemed seriously amiss. So she laid him down and began to do some sensitive cranial "listening" on his lumbar spine and sacrum. Suddenly he sat bolt upright on the table, and in a loud, clear voice said "I have to carry the spear!" He walked out, paying the receptionist on the run. The chiropractor knew he had found his own cure. She never saw him again.

### Time

In old Persia, a shaman and his apprentice are walking in the dusty foothills. Rounding the flank of the hillside, they see in the distance the stooped figure of an old man coming toward them. The apprentice, having studied hard with the shaman for ten years, is eager to show his skills. He bounds ahead of the shaman, and runs up to the old man. "Sir, I know what's wrong with you, I know, and what you need for what ails you is pomegranates!" The old man brushes him aside, irritated. He looks exhausted and despondent. Soon he reaches the shaman, who says, "Kind sir, you look tired. Pray stop awhile and share some tea – my eager apprentice here will gather us some kindling, and we can make a refreshment." The old man readily agrees to this warm offer.

It takes an hour to light the fire, unpack the kettle, suffuse mountain water from a spring half a mile away with tea chipped off his tea brick. Holding his own counsel, the shaman, by his very silence, allows the old man time to speak. It begins backward: where he is going today, which touches on his wife who died, to their wedding, to his father's farmhouse in spring. He tells his life story.

By the time they are packing up, ready to leave, the shaman turns to the old man and, in a soft, kindly voice, asks his permission to make a suggestion regarding his health. The shaman makes a deft, calming gesture with his hands; it is like a little ritual. The old man gratefully agrees.

"Sir, what you need for what ails you is pomegranates," says the shaman. The old man bows in gratitude, and gives the shaman three silver coins from his woven purse. He walks off, a different lift to his walk.

As soon as the old man is out of earshot, the apprentice, no longer able to contain himself, speaks up: "But I told him that. I told him that immediately!" "Yes," answered the shaman, "you were right, he did need pomegranates. But he needed pomegranates, and time."

## Treatment

### Overview

The "sacral" part of "craniosacral" work comes into play in the treatment of bad backs. The client who is in trouble is a sacred being who has lost touch with his spine, which is his core, his essence. In body language the spine is the primal structure, one of the very first to be formed after conception. Bone represents the immortal within us, and the spine harbors the core of our sense of permanence.

Begin your session by accessing "larger me" to discern the "big picture" of the client's life, for the spine is like the Red Road, the Native American term for the path through life. Spinal pain so often has its origins in soul confusion or soul loss. ("Soul retrieval" is a shamanic term that refers to the practice of returning to the time that the soul parted company with the body, and reconnecting the soul to the body by reexperiencing the primal trauma in order to exorcise its painful memory.) Your first three steps are to gain an understanding of who this client is, what really troubles him, and what is amiss anatomically.

- What distresses the soul?
- What is this? (A shot across his bows? A wake-up call?)
- Why did he need to break his back, or allow it to be broken?
- What does this pain represent in terms of his Red Road?,
- What is this not? (That is, rule out what is not present.)

Take a clear case history. Listen to every word said. What troubles the client most about this condition? Ask your own nagging questions; leave nothing out. Look for the "three causes," considering diet, posture, occupation, flexibility, sexual attitude, emotional issues, and the need for support in life.

Low-back pain limits movement. Consider asking the client if he feels limited in his movement or freedom by someone else, or by his own fears.[69] Ask him to give the first words that come into his head in response to the question "Who controls you?" Ask him what he would like to do about it, in ideal circumstances. Movement is totemistic within the dreambody; that is, it *means something* other than just simply being movement.[70] A movement in one place reflects the movement, or its lack, in another place, so watch the movement of the client's eyes as the questions register and the answers flash into awareness. Use peripheral vision to note secondary signals, especially of the feet. The feet often speak what the spine withholds.

Is his back giving out because his life is crumbling around him?[71] Is his back pain telling you that he has a "broken back" – something he is in denial of, with the pain acting to make him take notice? Has life broken him in two? Or, closer to the core, has he split himself in two?

### Treatment for a Bulging Disc

If the outer rings of the annulus fibrosis have torn but the nucleus remains encapsulated, lumbosacral traction with segmental craniosacral unwinding work to the lumbar vertebrae will usually allow the vertebrae to return to normal movement and position.[72] (Vertebrae tend to lock in the position they were in when the injury occurred: usually forward-bending and rotation.) Work with the psoas muscles, hip rotators, and coccygeus, and unwind the legs. Use the Sacral Steering Wheel and Sacrum Coupled with Symphysis Pubis techniques to release perineal tension. Consider prone perineal work for the same reason.

These injuries respond well because the nucleus has stayed in place. The client may come into the office in acute distress, yet skip out after one session of psoas release, leg and spine unwinding, and lumbosacral decompression.

In all types of low-back pain reducing obesity is an important consideration. But be careful – being mildly overweight is not necessarily bad for the back,[73] and by automatically encouraging weight loss you may not be perceiving the underlying cause of the back pain. Dieting also tends to make people miserable.

### Treatment in Disc Rupture

If the client has torn and ruptured a disc by bending forward and rotating at the same time, it is essential to return the vertebrae to the optimum alignment and movement when the time is right.[74] First, protective muscle spasm – self-splinting – has to be reduced. Consider the tonus of the iliopsoas and the related sacrospinalis, quadratus lumborum, latissimus dorsi, multifidus, and rotatores muscles. Work with the hip rotators and the muscles that attach to the sacral borders. This attention to the muscles facilitates emotional release, and insight. An adept combination of craniosacral work to the sacrum and low back, unwinding of the legs for the hip rotators, gentle lumbosacral decompression, and cephalad traction with the long levers of the arms often produces further insight and relief.

Bed rest reduces the self-splinting effects of local muscle spasm and often helps ensure successful craniosacral treatment. It may give the client the time and care he needs. The alternative to bed rest is careful, sustained movement, and attention to any underlying emotional issues.[75] Walking is probably the best exercise for disc injury; sitting in a chair is unquestionably the worst.[76] (Sitting cross-legged on the floor must also be avoided.) It will be obvious to you, but may not be to the client, that lifting of any kind is contraindicated. Coughing is best avoided – this is a time when cough-suppressant medication is often warranted.

When the nucleus has ruptured through the torn annulus and sciatic symptoms follow, treatment has to be more conservative. It is often possible to use osteopathic or chiropractic manipulation to return the extruded nucleus to its original place, which can bring about relatively rapid healing – a matter of three to four weeks may suffice. But there is also the worst-case scenario where axial compression has made the nuclear "cave" smaller than it was, too small for the nuclear protrusion to fully return into it. Then you have to wait for the body to begin breaking down and absorbing the extruded nuclear material, or refer the client for a surgical opinion.

While the tissues surrounding the fractured disc are healing, it is important to keep movement limited and sensitive in that area.[77] This allows for the maximum tissue health and elasticity to be retained. The deleterious effects of movement have to be weighed against its value in increasing blood supply and reducing muscle wasting. Individual advice based on a clear assessment of the degree of disc involvement is indicated.[78] Tailored exercise programs are excellent empowerments for the restless and self-motivated client.[79]

Pain killers do not heal. They provide a valuable function in dealing with distress, but are sometimes counterproductive, because they stop valuable feedback (pain) when the client moves incorrectly. Taken before a craniosacral session, pain killers may cloud diagnosis and interfere with good treatment. However, Valium or similar muscle relaxants, taken under medical prescription and supervision over a period of weeks in cases of severe pain and disability, do seem to be an asset: they slow workaholic people down, and enable them to rest.

The use of epidural injections of 2 percent procaine solutions in saline, administered by an expert physician, has been found successful in normalizing mild disc bulges and up to 60 percent of disc ruptures.[80] When craniosacral work is combined with epidural injections given by a licensed physician, it can be powerful medicine.

Surgical removal of the whole disc – a laminectomy – is better kept as a last-ditch option. C. N. Shealy calculated in 1973 that only one in ten laminectomies in the United States were justified at that time.[81] In its total laminectomy form, the operation has a failure rate of 10 percent to 20 percent, creating "23,000 cripples a year."[82] A partial laminectomy, to remove the bulge only, is preferable. Exploratory operations or laminectomies targeted to a specific disc based upon the pain distribution occasionally fail to find anything wrong, or have any effect. This is because some individuals have unique neurological pathways, where, for example, the fifth lumbar nerve is doing the job that would usually be carried out by the first sacral nerve. For various reasons, the surgeon may not explore the adjoining levels, and thus the operation fails.

I encourage my clients to try up to one year of alternative therapies before seriously considering an operation for a ruptured disc. When I worked in Santa Fe, a local orthopedic surgeon refused to perform a laminectomy until the client had tried at least one month of "conservative" therapy. When considering a laminectomy, keep in mind the failure rate. There is also the potential for future complications in that the neighboring discs are called upon to do extra work and can begin to bulge or tear a year or more later (especially if the client has not changed his lifestyle). At that point the client faces a slippery downhill slope. If he elects to have a second laminectomy – and many do – he ends up with further loss of motion and shock absorption, and a chance that he has now transferred the loads to other intervertebral discs or facet joints.

## The Dreambody's "Treatments"

Years ago, while teaching osteopathy in India, exhausted, alone, and careless (looking for a way out of an onerous schedule?), I tore my fifth lumbar disc. On the third day of bed rest, dozing at three in the afternoon, a dream came: I was in the jungle, walking with a friend. A Bengal tiger leapt out, claws extended, to seize me. In the dream, I jumped all the way across the clearing. What I actually did was drove myself, rolling, clear across the double bed, waking as I did so. There was a discreet and ecstatic snap. The pain, the muscle self-splinting, the full sciatica disappeared – everything was instantly gone. I thanked my dreambody, and its tiger.

## Other Treatments

All of the sacral techniques covered in the chapter "The Sacrum" are possible treatments, with the following considerations:

- Which technique, or combination of techniques would be most appropriate for this person?
- Where would an unwinding session fit in?
- What does he need?
- How can I provide that?

Remember to ask the client what he thinks is wrong. He will often know.

Consider using the CV4, since it can reduce muscle spasm in the low back and, via the core link, enhance sacral motion. Jaw release work also helps the low back, sometimes miraculously, by neurological reflexes and through deep energetic connections.[83] Unwinding work, or specific release work to the muscles, sutures, and joints of the stomatognathic system may all produce dramatic improvements in spinal pain, both in the low back and neck. (The thoracic spine often responds better to unwinding work with the arms and legs than to direct contact.)

*Lateral Thinking*   Sometimes what the client needs is most unexpected, meaning that you have to enter into what Edward De Bono calls "lateral thinking."[84,85] De Bono, a mathematician, was called in by a large company plagued by a high staff turnover rate. It had seemed that people were leaving in part because of the elevators – waiting for one to arrive took too long, and drove people to distraction. The wait was one of the most frequent employee complaints. De Bono was instructed to reprogram the operating software. He was not sure that this was the best approach, as it would be a long, costly, and perhaps unsuccessful "fix." He found another. He ordered full-length mirrors installed in every elevator lobby. Now instead of standing idly by, waiting for the elevators to arrive, employees were able to look at themselves in the mirrors. The complaints ended.

*Ice Packs and Hydrotherapy*   Applying heat to a painful back may feel nice and comforting, but an ice pack is more effective. Cold stimulates deep blood circulation around the disc, which speeds up healing, while heat tends to cause congestion and does not dull pain in the same way. Do not use an ice pack more than three times a day, or for longer than twenty minutes on each occasion – and never employ one if it increases the pain. The body responds to an ice pack in the following sequence: (1) a sensation of cold, which lasts from five to fifteen minutes; (2) numbness, from the prolonged exposure to cold; and (3) pain, the body's signal that it is time to remove the ice. Always stop the moment pain is felt from contact with the ice.

Having said that, a daily, hour-long soak in a very hot bath, keeping the spine in a slight natural backward curvature (lordosis), can be a valuable adjunct to bed rest, traction, manipulative therapy, and walking. It is technically inferior to the use of ice packs as a remedial action, but psychologically beneficial. Care needs to be used getting in and out of both bath and bed. The way most people get up – tightening their stomach muscles and jerking upright – stretches the posterior part of the discs explosively and leads to their gradual stretching and loss of tone, predisposing the individuals to disc fracture or rupture.

*Corsets*   The use of a corset specially designed for low-back problems can also be a valuable asset[86] for clients who absolutely must be at work tomorrow. Such corsets restrict irritating and unexpected movement and keep the spine erect, but they are emergency measures and no substitute for either bed rest, proper treatment, or conscious and constructive movement.

## Education

Once a disc has fractured to the annulus, that fracture will not heal. The client needs to understand that, while he may feel "100 percent" a few weeks after a bout of sciatica,[87] his spine is now more prone to injury than it was before. He therefore *has* to treat himself more carefully when it comes to weight lifting, posture, and soft beds. If he understands and accepts this, he can go off wind-surfing and otherwise lead a full, active life and rarely suffer a flare-up. It is a little similar to having a fractured cartilage in the knee: treated with care and understanding and not provoked, one can live with it perfectly well. If he does not accept it he may be in and out of the chiropractor's office for the rest of his life.

### Strength and Flexibility

Flexibility is more important than posture. Many clients want to know how to make their backs "strong" but, like the desire for immortality, the search for invincibility is doomed. There is no way to get the back muscles strong enough to overcome lax posture, carelessness, a loss of purpose or support in life, or the self-hatred that has its genesis in sexual inhibition. This matter necessitates clear understanding: in terms of both mechanics and muscle power, the back can never be invulnerable. It cannot absorb abuse and punishment without being damaged. Although there is no way to make the back indestructible, we can educate ourselves, and others, into making the back sensitive, responsive, flexible, and intelligent.

Our backs are an inherently unstable area of the body, in part because of the bipedal posture; in part because of the evolution of our large and heavy head; in part because of chairs, automobiles, soft beds, spectator sports, and an estrangement from the wild wilderness soul; in part because our psyche sometimes needs to quit and have some time out from standing up to the world ("I can't stand it anymore!!"), which is when psyche sends us to bed.

Strengthening the lumbar muscles rarely alleviates further back problems; it may, in fact, make matters worse.[88] If the muscles self-splint after a new injury, stronger muscles will create stronger self-splinting. This produces more severe pain and makes it harder for a practitioner to release the spasm prior to correcting the underlying vertebral displacement. As is often the case, acting out of fear causes trouble. Focusing on brute strength as the source of protection is more a cause of trouble than a prevention of it.

Vasily Aleksayev, the Soviet weight lifter, holds the world record in the snatch at 562 pounds (253 kilograms). In order to lift this weight above his head he took scrupulous care of his posture; if the lumbar spine is in a moderate lordosis it is virtually impossible for the disc to fracture or rupture. (Many weight lifters wear thick leather belts; these lend a modicum of support, but more importantly act as postural reminders.)

The Eastern model of a healthy body is based not on strength (the Western *idée fixe*) or trim appearance, but on flexibility and responsiveness.[89] There is an Indian observation that the strongest thing in the world is a blade of grass, because even when an elephant steps on it, it springs right back. Aikido, tai chi, yoga, and *chi kung* all employ careful and considerate techniques of how to use the body. In most forms of karate, for example, adepts are taught exemplary use of the back.[90] Nothing in tai chi is harmful to the back, and practice is excellent both to inculcate flexibility and as an exercise and meditation form. (The Shaolin monastic tradition of the martial art known as kung fu[91] taught novices to walk on rice paper laid on a coarse granite floor; once they could do this without wrinkling the paper, they moved to running across it; mastering that, they had to learn to fight on it. Such awareness of movement leads to excellent spinal mobility and posture.) Belly dancing represents an excellent Middle Eastern contribution to proper movement of the back, especially for postpartum women. The best Western equivalents to such dedication in the quest to master movement are ballet and fencing.

Whether the client has a bulging disc or a rupture, he needs to understand that doing something that is harmful to the back may not produce pain immediately. Objective guidelines are needed, since subjective experience is misleading. Basically, while recovering from a disc injury the client must avoid all forward-bending and all lifting of weights – even things as apparently inoffensive as purses.

Educate your clients while they are recovering that if they cannot reach the object to be lifted while in lordosis, they must find some other way to do it. When lifting, always separate forward-bending from rotation as the combination guarantees a fractured disc at some point.

### Patience

Men – and some competitive and impatient women – have to "try it out." Once the back starts to feel anything more than 30 percent healed, they start to test it. Men feel they have to test themselves – to see if they are *real men* once more (strong, capable, robust, able to carry a woman out of a burning house, that kind of thing). This is uniformly disastrous. Women, brought up with different conditioning and "hard-wired" with somewhat more self-caring genetic imperatives, seem able to be easier on themselves. (Perhaps this is all changing?) In any case, 75 percent of people with bad back accidents test their backs too soon, and suffer remissions.

*Charles, an author, was finally doing wonderfully. It had been a long slog, 3½ months of back pain. We had sessions twice, sometimes three times a week. Finally he was symptom-free – the dangerous time. I counseled him: "Just because it doesn't hurt doesn't mean it's better."*

*Four days later, a Sunday morning, he called me at home.*

*"I'm in agony ... can you come?"*

*"What did you do?" I asked on instinct.*

*"Well, I was feeling so much better, you know ... I woke up early this morning full of beans, so I went downstairs to fix breakfast for my wife. Once it was all ready, scrambled eggs, bacon, orange juice, coffee, the lot, I climbed back upstairs, set it down on the dresser by the door, and with a great flourish woke her up. A surprise! She looked so happy, I felt so well, I was so proud. I leapt on to the bed to join her, Superman-fashion. In mid-air I felt it go out. Oh my God, I thought to myself, here we go again!"*

There is a wonderful phrase in Chinese medicine, "going out onto the verandah." It applies to this "almost better" time. You have been sick and bedridden, perhaps it was your low back, and you feel like "the world has gotten you down." You wonder, often secretly, if you will ever be yourself again. Slowly, despite your doubt, things right themselves. One fine spring day you feel so good you can hardly believe it and you gingerly get out of bed and go out onto the verandah. And there is the whole world at your feet, bustling about, and you are filled with a new sense of joy and potential. You are ready to join in again!

But your back isn't. It is a difficult time to endure.

Another client had reached this stage, and his version of "walking out onto the verandah" consisted of moving the furniture around in his living room. It went fine. Then he turned to rearranging the bedroom. "Everything was great until that chest of drawers," he told me later that day. "I'd been in that damn room on my back for a month, and I never did like the drawers there. Promised myself, 'Tom, soon as you're better, you're going to move them so they don't block the swing of the door like that.' Down on my knees, shoulder against it to give it a good push, and *bam!* goddamn back went out again!"

Thus, educate your clients to recognize that healing is still going on long after the back pain or sciatica has disappeared. I advise allowing at least two weeks after the last awareness of pain before in any way stressing the area. If the client reinjures his disc before he has fully recovered, healing the second time around takes appreciably longer.

*Posture*

Once the client has recovered from an acute episode of back pain, it is more important than ever to pay attention to posture and what F.M. Alexander called "the correct use of the self."[92,93] Counsel clients to sit as little as possible, and stand (like John F. Kennedy) at work, or lie down. Teach the client to place his feet in a line beneath his buttocks (so that the lumbar spine can easily rest in an upright, gentle lordosis) when he absolutely has to sit. Teach him to stretch his large leg muscles – both the hamstrings at the rear and the quadriceps at the front – to free the lumbar spine of limitations imposed from the legs, so that it can "float in space" (as Moshe Feldenkrais espoused) and be able to cope with challenges without injury.

In 1973 I watched Moshe Feldenkrais at work.[29,30] A participant in the class, an Alexander Technique teacher, wanted him to define, once and for all, correct posture. But no matter how much he was pushed, Feldenkrais would not define it. He pointed out that there is no right posture, only the ability to move, to be flexible, not to get set in any particular pattern of use.

Reeducating clients to use and strengthen their leg muscles will transform the risk of exacerbating their disc injury from high to almost nonexistent. As discussed above, the insensitivity of our backs to muscular overuse is the result of an evolutionary parceling-out of sensitivity; thus, bending the back seems effortless, because we are so dimly aware of the muscle work going on. In our legs we feel strain immediately and stop using them, straightening up to rest. We don't feel the pain in our back muscles, except dimly, until it is too late.

Once a client understands that this insensitivity is not something to take advantage of, progress can be made and the legs can be put to their proper use. The legs have at least four times more muscle mass than the low back, so in lifting or moving weights it is wise to let them do the work. If your legs hurt, rest them until they can take it again. To use the back and bend forward to lift heavy weights just because it feels okay is asking for trouble. An old Jewish expression is apposite here: "You can do whatever you like, you just have to pay for it later."

*Kibadachi*, or the horse-riding stance used in karate, is one way to train the legs to take a flexible share of weight-bearing. Stand with your legs as if you were on the robust girth of a horse. Rotate your big toes all the way inwards until the lateral aspects of your feet are parallel to each other,

much as you might need to do if on a real horse that was galloping over uneven ground. Tuck in your pelvis. Use this posture when you have to lift a heavy weight. It will become second nature to do so in about six weeks if you practice *kibadachi* daily for five or ten minutes, keeping the knees bent the whole time.

The best way to get out of bed is to lie on one side first, then push yourself up with your hands. This way you can stay in lordosis and avoid both stretching and rapid pressure increase on the discs. Feldenkrais floor work teaches an even more elegant way to get up from laying down, based on spiraling up using the legs as long levers. This is well worth learning and teaching to your clients. It is simple, effective, and fun.

### Summary of Advice to Clients

Educate your clients that:

- An accepting, understanding attitude towards yourself helps.
- Getting impatient diverts needed energy away from healing.
- Trying to continue life as before means you have not gotten the point. Continue as before and you will get back pain as before, or a subsidiary symptom.
- Pain so often comes to teach us. Listen and learn.
- Quietly resolve not to make the same mistake next time.
- Devote ten minutes each day – less than 1 percent of your time – to exercises to strengthen your leg muscles: perform Feldenkrais exercises, or do some yoga in the correct posture. This will give you a much better chance of being not only pain-free but healthy. Take up tai chi or walking (the American Medical Association now advocates that you walk for a minimum of one hour per day in order to maintain basic health).[94]
- Practice, be aware, understand, be patient, and take your time. And watch out for Friday afternoons, "trinities" of stress factors, the accumulation of sexual longing or sexual repression, hurry, carelessness, and fatigue.

# 37
# *Headaches*

The first recorded description of headache – a migraine – was inscribed on a clay tablet in Mesopotamia some five-thousand years ago. Today, forty-two million Americans a year consult a physician for headache treatment.[1] Statistics show that 78 percent of women and 64 percent of men experience at least one headache a year and 36 percent and 19 percent, respectively, experience recurrent headaches.[2]

Headache sufferers seek out craniosacral treatment. Understanding the origin of a client's headaches means sensing how they fit into his world and how the world fits, perhaps too tightly, around his head. It means perceiving which of his attitudes toward himself (in particular) and life (in general) give him "a pain in the head." It has been proposed that there is really only one form of headache, but that its intensity varies from mild to excruciating. This chapter divides headaches into the most commonly recognized types: muscle-contraction, migraine, and cluster headaches.

## Muscle-Contraction Headaches

This is the simplest and most commonly occurring form of headache. The majority of people who suffer from muscle-contraction headaches are women, and 40 percent have a family history of headache.[3] These include the "Not tonight, dear, I've got a headache" types, where the cause is self-explanatory, to the social headache that excuses you honorably from the meeting you did not want to go to, essentially the same phenomenon.[4] Muscle-contraction headache tends to arise when there is a high degree of conflict in a social situation. Social pressure, including that of conditioning, tells the client to do something that his soul does not want to. He may not be able to verbalize a "no," but he can manifest a headache.

If these headaches become repetitive,[5,6] physiological and emotional change occurs, such as moodiness, withdrawal, hair loss, eye strain, chronic shoulder and neck tension,[7] and temporomandibular joint deterioration. "I want to bite but I dare not, so I bite down on myself instead." The body has to do something with the energy repressed by the freeze response imprinted on the temporomandibular joints, and tends to store it as muscle tension.

We need to talk after stressful events, like being berated by the boss. In ancestral terms, we would sit around the campfire at night and an individual, using great expansive and fierce gestures, would describe how earlier that day, crossing the vast savanna, he had met a saber-toothed tiger, in fact two saber-toothed tigers, and stood his ground. Raising a spear, he glared in their eyes and the tigers thought better of it and slunk off. The truth is always more complex, involving as it does aspects of our own behavior that we are ashamed of, confused about, or just do not understand. The truth may be that he wet his loincloth, ran the wrong way first and nearly got killed, and then by some miracle got himself up in a tree before knowing how he did it.

This verbal exorcism, a tribal rite of healing, is a natural antidote to stress and terror. We desperately need to "talk it out," to exorcise it. To better communicate the enormity of our panic we exaggerate, if not actually rewrite, the script. We glamorize our own role, deleting our stupidities. But we get it "off our chest" and out of a terrified nervous system. Our latter-day tribe (whether spouse, child, buddy, or bartender) hears us out, takes it all with several pinches of salt, sympathizes, and soothes our ruffled feathers. The sense of security that community gives us assuages our deep terror.

Put the same person in a situation where he can't talk – perhaps he feels humiliated and decides to keep quiet – and the event and fear he felt becomes a deep secret, a wound to the soul, an archaic wound buried in the body. His field changes, and a tight spiral of energy winds up around the masseter muscles, which have been ordered to "clam up." Six months later, his head starts to hurt from the pressure the hypertonic masseters are exerting onto the sphenoid via the mandible, zygomae, and maxillae. The muscle-contraction headache may begin a process of self-punishment, like banging his head against the wall in an effort to free the sutures. A year later the individual may develop temporomandibular joint pain, five years later cervical arthritis. Ask such a person what troubles him and his field suddenly goes all funny: it clamps down. This is where you see people instinctively shaking their heads when you ask what is wrong. (The shake itself is an instinctive effort to free "the mechanism.") They clam up and cannot tell you. They have been clamming up for so long it seems they cannot break the pattern, but the headache is doing its work, and forcing them to wait. Wait for them to begin to talk and soon the truth and storytelling come out, perhaps all mixed up, in a never-ending flood of disclosures.

The jaw, in particular, may hold tension. Prognating the jaw is a primary fight signal: it shows our readiness to fight and to bite.[8] (We had a mean array of teeth 10 million years ago![9]) Talking about a traumatic event afterward not only eases the psyche, it gets the tense jaw and masseter muscles unwound and loosened up too.

Postural patterns in response to stress include the submissively lowered head (which acknowledges shame but also covers the vulnerable throat); the tightened fists that eventually become arthritic; and the neck that was ready to jut forward to fight, but was reined in, and kept reined in, leading to chronic suboccipital restriction, tinnitus, and atlanto-occipital joint compression. Shoulder muscles that were primed to punch tend to never let go of their preparatory tonus unless given real permission and opportunity to relax, such as with craniosacral touch, a movement meditation like tai chi, or Continuum floor work. They lead to more stiffness and eventual local arthritis, and further deterioration in mobility at the cranial base via the trapezius, levator scapulae, and sternocleidomastoids.

Muscle contraction headaches tend to occur between four and eight in the morning and four and eight in the evening (an easy mnemonic),[10] times when the psyche is closer to the surface, communicating its needs and dissatisfactions in an inimitable way.

### Other Causes of Muscle-Contraction Headache: The Constant-On Engram

The innervation pattern to a particular area at a particular time is called the "engram," derived from the Greek word for "a trace." The brain fires signals to muscles on an on/off basis. Like a light switch, the chemical-electrical-neuro-transmitter current to a muscle is either on or off; there is no in-between. In a "constant-on engram," the current is switched on, there is constant firing, and the muscle contracts continuously. The healthy rhythmic, or intermittent, contraction pattern is displaced and an emergency pattern instituted.

An overloaded nervous system produces a constant-on engram and results in mandibular tension through the following mechanisms. The nucleus

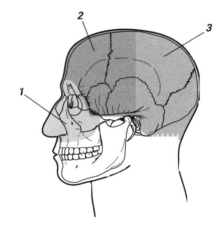

*Headache distribution*

*1 Headache originating in eyes or sinus network*
*2 Headache originating in cerebral arteries, meninges or cortex*
*3 Headache originating in cerebellum or cervical spine*

for the motor division of the trigeminal nerve is in the part of the brain stem called the pons, extremely close to the reticular activating system – which it had to be in our earlier evolution to allow us to bite an adversary instantly in the event of a surprise attack. In a very stressful lifestyle, especially one encompassing multiple kinds of stress – airline travel, changing time zones, social pressure, a disjointed sleep schedule, care deprivation, and alcohol, caffeine, and sugar abuse – the reticular activating system becomes hyperactive; overloaded, some of its electrical excitation begins to spill over into the trigeminal nerve motor nucleus. This stimulates the muscles controlled by the trigeminus, especially the muscle groups for the lower jaw, which then go into the "constant-on engram."

This becomes a vicious circle. The already overloaded reticular activating system is further stressed by the new pain in the jaw, which stimulates more of its electrical activity near the trigeminal nucleus. The jaw muscles tense even more, the temporomandibular joints are compressed and become painful, and associated muscles (such as those at the back of the neck and the front of the throat) also tense. Muscle contraction headache and temporomandibular joint and neck pain begin, all adding to the overload on the reticular activating system. To make matters worse, the primitive automatic response to pain is to tighten up, which in this case only worsens the pain. Unless some dramatic change occurs, such as a vacation or the forced recumbency of a migraine headache, the situation tends to self-perpetuate. The dreambody's way out is to make you collapse and go to a safe warm bed.

As we have seen in Chapter 27, in acupuncture frontal headaches are also considered to have possible large intestine involvement.

### Types of Muscle-Contraction Headache

**I: The Secret Headache** Headache also occurs long after physical trauma, especially if the person could not talk about the trauma in a meaningful and cathartic way. I am thinking here of a German woman who, twenty years previously, when she was just eighteen, had left home at four o'clock one morning with three friends to go to the Nürburgring to see the Grand Prix. The group's driver had taken methedrine ("speed") to stay awake, and under its influence got into a race with another car on the deserted pre-dawn roads. Approaching a metal bridge over a river, the driver lost control and the car flipped and crashed into the pedestrian guard rail – the only thing that saved them from drowning. The car was totaled. The woman in question had only a small cut on her occiput but was in deep shock, hardly able to stand. Her main concern was that her mother would find out about the accident – she was starting to break away from home, and these friends were precisely her way out. She knew her mother would blame the accident on her friends, so as she made her way home by bus she bottled it all up so that her mother would never know what happened. Unable to tell anyone about her experience, she held a psychological scar and began a cycle of headaches instead.

Twenty years later in a craniosacral class, someone touched her occiput, and the whole thing came back, smell first, then visual recollection: the downhill slope to the bridge, the wet road, the dark, the music inside the car, the smell of Gauloise cigarettes, the excitement of the pre-dawn race, and then that awful crash. With her injury physically touched, she rejoined the trauma, but this time could also talk it through to release it from her body. She could tell twenty people about it, as if around the campfire. Four years later her headaches have almost disappeared.

**II: Membrane-System Headache** One woman suffered a severe whiplash injury when she was sitting in her car at a traffic light in Texas and another car hit her at speed from behind. While she did not lose consciousness, she was concussed and a blinding headache took hold within several hours. Two days later, the headache subsided, but was followed within hours by the gradual onset of low-back pain. For two years she sought out many different treatments for the back pain, but nothing worked. After our first craniosacral session, I felt that something crucial had moved into place in her low back. When she got up off the table at the end of the session, she remarked, "Why, this is wonderful. My back is free of pain." Very encouraged, she sailed across the room. I still remember how she reached for the door handle and suddenly something caught in her. I saw her field collapse. She turned around slowly, eyes wide, and said "The headache is back."

This is an unfortunate example of the accommodation that the dura and reciprocal tension membrane make to trauma. An area of very high survival importance – the cranium – managed to displace its dural trauma to an area of much lower survival importance – the lumbar spine.

**III: Physical-Abuse Headache** During a slide show on the sphenoid during a craniosacral class in Zürich, a delicate forty-year-old blonde, who had suffered from headaches of no known cause since childhood, found these words coming into her consciousness: "If a mother knew how delicate the head was, she would never squeeze there." She noted to herself that this was a funny thing to think, but then let it go as a curiosity, and thought nothing more of it. Then, later that day, laying on the table with her partner touching her sphenoid, she went pale and began to get distressed. Her head started to hurt. The partner called me over, and I took over with the assumption that the partner had faulted the sphenoid.

"She's pressing too hard," the student said as I began to touch her sphenoid extremely gently. "She's pressing too hard," she repeated. I was slow on the uptake, and did not realize for a few minutes that we were not in present time; it was not her partner who was pressing too hard, but her mother, and the time was not now, but thirty-seven years earlier. She followed her own desire to move and began thrashing her head back and forth, and screaming, transfixing a heretofore silently meditative class. The screaming went on for almost an hour, her voice alternating between that of a three year old and that of a mature woman violently angry at the abuse she had received.

By the time the storm had passed, she was pale, trembling, sweating, and limp from exhaustion. It had all come back to her: how her mother had tortured her before the age of five by squeezing her temples, her tiny head fit to burst. She had suppressed the whole memory. All she knew in ordinary time was what an aunt had told her – "When you were a little girl you never looked happy, you were always frightened, and you were sick a lot.... Your mother kept postponing leaving you with us."

I suggested she take the rest of the day off, perhaps write down what had happened, be quiet, find a good friend to sit and talk to. She gave me permission to share with the class what had happened; it had affected us all very deeply, the pain in her screaming was profoundly real. At four o'clock that afternoon, she came back carrying a very large Swiss chocolate cake for the class, beaming and happy, an enormous weight lifted from her psyche, a band of pressure permanently gone from her head.

Trauma to the head does not always leave headaches, but if unresolved and suppressed it can drain the field, and lead to a flat, dull life.

## Migraine Headache

An estimated 8 million Americans[11] suffer from migraines, which are commonly known as "sick headache." Fifteen percent of those under the age of forty suffer from migraines,[12] and although some people experience headaches only rarely, others have symptoms that can last several days several times a month, or even per week, making it difficult for them to hold jobs. Most people who get muscle contraction headaches also suffer from migraines.

Migraines come in a thousand different forms. One client said to me, after reading Oliver Sacks' exhaustive and definitive book *Migraine*,[13] "That fellow Sacks didn't know the first thing about migraines. He didn't describe anything remotely like *my* migraines."

Basically, migraines are a hemicrania, or "half-head" headache. Among sufferers, 60 percent to 80 percent have family members in concurrent or successive generations who also have migraines.[14] About 50 percent of sufferers have a two- to four-hour premonitional period before the symptoms appear, during which time they experience vague effects, such as a mild increase in sensitivity to light, loss of appetite, a feeling of being ungrounded, or mild dyslexia. (Craniosacral work is most effective at this stage of the migraine.) Twenty percent of sufferers see an "aura," or light display of some kind.[15] The actual headache is accompanied by a throbbing pain, nausea, and light and noise intolerance.

We have relied on our left hemisphere for hundreds of thousands of years, with the result that it is appreciably larger than the right,[16] making our whole nervous system fundamentally slightly out of balance, and therefore easily destabilized. Epilepsy,[17] migraine, and cluster headache sufferers all exhibit markedly increased left-brain activity, leading to distress on the same, or opposite, side of the head, depending on exactly which brain tissues are affected and the individual's specific compensatory habits and neuromuscular patterning.

Migraine is an extraordinarily sensitive psychogenic illness. This is illustrated by the fact that up to 40 percent of people with a migraine get better when given a placebo.[18] Some 30 percent of those who go to see their doctors while suffering from a migraine attack get better during the visit, before any treatment is administered.

### Migrainous Intensity

Intensity is a good key word to remember in the understanding of all forms of headache, but especially in migraines. Sufferers are often intense people who have forgotten how to play, whose intensity manifests in the way they excel in life, the way they make a living. Sometimes they become so focused on their work that it is almost the only way they function – as if the brain were a computer running their lives with only one program, the "work diskette." In order to change the migraine pattern you have to work with the client's relationship to his own intensity. The "migraine personality" is said to be perfectionist, obsessive, and possibly compulsive, sensitive, tense, meticulous, ambitious, and usually highly intelligent.[19,20] (All such classifications are somewhat inadequate, since they fail to do justice to our individual complexity, but they are a good place to start.)

### Types of Migraine Headache

*I: Saturday-Morning Migraines*  One of the most interesting forms of migraine is known as "the Saturday morning migraine." These occur in people who work very hard from Monday to Friday, riding roughshod over their own sensitivity, and need for rest, during that time. They are pushers, and often perfectionists. When Saturday morning comes around and they finally put their feet up, switch on the television, and open a box of chocolates – *wham* – on comes the headache. "Why me?" they say to themselves, seeming to negotiate their way through some feelings of guilt. "I've worked so hard all week, don't I deserve some rest?" They assume that the headache has something to do with the chair, or maybe eyestrain from watching television, or perhaps the chocolates. But what is really happening is that the dreambody is taking charge. It is not a question of the dreambody getting even: I don't think it is interested in revenge,[21] but it is certainly interested in balance,[22] in seeking an optimum homeostasis. What can it do with a personality who has been running full-on for five days, whose bloodstream is awash in caffeine, sugar, and adrenaline breakdown products? Well, fasting for twenty-four hours with complete bed rest in a nice quiet darkened room will do the job just fine, and a migraine ensures it.

**II: Menstrual Migraines** Thirty percent of women who suffer from migraines get their first migraine with their first period. After puberty women get two to three times as many migraines as men, while prior to puberty the numbers are the same. At least 60 percent of women suffering from migraines seem to do so solely as a result of changing levels in their sex hormones. (In body language, hormones seem to equate largely to feelings, so a woman's feelings about her own sexuality and fertility are obviously involved. Hormonal fluctuation does not occur in some mysterious void; it is both affected and driven by emotion, by the need to give and receive love, and by intent and attitude.) For these women, headaches occur only in relation to their menstrual cycles,[23] or while under treatment with sex hormones. Women who are prone to menstrual migraines may not get a migraine with each period, however.

Menstrual migraines seem to stem from an abrupt drop in blood estrogen levels, which also produces fluid retention and breast tenderness. Estrogen-based oral contraceptives may set off, or exacerbate, menstrual migraines. The medical administration of estrogen for other purposes worsens headaches in 50 percent of female migraine sufferers.[24] Elevated prostaglandin levels are also implicated – prostaglandins increase the nervous system's sensitivity to stimuli like pain, light, and noise, so that normally comfortable sensations become unbearable.

Most menstrual migraine sufferers find great relief during pregnancy, when blood estrogen levels remain continuously high. At menopause, they enter a changing of the ways, where the migraines may disappear forever, or become more severe.

### The Chemistry of a Migraine

The understanding of headaches has been deepened by the work of brain and orthopedic surgeons, who have documented the sensitivity of soft tissues in the spine, the dural membranes, and the brain tissue itself.[25] The actual chemical sequence that leads to a migraine has been less amenable to discovery. It seems to begin with a local scarcity of serotonin (a neurochemical), itself probably initiated by stress, with a resultant dilation of the superficial temporal and middle meningeal arteries. During the migraine itself, cell receptors for serotonin turn on and serotonin begins to overwork, and therefore be consumed faster.[26] Serotonin also inhibits the release of endorphins, our natural pain killers. Local hyperactivity in the cerebral cortex seems to cause additional, sometimes isolated, chemical changes that affect the parts of the arachnoid and dura mater that are pain-sensitive, inflaming them and leading to trigeminal nerve pain, and modified trigeminal functioning, whose effects include further changes in blood-vessel dynamics.[27]

Once the migraine biochemistry has kicked in, a wide variety of symptoms begin to occur. These may begin with the appearance of the "aura,"[28] which is some form of disturbance in the visual field. It may be a halo appearance of light at the periphery of the visual field, a borealis-like shimmering in the sky, or partial blindness. One man I worked with would sit down for supper but not be able to see the plate right in front of him – there was only a black hole.[29] The aura is often followed by hypoglycemic symptoms, or a feeling of being on the verge of mania, as if you'd drunk too much coffee. Nausea, vomiting, cold sweats, and pain – typically in one-half of the head – mark the arrival of the full migraine. This is usually accompanied by photophobia (increased sensitivity to light), ultra-sensitivity to noise, and an eerie and pronounced change of mood. For some people the first sign of migraine is vertigo; a cranial nerve is still affected, but rather than visual symptoms, it is balance that is affected.

It is interesting that these latter symptoms are very like the experience of having a hangover, pointing to similar liver and water balance involvement. Whether the migraine is due to intensity, the Saturday morning effect, or menstruation, it often has a strong dietary component. Caffeine, alcohol (especially red wine), aged cheeses, milk, overripe bananas, and anything made from cocoa all may predispose a person to, or bring on, migraines. Some people are also sensitive to lima beans, figs, onions, potato chips, MSG, and birth control pills. Others have their own "pet" triggers, such as the smell of gasoline, or cigarettes.

As the French will tell you, the liver is both the seat of the soul and the foundation for robust health. They have a point: the liver and its close associate, the gall bladder, seem to be the parts of the body most associated with biliousness and malice. Unexpressed resentments and anger are definitely part of the migraine makeup, especially to be suspected in people who make a great show of being nice and polite but are in fact emotional "holders." Holders make excellent soldiers: the most common illnesses suffered by U.S. infantrymen[30] are migraine, cluster headaches, and kidney stones. Liver dysfunction is reflected in right-sided headaches, right-sided sinusitis, and pain in the right leg.

Be watchful of the client who is unable to express his anger; particularly watch for the "flat affect" – the monotonous verbal delivery of someone who seems to be operating on a limited emotional plane. Folk wisdom has it that:

- Underneath the dutiful person is the angry person.
- Underneath the angry person is the fearful person.
- Underneath the fearful person is the guilty person.

When we are deeply connected to our emotions and feel able to express them, and not be holders, we communicate our feelings effectively and appropriately. This clears the dreambody of the tendency to accumulate the tension that leads to a headache. Margaret Thatcher, accused by a British member of parliament in early 1993 of making "an emotional outburst" in response to genocidal events in Bosnia, replied forthrightly: "I'm very proud to be an emotional person. Everyone should be connected to their emotions!"

Skipping meals, becoming dehydrated, and having an irregular sleep schedule all predispose a person to migraines, as does air-conditioning – especially arid aircraft air-conditioning – and most types of fluorescent lighting. Hence, airline flight attendants are particularly susceptible.

### Treatment

Migraine is one of the areas where craniosacral work really excels. Specific work with the sphenoid,[31] maxillae, and mandible represents the most powerful way to both prevent and interrupt migraines. Maxillary position and motion,[32] or its absence, seems to have a leading role in migraine causation, making Sutherland's Grip the best single craniosacral treatment for migraine. It is a good idea to teach your clients how to do this on themselves as a self-help tool.

Gentle manipulation of the cervical spine, performed by appropriate health-care providers, relieves migraines in a minority of clients.[33] For similar reasons (probably to do with internal carotid artery sympathetic innervation), deft craniosacral work to unwind the mandible and upper neck is always worth trying in the first two hours of a migraine.

Most migraine remedies on the market are not reliably effective and tend to have strong side effects, such as sedation and nausea. They do not address the underlying biochemical mechanisms of migraines, nor the psychological components. Narcotics are sometimes used to blunt migraine pain, but they cannot stop it. Sumatriptan, a drug introduced in 1991 that is chemically related to serotonin, seems to act by returning the dilated arteries to normal; it, and the ergotamines (which also work on brain receptors), are the only medications that can stop a migraine after it has established its grip. Sumatriptan can even dispel a migraine in its fourth hour, which is long after craniosacral work is likely to be effective.

Biofeedback is a valuable addition to the preventative treatment of migraines.[34] When experimental subjects using biofeedback technology master the ability to increase blood flow to the head, they find that they can stop a migraine attack in its tracks. It has been reported to me by several students that sexual activity, especially orgasm,[35] often averts an oncoming migraine; the mechanism by which this works is probably similar to the mechanism mastered in biofeedback. Researchers have also had success reducing migraines by limiting sleep to 7.5 hours.[36]

## Cluster Headaches

Cluster headaches tend to occur two to three hours after the sufferer has gone to sleep or two to three hours before he would normally awake. He is woken up by intense pain in one eye, usually brought on by alcohol consumption. Cluster headaches create pain so severe that sufferers consider, and occasionally commit, suicide. The headaches are so named because they occur in dense clusters, with two to five headaches a day for up to six months at a time, and in rare cases the headaches last up to a year.[37] This devastating period is usually followed by a much longer pain-free period, sometimes as long as two years. Unlike migraines, cluster headache pain may subside after a very short period, thirty minutes if the individual is fortunate, up to three hours if not.

Learn to distinguish migraines from cluster headaches. The typical migraine sufferer finds a quiet, dark place, lays down, and feels horrid, but knows that within twelve to thirty-six hours it will be gone. The cluster headache sufferer is in such acute agony that he (90 percent of the sufferers are men) will pace about the room, unable to sit or lie still, and may even bang his head against the wall (or solid iron objects like fire escapes) in an effort to shift the pain or distract one part of the brain by hurting another.

Some sufferers have cluster headaches that mirror muscle contraction headache patterns, with a marked diurnal (twice-daily) pattern. (Migraines have no such pattern.) There is no "aura" in cluster headache, but the superficial temporal artery does dilate, as in migraine. Cluster headache pain is described as piercing, burning, or stabbing, steady and intense; migraine pain as throbbing or pulsating. In 90 percent of cluster headache sufferers there is no family history of the headaches; in migraine there is almost always a family history.

In cluster headache, the pain is usually most intense in one eye, just behind the eye, or at the greater wing of the sphenoid on the same side. It occasionally radiates down into the neck, around the eye, or into the jaw. In migraine, the pain usually localizes on the forehead or temple, but occasionally the head is hurting so unpleasantly that it is hard for the sufferer to tell which part is most affected.

During the cluster headache attack, one side of the face weeps. The skin sweats, the eyes water, the nose runs, and the mouth salivates. The eyelids of the affected side swell, and the sclera reddens. It is as if the soul, unable to do it in the ordinary way, has found a way to cry. The denied part of the psyche can finally come out and express its displeasure. Cluster headache brings with it sinus congestion as part of the weeping face phenomenon.

Drinking red wine during a cluster headache episode will definitely make things worse. During the pain-free months, it seems to be no problem, but the liver may be becoming congested, contributing to the onset of the next episode.

Ninety percent of cluster headaches occur in men, 60 percent of migraines in women. Most cluster headache victims are heavy smokers and many are heavy drinkers. They almost always deny both, with justifications to the effect of the following:

*Well, yes, I have a tequila sunrise when I get up, but lots of people do that. Okay, yes, sometimes two. Mid-morning, a stiffener like a shot of whiskey, but most of my friends in business do the same. And there is nothing wrong with a couple at lunch, especially business lunches, is there?*

*Cigarettes? Well, yes, I do smoke a few. Maybe a pack a day. On weekends. During the week I smoke a little heavily, the pressure you know, and everyone else smoking makes matters worse.... Yes, come to think of it, it does rise to two or three packs a day. But not always.*

There is no comparable drinking and smoking pattern in migraines sufferers, although liver overload plays its part. Consider the high incidence of cluster headaches in the U.S. infantry as a clue to the type of men who suffer from it. Cluster headache men have typical one-liners, delivered with a particular, almost military, clipped intensity:

*I had almost achieved everything in my life that I always wanted, when these damned headaches came along and screwed it all up!*

*Everything I have ever set my mind on achieving, I have achieved. (This delivered with awesome ferocity.)*

*"If I could only get rid of these headaches, my life would be freed up a lot." ("Freed" is the key word for understanding and treatment – free the sutures, free the driven attitudes, free the imprisoned person.)*

### Types of Cluster Headaches

*I: Macbeth Types* There is a distinct psychological profile to the cluster headache male. The first headache tends to be between the ages of twenty and forty, although occasionally much younger or much older. These men tend to be "Macbeth type" – that is, basically affable, reasonable, easygoing men who have bonded with women who are extremely ambitious, and project their ambition onto their spouses. Think of a recent American president and his petite but very willful wife. The cluster-headache sufferer tends to have a large-boned, ruddy complexion, heavy facial features, a pronounced nose, *peau d'orange* (orange peel) skin, and many small broken blood vessels on his face. They are often led into the therapy room by a small, petite wife who does not volunteer to leave. Sometimes a "cluster head" individual is lean, hard-looking, and in extension (tall and thin). The head has lost its fluid, flexible softness; it has become an armor. Tender psyche has had to hide deep inside.

*Driven Men* If sufferers of cluster headaches are not the "Macbeth type," they tend to be driven, highly ambitious, and hard on themselves ("hard-headed"). Their life has been a tremendous push, brought up short by the appearance of their headaches. These are goal-oriented people with tendencies to compulsiveness. Or they may be like the migraine personality – conscientious, persevering perfectionists, highly self-sufficient, responsible, and resourceful – but are also tense, overwrought, and often caught up in denial. They tend to say things like:

*Oh, yes, I get to bed early, keep regular habits. But then I lie there and get to thinking, you see. I look over to the far side of the room and see the video machine, and I remember about the*

| A Comparison of Headache Symptoms | | |
|---|---|---|
| | **Cluster** | **Migraine** |
| **Nature of pain** | Steady, intense, piercing, boring, or burning pain | Throbbing, pulsating pain at the temple or on one side of the head |
| | Located either in the. eye, forehead, or temple, sometimes radiating down into the neck, around the eye, the region behind the orbit, or into the jaw | Exacerbated by exercise |
| | Not exacerbated by exercise | |
| **Duration** | 15–90 minutes | 2–72 hours |
| **Who has them** | Much more common in men (90%) Heredity is not a factor | More common in women (60%) Heredity is a factor |
| **Attack pattern** | Typically, two or more times a day for a period of three to sixteen weeks, usually followed by pain-free periods of months or years | Not usually clustered; attacks may occur anytime, and pain is often present on awakening |
| | Attacks often early in the in the morning, or two to three hours after retiring | Also "Saturday morning" migraines, "menstrual migraines," and those related to diet |
| | Other patterns include pain between four and eight in the morning and evening | |
| | Typical clusters occur once or twice a year | |
| **Advance warning** | None | Often visual, nervous, or mental symptoms, like dyslexia, or seeing an aura of flashing light |
| **Other common signs and symptoms** | Sinus congestion or stuffy nose, unilateral or bilateral facial sweating flushed facial appearance, *peau d'orange* (orange peel) skin | Nausea and vomiting, phonophobia (intolerance of noise) and photophobia intolerance of light), pale facial appearance |
| **Diet** | During headache, red wine brings on an attack; at other times can seemingly drink it with impunity | Rich diets predispose to migraines: cheese, liquor, chocolate, and red wine |

**Note:** Persistent headaches are a common symptom of brain tumors, especially those headaches that occur at night or upon awakening. Clients exhibiting such headache patterns must have the possibility of tumor ruled out – without delay – since prompt diagnosis and treatment is often lifesaving.

*reprogramming I promised my wife I'd do. So I get up, just a few minutes you understand, and set it up for her. I turn it on to check that it is working all right, and there just happens to be a program on the stock market, so I watch that. Then it's one in the morning and I remember that I can get the BBC on shortwave, so I listen to that while I see if I can catch up with my reading on the latest in laptops. One thing just leads to the other. My mind never stops. Sleep? Well, I suppose from three till six. But that's often enough for me. There is so much to do before I leave for the office.*

If they are fun-loving types, those with cluster headaches take their fun to extremes, like one client who is a surfer and seems to *have to* travel the world in search of the perfect wave. (Not such a bad way to live!) But some element of easy-come, easy-go is missing; there is a relentless compulsion to it. Being overly self-sufficient is a component of the cluster headache personality type.

One client I worked with who suffered from cluster headaches had a difficult time at grade school; reading and learning were difficult for him, so he did what he was good at – working with his hands. He achieved real mastery with craftsmanship. He said to me, "Whatever I have ever set my mind to achieving, I have achieved. I've found my own way in life, and I've done very well! Now, I want you to tell me how I can get rid of these damn things once and for all. I will do anything to be free of them."

I suggest learning meditation, indicating that perhaps this would begin to soften his driven lifestyle.

His response: "Well, but why? Why should I meditate? What is it good for?"

I suggest that it is good for the soul.

"Nothing airy-fairy about me, mate," he replied. "I don't believe in the soul. There is no soul. Prove to me there is a soul!" he replied, his face instantly reverting to its rigid and mask-like defensive look.

# 38

# *Brain Tumors*

The incidence of brain cancer has risen more than 20 percent in the past twenty years.[1] People who have brain cancer or tumors seek out craniosacral treatment, so it is advisable that you keep abreast of the latest developments to enable you to be of the greatest service to your clients. To deepen your understanding of tumors, read the scientific and medical literature, talk with oncologists and other health professionals, and learn what treatments are available.

Beginning in the early 1980s, the Center for Disease Control in Atlanta, Georgia began to track an exponential increase in the incidence of certain types of brain tumors in certain age groups in the United States.[2] For instance, central nervous system lymphoma increased by 300 percent in the ten years from 1980 to 1989. In the twenty-one years between 1968 and 1987, deaths from brain tumors in the United States and western Europe rose 200 percent in people sixty-five years of age and older.[3] Only a small part of this recorded increase was due to AIDS, and to improvements in the technology of diagnosis and detection.

Powerful emotional forces – such as devastating loss and repressed anger – also seem to play a part in cancer formation, and loss of purpose in life, especially if it is associated with loss of spiritual purpose and vision, or the loss of one's life dream, may prepare the ground for tumor formation. Typically, there is a seven- to ten-year delay between the stressful event and the detection of the tumor. Changes in factors such as diet, smoking, and the electromagnetic environment may take up to forty years to manifest as a brain tumor.[4] On the positive side, medical science has now proven that regular exercise leads to a reduced rate of all types of cancer.

The dreambody loves to grow, to evolve in heartfulness and spirit. There is often sense to be made of the hypothesis that when we stop growing, errant cells within the body start growing for us. There is another level of truth acknowledged in the expression "there are no accidents" – that everything is ordained, or karma, or "written." But there are also accidents – life, and cellular physiology, is too complex for there not to be.

During the heated debate over Ronald Reagan's Strategic Defense Initiative, popularly known as "Star Wars," a senior engineer from Bell's major telephone research laboratory gave evidence that in a large city with over five million telephone receivers there was an average of one or two truly "phantom" calls per day – that is, calls were made to a telephone number that no one had dialed. Factored into the projected complexity of the Strategic Defense Initiative, phantom electronic events would produce crucial and disabling errors. Applying this to the body, itself an electric medium,[5,6] you can only wonder at the cellular errors produced by a cranial "telephone exchange" consisting of 100 billion cells.

## Factors in Nervous System Disease and Tumor Formation

Here are some of the known factors that may predispose a child to neurological injury, or brain tumor formation. The same predisposing factors can likely be considered ingredients in the incidence of brain tumors in adults.

### From a Child's Father

The male reproductive tract is exceedingly vulnerable to poisons and radiation because it is composed of cells with a very high level of metabolism. Mutagens easily damage their genes or that of the sperm traveling in it. Lead, industrial solvents like benzene, toluene, paint thinner mixes and carbon disulphide, pesticides like DBCP (dibromochloropropane) and Kepone, marijuana, large amounts of alcohol, and ionizing radiation all are known to damage sperm production, viability, and integrity.[7]

Common sense and some scientific evidence tells us that a father's exposure to toxic substances may increase the mother's risk of miscarriage and stillbirth, itself commonly the result of abnormal fetal development. Men whose work exposes them to any of the substances just mentioned are likely to have children with a higher incidence of brain tumors. The link between the father's exposure to ionizing radiation and an increased rate of leukemia in his children is well-researched, with studies dating back to the aftermath of the atomic bomb explosions over Hiroshima and Nagasaki. Childhood leukemia is also higher in children whose fathers work with, or are exposed to, solvents, petroleum products, and spray paints.[7]

From the toxins and mutagens mentioned, we can deduce that children may face a slightly increased statistical risk of brain tumors and cancer if their fathers work with chemicals. Thus, professions at risk would include auto mechanics, machine repairmen, metal processors, and also workers whose jobs expose them to higher-than-average levels of electromagnetic fields or radiation.[8] Farmers who are exposed to some types of herbicide have six times greater risk than the average person of developing certain cancers. Ham radio operators suffer from a significantly increased incidence of acute myeloid leukemia.[9] For instance, in one study the children of male anesthesiologists were shown to be 25 percent more likely to have major malformations like spina bifida, heart defects, and cleft palate than the children of male surgeons. They share the same workplace, but are in different proximity to certain potentially harmful chemicals and gases.

Similarly, an unusually high rate of miscarriage has been noted among the wives of dentists who use nitrous oxide, and the wives of men who smoke heavily. Babies whose fathers smoke a half a pack of cigarettes or more daily are more likely to die at birth than babies with nonsmoking fathers. But cigarette smoking by fathers may have even more subtle and delayed effects on a child's brain development. In a study published in 1992 in Canada,[10] children whose mothers were exposed to someone else's cigarette smoke during pregnancy had lower scores in speech and language development, motor skills, mathematics, and intelligence and behavior during the early school years. It is well-established that alcohol consumption – even small amounts – by the mother during pregnancy carries with it an increased risk of brain damage for the child, and alcoholism in the father also seems to be passed along in nervous system damage to the child. Laboratory rats sired by fathers who regularly consumed large amounts of alcohol showed basic flaws in their ability to learn simple tasks.

### From a Child's Mother

Since women work in all of the professions mentioned above, they and their children are similarly at risk. Pregnant women who work as telephone operators and sit all day in front of computer screens have been shown to have a higher incidence of miscarriage than telephone operators in older exchanges that lack computer screens.

The role of cigarette smoking and alcohol consumption in birth defects and developmental difficulties is thoroughly established and cannot be overemphasized. Fetal alcohol syndrome is a condition where the alcohol content of the mother's blood is sufficiently high at critical moments in the embryonic and early fetal stages of gestation that severe brain and cranial bone abnormalities result. Microcephaly (abnormally small-brained) and anencephaly (the complete, or almost complete absence of the cerebral hemispheres) result. Prescription medication is tested to ensure that it does not harm the infant, but careless or desperate mothers may still take a medication that is contraindicated during pregnancy. All of these factors increase the chance of tumor formation in childhood or early adulthood.

### The Home Environment

An issue of contention is whether exposure to electromagnetic fields, as emitted by many household appliances and overhead power lines close to a child's bedroom, causes an increased incidence of leukemia.[11] Common sense says it does. The fifty-hertz cycle of household electricity happens to be exactly the same cycle that the body uses for its own field.[12] Swedish studies associate the presence of leukemia in children with the proximity of two or more high-tension electrical wires passing within yards (meters) of the child's bedroom on different sides.[13] One wonders at the effect such electrical fields may have as precipitating factors in those who are particularly sensitive to them,[13] whether genetically or energetically.[14] What are known as "small-gauss fields" – extremely fine electromagnetic radiations – clearly cause cell mutations in experimental animals within just a few days of exposure. Certain types of microwaves also cause similar cellular changes.[15] In response to such research, the American Physical Society announced in 1995 that "it can find no evidence that the electromagnetic fields that radiate from power lines cause cancer."[16,17]

The use of common kitchen appliances, such as the tabletop toaster, leads to the creation of intense local electrical fields, which again radiate electrical waves at fifty hertz. The hand-held hair dryer, using up to two-thousand watts of power, emits an intense electrical field in immediate proximity to the brain. While there are no definitive statistics on hair-dryer use related to the incidence of brain tumors, one cannot help but have reservations. Cellular telephones, another electromagnetic source, emit radio waves from their antennae (which, in a car, may be located close to the driver's or passenger's brain), but the evidence accumulated to date suggests that they are innocuous. Research by Genevieve Matanoski of Johns Hopkins University found that the incidence of all kinds of cancers is higher in field workers who work on or near power lines.[18]

## Working with Clients with Brain Tumors

Working with brain tumors represents one of the most challenging facets of craniosacral work. The cranial wave reflects the presence of tumors through its "feel" (piezoelectric qualities) and its motion (mechanical constituents). The best combination of therapies in working with brain tumors is founded on medical diagnosis and the use of radiation or chemotherapy, supported by the adept use of acupuncture, biofeedback, craniosacral work, macrobiotic or traditional Chinese medicinal diets, and meditation.

For visionary craniosacral work, begin by focusing on the client's whole field, then discern the cranial energy field. What is happening for this person now? Sit and meditate with him. Do a meditation on the client's seven soul centers, paying particular attention to the upper three. Scan the cranial bones one by one, taking note of any deviations in the membrane system, and brain structures. Wait until you get a clear image of the location and situation of the tumor. Talk to the tumor, get a sense of its needs. Love it. Ask it why it needs to be there.

Love is the strongest healing energy of all. In treatment, prayer can be harnessed to love, and used as a healing agent. It is a kind of tunnel vision thinking to pray for the dimunition or disappearance of the tumor; the higher way is to pray for the greatest good to come about, whatever that may be. This may encompass praying that they may be able to fulfill their agenda, or to share the gifts they came here with. Both prayer and meditation are powerful healers: they enable our soul to communicate with our heart. They also allow the collective soul – the long wave[19] – to communicate with our heart. A five-year-old, asked if she knew the difference between prayer and meditation, answered without a moment's hesitation: "Prayer is when you speak to God, and meditation is when God speaks to you."[20,21]

Meditation can be taught to the naive client, or their existing practice deepened through your presence. Healing rituals known in shamanism as "rites of intensification"[22] can be employed to assist the client in becoming more aware of the forces in their field that may be contributing to their condition. Eating a low-fat diet, and everyday practices such as walking (or more robust exercise) have been proven to lead to reduced rates of all types of cancer. They may well help in tumor control.

Any craniosacral technique that takes pressure off the brain is likely to produce relief in clients with brain tumors. Any technique that increases pressure to the brain, such as the Square Ashtray or CV4, is likely to make matters worse. Scan for other "negatives" – things not to do. Sometimes even mild compressive techniques, such as Temporal Palming and Sphenobasilar Decompression, aggravate.

Open the sutures of the head, reduce mandibular compression, and improve cranial energy flow with directed energy work. Perhaps employ deep lymphatic drainage to the anterior triangle of the neck, scalene muscle release, and extensive work with the muscles of mastication – all to optimize cranial hydraulics and mechanics. Consider giving several "Windows to the Sky"[23] sessions to further release the cranial base, and to induce insight and reverie.

# PROTOCOLS AND TESTS

# 39
# *Craniosacral Protocols*

The following chapters provide a short selection of craniosacral protocols, or treatment sequences, that are learning aids designed to help the student practitioner get started. They also guide the more experienced practitioner through novel and complex learning curves, such as the Lateral Structures Protocols or the Windows to the Sky series. As such, protocols are not meant to be strictly adhered to, but rather used as guidelines on which to base future development. They are not a craniosacral Ten Commandments.

*The chapter "Introduction to the Techniques" provides important guidelines on how to conduct a craniosacral session. Please familiarize yourself with its contents before using any of the protocols.*

## The Logic of Protocols

Protocols exist for specific anatomical and physiological reasons. For instance, in Chapter 40, Familiarization, we start with the sacrum because it is the foundation of the cranial "mechanism" and the anchor of the spinal dura. If the foundation is imbalanced, or moves improperly, the pinnacle of the structure cannot be in balance. From the sacrum we move to the occiput and perform a CV4, which helps release the atlanto-occipital joint, free and balance the membrane system within the head, and optimize muscular tonus throughout the body. These changes help deepen all our subsequent work. Two steps later we perform a Temporal Auricle Decompression, which helps free the temporal portion of the squamous suture with the parietal bones. Having released the temporals from the parietals, we move next to

release the parietals themselves, which will move much more readily as a result of the temporal preparation, and so on.

There are many different ways to achieve a given end – for example, to release the squamous suture. After working with the "Familiarization" protocol for a while, you may suddenly have the instinct not to do a Temporal Auricle Decompression with a specific client. Since you understand that part of the reason it preceded the Parietal Lift was to release the squamous suture, you can now devise a new way to achieve the same result. You might use a unilateral hold, such as the Temporal Cross-Check, or Release of the Posterior Fibers of Temporalis, or perform a mandibular compression technique. You have begun to perceive and respond to the client, rather than squeezing him into a set protocol.

## Foundations and Principles

The ability to sense the cranial wave is the foundation of this work. Meditate to inculcate stillness within you. Sit quietly with your clients before you touch them. Ask for inner permission to touch the head before you do so. Then place your hands on the head and wait until the cranial wave makes itself felt.

Sense many people's cranial waves, especially those of infants and people who have survived head injuries. These heads, demonstrating the extremes of cranial movement, enable you to understand a normal cranial wave better. Infants' heads move the most, and the most fluidly. After head injury, cranial motion patterns become disturbed or frozen in ways that are distinctly different from normal. Feeling one post-trauma head will help you identify others.

All craniosacral techniques and protocols are based on the ability to sense the cranial wave. It is vital that your hand contact remains a sensitive one. You need to be able to feel the cranial wave formations throughout the duration of your contact. If, because of your own posture, or because of the weight of the client's body, your hand becomes numb, then obviously you can no longer feel his cranial wave. More than this, you need to have continuous sensitivity to the response of his cranial wave to your contact. You need to be able to feel, moment-to-moment, how the part you are touching responds to your contact, and then respond to that response, and so on. As you do this, you need to pay attention to your own posture too: the more mobile your body is while you touch his, the greater liquidity of movement is transferred to him. But even if you have difficulty feeling the cranial wave, don't give up. The important thing is sensing where the bone (or whatever tissue you are tuning in to) *wants to go* – this is the first principle of treatment. From that we move into realizing where it does *not* want to go, which is the second principle. If you can sense both of these things, you can begin to work effectively, and safely. You can certainly begin to practice the familiarization protocol. Keep working with it until you can sense when the cranial wave peacefully quits on you – the still point, which is the third principle that you need to work towards sensing. The fourth principle is the archaic wound, which feels altogether different from a still point, because there is nothing peaceful about it at all – it is more like the part has gone deathly quiet because it is afraid it is going to get hit by that truck again. You have moved it into the same position it was in when it was hit, and it freezes in fear.

## Development and Destinations

If you can "sense" these four principles, then you have moved beyond the foundation of your craniosacral practice and are beginning to attain to an intermediate level of skill development. If you cannot, this is what to practice on. Remember that the key to palpation and healing lies in your own inner meditative state, especially when you are having difficulties sensing the wave, or one of the four principles. The more deeply and easily you can move into an altered state of consciousness, one where your perception of time slows down, the more you will sense nuances within the cranial wave. The mastery of these four aspects of the cranial wave represents your midpoint goal in craniosacral skill development. Consider these protocols as challenges to help you develop your skill.

The high art, the destination point in the development of your skill, lies in sensing exactly what the client needs, and inventing the appropriate technique. Exemplary craniosacral healing work does not lie in applying a specific technique or sequence of techniques to an individual client, but rather in responding, moment by moment, to changes in the client's field of consciousness. The body is the conscious medium. In craniosacral work, we sculpt it at the deepest of levels.

Use these protocols as starting points; do not become wed to them. Once you understand the anatomical and energetic reasons for their existence, you can begin to modify them according to the individual client's needs. After some months or years of practice you can go beyond them altogether, into the real work.

# 40
# *Familiarization*

This protocol is designed to provide a simple yet systematic sequence of contacts with the principle bones of the neurocranium, and the viscero-cranium. It allows you to begin sensing and balancing the reciprocal tension membrane. Repeating this many times will begin to lay the foundation in practice that is essential for gaining expertise in craniosacral work. A complete protocol, done with care, focus, and love, that is, with craftsmanship, takes from sixty to ninety minutes. Technique descriptions can be found in the relevant bone chapters, as indicated below.

## Protocol

### *Start*

- Center
- Ground
- Perceive two places to initiate contact

### *Sacrum*

Use one of the following:

- Sacrum Prone Technique
(The Sacrum, p. 75)
- Sacrum Outside-Leg Technique
(The Sacrum, p. 80)
- Sacrum Inside-Leg Technique
(The Sacrum, p. 80)

### *Occiput*

Use one of the following (see contraindications for CV4 under Chapter 23, The Occiput):

- Occipital Eight-Finger Hold (The Occiput, p. 92) in clients where a CV4 is inadvisable, or
- CV4 (The Occiput, p. 93) for neck traction/release, diagnosis of fault patterns within the head, still point induction

### *Sphenoid*

- Sphenobasilar Decompression
(The Sphenoid, p. 113)

### *Temporals*

Use both of the following:

- Temporal Three-Finger Contact
(The Temporals, p. 126)
- Temporal Auricle Decompression
(The Temporals, p. 126)

### *Parietals*

Use both of the following:

- Basic Parietal Hold (The Parietals, p. 136)
- Parietal Lift (The Parietals, p. 136)

### Frontal

■ Frontal Cup and Straddle
(The Frontal, p. 146)

### Zygomae

Use all three of the following:

■ Zygomae Three-Finger Palpation
(The Zygomae, p. 165)
■ Zygomae Lateral Release: Decompression
(The Zygomae, p. 165)
■ Zygomae "Bicycle Handlebars" – Unwinding
(The Zygomae, p. 165)

### Maxillae

■ Maxillary Lateral Decompression of the
Medial Palatine Suture (The Maxillae, p. 175)

### Mandible

■ Mandible Thumbs-Internal Technique
(The Mandible, p. 198)

### Completions

Use one, two, or all three of the following:

■ Ventral Sacred Energy Vessel Hold
(The Sacrum, p. 83)
■ Clear the Confusion (The Frontal, p. 145)
■ One or more closing contacts of your choice

# 41

# A Sequence of Techniques for Headaches

This itemization gives the principle techniques to consider in the treatment of most forms of headache. They are described in the sequence that selected, individually appropriate holds might be used in treating a client with a muscle contraction or migraine headache. Choose not more than eight or ten techniques for any one session. If you select the right technique, just one may do. Note that as part of the treatment of headache, the presence of severe eye strain, heat stroke, a cerebrovascular accident (stroke), high blood pressure, or a brain tumor needs to be considered, and may need to be investigated by the appropriate specialists.

The Windows to the Sky sequence may also be considered for the treatment of the energetic and spiritual components of headaches. It often proves effective when the more mechanical craniosacral techniques are not. Last, remember that studies find that up to 40 percent of headaches respond favorably to the presence of a physician or to placebos; thus, as a healer, your attitude and the way you "hold space" for the client may play a crucial role.

## Protocol

- Unilateral Flexed Knee Perineal Work (Sacrum, p. 74)
- Unilateral Piriformis and Coccygeus Release (Sacrum, p. 78)
- Sacrum Outside Leg Technique (Sacrum, p. 80)
- Occipital and Sacral Coupled Hold: Core Link Appraisal (The Occiput, p. 90)
- Wind Palace (GV16) (Last paragraph of Wind Palace contact in Windows to the Sky, p. 259)
- Masseter Release – Three Approaches (The Mandible, p. 194)
- Suboccipital Hold (The Occiput, p. 91)
- The CV4 (The Occiput, p. 93)
- Occipital Approach to the Transverse Sinus (The Occiput, p. 94)
- Mandible Thumbs-Internal Technique (The Mandible, p. 198)
- Lateral Pterygoid Release: Oral Approach (The Mandible, p. 196)
- Frontal Anterior Decompression (The Frontal, p. 144)
- Sutherland's Grip (The Sphenoid, p. 114)
- Zygomae and Nasal Oral Index-Finger Technique (The Zygomae, p. 166)
- Zygomae Oral Anterior Decompression and Unwinding (The Zygomae, p. 166)
- Sphenobasilar Decompression (The Sphenoid, p. 113)
- Sphenoid External Coupled Contact with Mandible (The Sphenoid, p. 116)
- Release of the Posterior Fibers of Temporalis (The Mandible, p. 197)
- Parietal Lift (The Parietals, p. 136)
- Ethmoid and Sphenoid Oral Thumb-Based Perpendicular Plate Release (The Ethmoid, p. 154)
- Palatine Decompression (The Palatines, p. 180)
- Incisive Bone Decompression and Unwinding (The Maxillae, p. 174)
- Temporal Palming: Lateral Structures Quad Spread (The Temporals, p. 127)
- Oral Coronal Shear Test (The Sphenoid, p. 115)
- Clear the Confusion (The Frontal, p. 145)
- Frontal-Zygomae-Mandible Triple Spread (The Frontal, p. 147)

# 42
# *Cardinal Eight Protocol*

This is an intermediate level sequence of techniques that combines directed energy work at specific energetic or acupuncture points with compound coupled craniosacral techniques. The name "Cardinal Eight" refers to the ability of these techniques to interface with the cardinal aspects of the cranial mechanism and field. Half of these methods appear in the techniques sections at the end of the individual bone chapters (with notations below on where to find them); the remaining four are given here for the first time. We develop our skill best when we move incrementally, using some known techniques and expanding our skill level by interlacing these with some new ones. It also helps balance the client's "mechanism" to use some symmetrical techniques with some asymmetrical ones, and some mechanically-oriented techniques with some energetic – it gives the work depth and scope.

This protocol works well in muscle contraction and frontal headache, whiplash injury, and cervical spine hypertonicity. It is also profoundly balancing, and usually euphoric.

## Protocol

- Hypnagogic Points at Axis (below)
- Mandible Compression
(The Mandible, p. 200)
- Sphenoid External Coupled with Unilateral Mandible Contact (below)
- Incisive Bone Decompression and Unwinding (The Maxillae, p. 174)
- Occiput and Viscerocranium (below)
- Passive-Interactive Square Ashtray
(The Temporals, p. 129)
- Zygomae Lateral Release: Decompression (The Zygomae, p. 165)
- Middle of Man (below)

## New Techniques

### *Hypnagogic Points at Axis*

Locate the posterolateral prominences over the lateral masses of the axis (second cervical vertebra), feeling for the little energetic whirlpools on each side that seem to suck energy inward. The pressure to apply here is in the order of ⅓ to ⅔ ounce (10 to 20 grams), minimally anterior but largely cephalad in intention. This technique will tend to put the client into an altered state of consciousness quite quickly – he drops into a deeper state more conducive to reverie and insight, the hypnagogic realm.

### *Sphenoid External Coupled with Unilateral Mandible Contact*

Begin with the standard mandible contact (see Mandible Thumbs-Internal technique) and wait. When you feel the cranial wave patterns, begin interactive or unwinding work to release the viscerocranium, and then mediate to the falx via the temporomandibular, and also through spontaneous decompression of the maxillae/palatines/sphenoid. Test the range of mandible motion and the ease of motion in prognation and retrusion, lateral glide to each side, trituration (rotation), and decompression. Next move to interactive work and sense the unwinding patterns of the mandible. Remember its broad representation in the cerebral cortex, where the neurons that activate its sixteen muscle groups interface with half of the motor neurons in the cortex.

Assess which side of the jaw is tighter. Retain your contact on the tighter side – one thumb on the occlusal surface of one side of the mandible – and move to a spanning contact over the greater

243

wings of the sphenoid with your free hand. Three-dimensional, asymmetric techniques like this give great capability to unwind and normalize "the mechanism." Use it to balance and unwind the lateral structures, such as the temporalis, masseter, and lateral pterygoid muscles, the sphenoid sutures, and both temporomandibular joints. You might also use it to create space for the palatines, vomer, and zygomae.

### Occiput and Viscerocranium

Sit to one side of the client's head and cup the occiput. Once you have a stable contact with the occiput, place your free hand in a spanning contact with the external surface of the mandibular body. Once you have balanced the mandible and occiput, move the viscerocranial hand to your next contact on the external surface of the maxillae, and so work superiorly and laterally to zygomae, frontal, and finally sphenoid. Balance each bone with the occiput until the anterior half of the head is perfectly balanced with the posterior half (the latter represented by the occiput)

### Middle of Man

Middle of Man is an acupuncture point (Governor Vessel 26) located in the deepest part of the curve of the anterior nasal spine. Take a contact with the fingernail of one middle finger, and span the greater wings of the sphenoid with your other hand (see the lower photo on page 260).

Your target structure is the hypothalamus, the "brain of the brain." This is the brain structure where our sense of identity seems to reside. Vector *chi kung* energy down your middle finger, which is pointed straight at the hypothalamus. At the same time, direct energy from one greater wing to the other, with your focus being to have both vectors of energy intersect at the hypothalamus, bathing it in energy, and "lighting it up."

This is an excellent way to end a session because it helps bring the client's awareness to his center, his "cerebral home."

# 43
# *Lateral Structures Protocol*

This thirteen-step lateral structures protocol forms a useful foundation to practice perceiving, sensing, and understanding the head in a three-dimensional way. It is designed especially to create lateral space within the head, free energy flow in the reciprocal tension membrane, and open up the interface between neurocranium and viscerocranium. It will help you to begin to deepen your ability to see how the internal structures interrelate. Practice this protocol until you are thoroughly familiar with it.

As in the prior protocol, new techniques are introduced here to supplement those already introduced. Descriptions of the techniques that have been introduced earlier can be found from the page notations below.

## Protocol

■ Scalene and Temporal Hold, Head Turned to One Side (The Temporals, p. 127)
This begins to free the cranial base musculature, and thus enhances cranial motion.

■ Wind Palace and Glabella
Move into a Wind Palace (the acupuncture point Governor Vessel 16) contact, placing two fingers on the midline between occiput and atlas (the first cervical vertebra), and couple this with a second hand spanning the nasion/glabella (inner-eye soul) area and also contacting bregma (the crown soul).

This technique begins to open the channel of the inner eye, energizes the falx cerebelli and falx cerebri, and helps free the atlanto-occipital joint.

■ Wind Palace and Middle of Man
This facilitates the opening of the Governor Vessel meridian again, evaluating the field at both Wind Palace (Governor Vessel 16) and Middle of Man (Governor Vessel 26). Contact Wind Palace as just described, above. For your Middle of Man contact, make precise fingernail contact in under the nose. Impart a cephalad intention at both contacts.

This is very good for releasing the head from the neck, and the maxillae from the mandible. It also accesses the hypothalamus.

■ Zygomae Lateral Release: Decompression, and Zygomae "Bicycle Handlebars" Unwinding (The Zygomae, p. 165)
These two techniques take advantage of the zygomae's role as "governor" of some of the next structures we are going to seek to free and balance – the sphenoid, maxillae, and temporals. You may choose to use a third technique and go inside the mouth for lateral and anterior decompression of the zygomae.

■ Ethmoid Pinch
This is a sequential, coupled hold that begins by taking the frontal into anterior decompression by way of spanning the lateral orbital notches; track its release. The ethmoid cannot free until the frontal has disengaged. Locate an opposed finger and thumb as near to the ethmoid as possible, directly anterior to the medial canthus of the eye.

This releases the ethmoid to move anteriorly and frees up its control over the inferior-lying vomer.

■ Ethmoid and Sphenoid Oral Thumb-Based Perpendicular Plate Release (The Ethmoid, p. 154)
Use this for vomer diagnosis and decompression. Decompress first in the caudad plane, then in the anterior plane.

■ Sutherland's Grip (The Sphenoid, p. 114, and The Maxillae, p. 174)
Take both the sphenoid and maxillae into anterior decompression. Intend to free the sphenobasilar joint with the sphenoid contact and the maxillae from the palatines (and therefore also free the palatines from the sphenoid) with the oral contact. Anatomically speaking, the sphenoid will free more readily if it is taken into flexion, which will rotate the pterygoid processes away from – posterior to – the palatines. This is a powerful corrective technique for most kinds of sphenoid lesion, and one of the most effective ways to separate the front half of the head from the back half.

■ Mandible Thumbs-Internal Technique, Palpation and Unwinding ("The Mandible," p. 198)
As we have already normalized the maxillae in relationship to the sphenoid, we use this technique now to move into normalizing the mandible. Work to release the viscerocranium (and mediate to the falx) via the temporomandibular joints. The very fact of introducing freedom at the temporomandibular joints may permit spontaneous decompressions of the maxillae, palatines and sphenoid. Test for decompression, prognation, retrusion, lateral glide to each side, trituration (rotation), and compression; then move to unwinding.

■ Temporal Palming: Lateral Structures Quad Spread (The Temporals, p. 127)
This mildly compressive technique frees up some of the stomatognathic system musculature, and releases sutural pressures on the temporals.

■ Square Ashtray (The Temporals, p. 128)
This is used for profound balancing of the temporals and tentorium. *Caution:* Do *not* use this technique on a client who is free from inner-ear disturbance. (Only use it in clients with symptoms of temporal bone imbalance.)

■ Temporal Oscillation (The Temporals, p. 129)
Use this to "lubricate" then free the squamous sutures. Use this with extreme care since the possibility of destabilizing the normal pattern is immediate.

■ Passive-Interactive Square Ashtray (The Temporals, p. 129)
You can strongly interact with the tentorium on an energetic level with this technique.

■ Directed Energy to the Mammillary Bodies (The Temporals, p. 130)
This may enhance the client's sense of well-being.

■ Temporal Auricle Decompression (The Temporals, p. 126)
This works as a final temporal assessment to ensure that the bones have not been impacted by the last technique. "Box the compass" by checking each plane of motion sequentially, teasing out the last threads of adherence or imbalance in the structural interrelationships. This technique works in a plane that the earlier temporal contacts cannot fully access.

■ Clear the Confusion (The Frontal, p. 145)
Having spent so much time on the lateral structures – especially interfacing with the tentorium – it is an appropriate completion to honor the falx. Access the pituitary, hypothalamus, thalamus, and pineal structures by changing your intensity, vector, and monitoring changes in the field, as you sweep cephalad. This serves to release a heightened accumulation of energy in the lateral areas of the head, bringing balance back in to the center.

# 44
# *Techniques*
# *for Unwinding*

Your first contacts in an unwinding session may be anywhere on the body, and in any combination. The Way lies in not repeating the same contacts – respond to the differences in people, don't try to make different people fit the same technique. Being present, and not trying, are the keys to achieving this.

Doing unwinding work on a floor mat allows for deeper regressive states – the client has no fear of falling off the table, and you have no fear that the table may fall over. Being on the floor brings with it a sense of returning to a primal, or pre-walking, state of consciousness. There is a rich sense of earth energy all about. You can often access the child, and work with vulnerable states of consciousness better than you can on a massage table. Much can be revealed in such innocent states of being:

*If I defend myself, I will be attacked.*
*If I can learn what my defenses hide, no one will need to attack me.*
*If I master the art of genuine defenselessness, I will be strong*

Your intention in unwinding work is to begin reversing the incoming forces that overcame the client's ability to absorb, deflect, or assimilate trauma. Let the cranial waves lead you. Stay as long as needed on each contact. Monitor your own breathing patterns, and take deep sighing breaths to stay open, free, and accessible.

Here are two suggested sequences for unwinding work. Start with a protocol, but listen to how the body wants to move – if it moves into its own pattern, jettison the protocol, and follow the lead of the dreambody.

## First Protocol

■ Feet

Begin with a bilateral contact to the calcaneal and lateral aspects of the feet – a superb initial contact. It allows you to tune in to leg, hip, and iliopsoas status, then spinal and finally sphenoid status. Support both feet off the table surface with hands cupped around the calcaneal bones.

Tune in to the movement patterns. The challenge is to realize that the two legs may need quite different unwinding, and to begin to supply this.

This contact may evolve into interactive work – you may find yourself using direct action or opposite physiological motion to release a knee, or the hip rotator muscles. Move to a unilateral hold, or stay with the bilateral, as seems appropriate.

■ Sacrum

Choose from the Outside-Leg Technique (p. 80), Inside-Leg Technique (p. 80), Sacral Steering Wheel (p. 81), and Occipital and Sacral Coupled Hold: Core Link Appraisal (p. 90).

Sacral Steering Wheel work uses both hands in under the sacrum, with a transverse supportive contact. It allows for full control of the sacrum's motility patterns, with fingertips overlapping the sacral border away from you, allowing contact with some gluteal, piriformis, and coccygeal muscle fibers. This is an excellent technique for the indurated, resistant sacrum.[1] Wait for the cranial wave formations to declare themselves before moving to assist it.

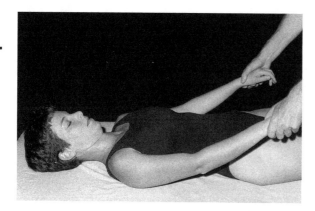

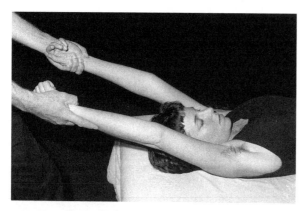

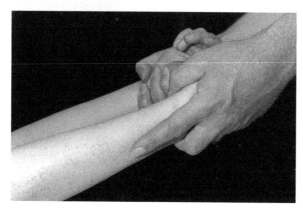

■ Arms

Begin with choosing to take the hands either pedad or cephalad. If pedad, stand to one side of the client's knees and take up a "wrist trap" contact with one, or both hands. Begin to decompress and unwind pedad. If cephalad, sweep the arms up, perhaps over the heart, and make micromovements until you find the still point in the arc. Use a wrist trap, central three-fingered grip, or place your index finger down the central midline of the forearms. Go to a unilateral contact when appropriate, and if you begin to discern a cranial connection with the arm, use the sphenoid access contact through the elbow.[2]

■ Neck

The best way to truly unwind *everything* in the neck is to bring your client's shoulders level with the top of the table so that his neck and head are in "outer space," and are entirely free to move in any direction. It is surprising how powerfully, and how often, the head and neck want to unwind in the posterolateral planes. Perhaps this is because of the prevalence of whiplash injuries. It is certainly often a distant echo of birth traumas....

Assume a strong, wide, and competent stance. Bring flexibility into your knees. Take up a bilateral cervical contact, or support the entire head. Wait until you feel the patterns declaring themselves, then move in and assist them to do what they cannot quite do alone.

As long as you do nothing jarring, this is an optimum way to initiate cervical and membrane system unwinding. The vertebrae love to rotate, to side-bend, to flex and extend. Discern which motions the neck innately wants to enter into, then help them discover those movements in safety, slowly.

■ Temporal Palming (The Temporals, p. 127)
as a Cranial Unwinding Contact

Now sense the brain's position in its watery, high-domed cavern. Take a Temporal Palming contact, making sure you have your thumbs in zygomatic contact, and possibly your pinkies on the occiput for further stability and competence in technique. A refinement of this technique is to put your own inner eye (glabella) over the client's, when this seems both needed, and acceptable to them.

With inner-eye contact, and with the client's head resting on the table surface, there is now a point of contact with all four major poles of the membrane system. End by moving your inner-eye contact up to the forehead hairline while bringing your temporal fingers to the crown. Come off contact at the crown at the same moment your forehead leaves the client's.

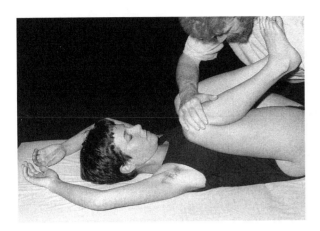

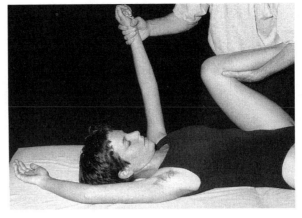

**Far left:**
*Fetal curl
and sacrum*

**Right:**
*Unilateral
Arm and Leg
contact*

## Second Protocol

■ Mandible Thumbs-Internal Technique,
Palpation and Unwinding (The Mandible, p. 198)
Sit or stand at the head of the table and begin
mandibular release and unwinding with your
thumbs on the biting surfaces of the lower teeth.
Maintain this contact through full neck unwinding
until you reach a deep still point.

■ Fetal Curl and Sacrum
A provocative initiation contact, but one you will
find arising spontaneously from the bilateral foot
contact of the first series: the dreambody loves this
shape. Take a primary contact with the client's
fully flexed knees, and a secondary contact on the
sacrum for root soul connection, and spinal column unwinding. Take care to maintain a strong leg
base for yourself. This hold occasionally evolves
into a side-lying, full fetal curl, regressive contact.
Stay focused on your breathing, and be sensitively
silent; there is every chance that the client can
transit a deeply healing space.

■ Unilateral Arm and Leg Contact
Choose a side, and notice why. Stand at your
client's mid-thigh level. Take a leg contact under
the flexed knee, and bring the knee against your
own hip. Collect the hand and arm on the same
side with a wrist trap, three-fingered contact, or
open-palm grip. This hold requires a lot of practice
and responsiveness, because the arm and leg feel so
different, and have different needs. When you have
finished with this side, sense whether the other
side needs the same contact.

■ Center of Centers: The Heart
This contact may be taken in a variety of ways,
such as:
   ■ Standing to one side, take an encompassing
   contact with one hand above (anterior to) and
   one below (posterior to) the heart. Stand, taking a very long stance at the client's head.
   Place your anterior hand midway down the
   sternum. Use your perceptive capabilities to
   sense the position of the heart within its
   warm, pillowy cave (just as you would the
   hemispheres of the brain within the cranial
   vault). Now go into unwinding until you find
   the still point, until you feel the heart shift
   and settle and relax, as it finds its central
   place of rest.
■ Access the heart with your palms on the
"yin surface" (hairless, soft-skinned, medial
aspect) of the upper arms. Rest the client's
arms on the table surface to either side of the
head. Point your own fingers directly towards
their heart.
■ Make a fingernail or fingertip contact with
Little Rushing In (Heart 9) at the lateral and
proximal border of the fifth fingernail bed.
■ Access the heart from the "phoenix" position, with the client's hands swept up and out
above his head, unwinding from there.
■ Access the heart via the Ventral Sacred
Energy Vessel Hold (The Sacrum, p. 83). Sense
the heart in its pillowy cave, and bring it
exactly in the middle.

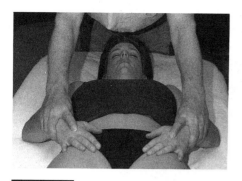 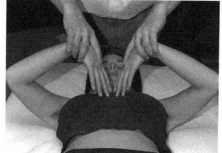 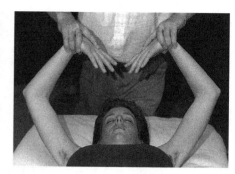

*Accessing the heart from the "phoenix" position*

■ Head

We are coming full circle. Having begun with the mandible, and released the temporomandibular joint and neck, we are now fine-tuning the cranial bones themselves:

■ Pole Work with the Membrane System
CV4 (p. 93) (posterior pole); Clear the Confusion (p. 145) (anterior pole); and Temporal Palming: Lateral Structure Quad Spread (p. 127) (lateral poles). With each technique you are accessing the major poles of attachment of the membrane system; with each contact, sense its needs for unwinding, stabilizing or decompression.

■ Frontal-Zygomae-Mandible Triple Spread (The Frontal, p. 147) This technique encompasses both neurocranium and viscerocranium, and completes the balancing of the head. Sit comfortably at your client's head, and place the pads of your central three fingertips on either side of the mental protuberance. Place the distal part of your palms on the raised prominence of the zygomae, and the heels of your hands on the frontal. Tune in to all six contacts – three with each hand – and begin to balance the viscerocranium and neurocranium.

■ Crown Soul – Directed Energy Work
End by making thumbnail or central three fingernail contact with the crown soul at vertex (Governor Vessel 20, One Hundred Meeting Places) – and vector energy down the "red road" of the spinal cord to the coccyx and root soul.

This final contact takes the work into the realm of the pure energy of the spirit.

# 45

# *Windows to the Sky*

When sensitive people are touched at certain acupuncture points they feel transported to an older realm. These acupuncture points are places of deep change; accessing them can quickly make things different for the client – how he feels, how he looks, how he experiences himself and his world.

The Windows to the Sky points are highly evocative locations that are especially good in taking clients into the hypnagogic realm, through out-of-the-body experiences, and into past-life regressions. They are used by past-life therapists to facilitate their work; for instance, at The Light Institute in New Mexico, Chris Griscom uses a combination of craniosacral work and the Windows to the Sky points to induct clients into previous incarnations. Many bodyworkers use them instinctively to calm, to deepen, and to facilitate unfolding.

This work represents one of the highest applications of sacred touch, both for the enhancement of spiritual clarity, and for grounding those clients who are "too much in their heads." As they are powerful access places, the Windows to the Sky points need to be approached with great respect. It is important not to push people beyond their limits.

## Appropriateness

Jack Worseley, an authority on five-element-theory acupuncture, believes in using these points only if the client "asks" for them. Asking in the Chinese model means that he describes particular bodily sensations or life experiences that indicate a need for attention at some, or all, of these points. This asking may also take the form of a poignant dream, or an expressed need to see something in his life more clearly – when he is on the verge of some understanding, and needs a window on to it. Just as work with the sphenoid can open the inner eye, opening one of the window points may allow him to see more clearly.

Think of using these points when someone asks about what happened to who he used to be, to his old resolve. Listen for key words, for spiritually or emotionally loaded sentences, where the client explains that he can sense the need for action, but realizes that for some unfathomable reason he is not taking that action. Use this sequence in cases of despondency, when the client knows that something is amiss but cannot discern what, which in normal times he could "shake himself out of it." This awareness of dysfunction coupled with the inability to do anything effective about it is a hallmark of the need for window work.

Another time to use the sequence is when the client's actions are not in line with his purpose or principles in life *and he is aware of it.* This last is the key distinction in using windows work – awareness of dissonance between action and purpose. The window allows him to see what he needs to do in order to return to his natural level of integrity.

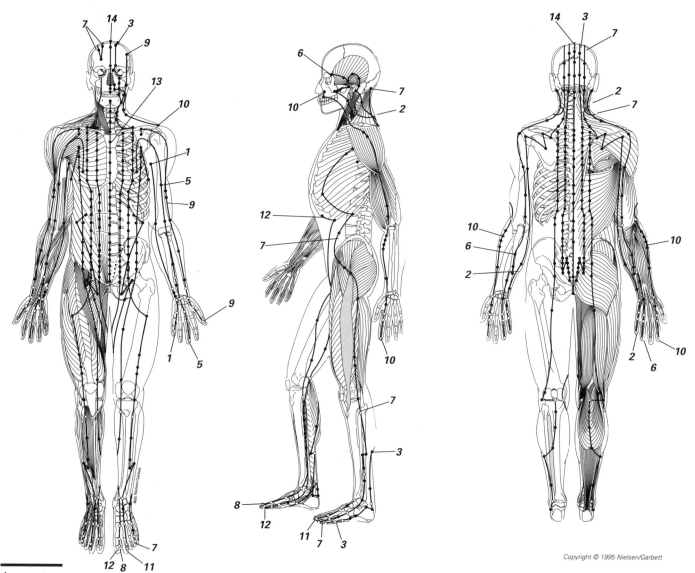

*Acupuncture meridians and vessels*

**1** *Heart*
**2** *Small Intestine*
**3** *Bladder*
**4** *Kidney*
**5** *Heart Protector*
**6** *Triple Warmer*
**7** *Gall Bladder*
**8** *Liver*
**9** *Lung*
**10** *Colon*
**11** *Stomach*
**12** *Spleen*
**13** *Conception Vessel*
**14** *Governor Vessel*

## Trinity

In Chapter 36, Bad Backs, I discuss the importance of assessing the three cardinal components of an illness. In "windows" work we also look for three indications. In this case, the first is that the client has physical symptoms in his head or heart, such as a hearing loss, or pain described as being behind the heart. The second is that there is something missing in the "heavenly" aspects of his spiritual life, or he feels a general spiritual dullness, which may extend into a sense that something is not connected in his life. (This is similar to the effects of a sphenoid lateroflexion lesion.) The third component is that he realizes that his recent life actions are not in accord with his beliefs, but as yet has no control over the pattern. When these three factors combine, windows work is indicated.

## Heaven and Earth

The trunk of the body is earth and the physical; the head is heaven, the spiritual realm. The neck – where all of the classical windows points are located – is the junction between heaven and earth. It is the earth's window to heaven. The window points are mainly used to treat head symptoms, or to connect the head with the heart.

Sometimes we need an opening in the neck, sometimes we are too open and need a window closed, so that we can be more "earthed." These points may be stuck open, or stuck closed. This series of points is therefore very important in visionary craniosacral work.

## Point Location

As an initial landmarking aid to locating the throat points, look at the client's neck as he lies supine and note the exact location of the most prominent part of the Adam's apple. Draw a line of sight posterior to the sternocleidomastoid muscle, and note the anteroposterior depth of it. Stomach 9 is located on the anterior face of the sternocleidomastoid, Large Intestine 18 on its middle (lateral) face, and Small Intestine 16 on the posterior face. The line of these three points makes a very slight curvature, with its posterior point marginally more superior than its anterior.

This is a suggested sequence for a Windows to the Sky session. The focus, timing and channel of consciousness in which you work is as important as getting the location of the points right. The effectiveness of this work turns upon its appropriateness – as indicated by the client's need for it – the quality of your presence, and the clarity of your intent as you touch each point.

■ Thoracic Pump, Ribs 2, 3, 4
This is a preparatory technique prior to beginning windows work. Begin with a heel-of-hand contact with both hands to the anterior aspects of the third and fourth ribs, just lateral to the breastbone. Instruct the client to begin taking consecutive deep breaths. Follow the first three or four breaths with ever deepening pressure: allow him to breath in, but make him work against your resistance so that it is hard work. Upon the onset of the fourth in-breath, suddenly release all pressure and come off-contact (be sure not to jerk). The unexpected suddenness of the maneuver causes a sharp in-breath, often marked by a muted gasp – a kind of implosion sound – from the air rushing in through the throat. This prepares the neck and cranium for Windows to the Sky, work by releasing venous and lymphatic back pressure, "emptying" the head.

■ Room Screen, Stomach 15, Ribs 2-3
The point name is also translated as Roof Screen; like the last technique, this is not a classical window point, but rather a sequence initiation technique. Sit to the client's left and place your left hand transversely under his left scapula, supporting it entirely up off the table surface. Place his left upper arm or elbow on your left forearm, so that his left arm, ribcage, and shoulder girdle are completely separated from the table surface. Now place the heel of your right hand over the anterior prominence of the humerus and locate Room Screen (Stomach 15), which lies between the second and third ribs, directly superior to the nipple. Begin hypnagogic-level, gentle lateral traction of the

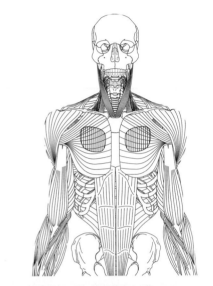

*Thoracic Pump, anterior view*

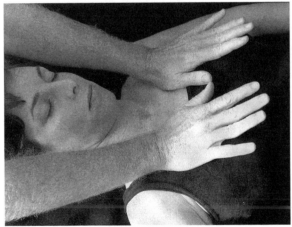

*Hand location for Thoracic Pump*

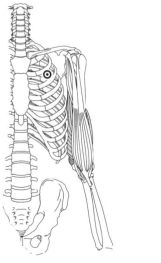

*Room Screen, ST15, anterior view*

shoulder, while deepening energetic access through Room Screen. Send your finger energy deep inside the cave of anahatta, the heart soul.

Room Screen is a controller of the spaciousness of the spiritual heart. Moving the shoulder (the wing – see below) and opening the space of the heart makes the client ready for flight into other realms, where nothing exists, and everything becomes clear.

■ Heavenly Palace, Lung 3, Rib 6
The point Heavenly Palace is also known as Celestial Mansion. "Heaven" represents divinity, clarity of vision, and the sense of spirit. We use heaven points when the client lacks contact with his own divinity or clarity of purpose. A "palace" is a place we enter rarely, a magical and special place barred by guards. You can ask to be admitted, but you must be let in. This point is also used in the treatment of frozen shoulder, in which case it tends to be acutely painful.

Bring an arm by your side. Note where the axillary crease ends inferiorly. Bring your other hand across your chest and measure four finger-widths from the inferior crease down toward your elbow. Heavenly Palace is located at this level, on the lateralmost part of the biceps brachii. It is sometimes described, delightfully, as a point that you can only just touch with the tip of your nose.

The arms are part of the heart soul, and can represent our wings (feathers are highly modified bone[1]). The biceps and the deltoid are our two most powerful "flying" muscles. With this contact, your intention is to invoke the bones' potential to be feathers. Use a light but thoroughgoing contact to facilitate flight out of present-time reality, and into another realm.

■ Heavenly Pond, Heart Protector 1, Rib 5
This point is also known as Celestial Pool. The "pond" represents a source, resource, or reservoir of energy for the spirit. Some of these reservoirs are larger, such as Sea of Chi (Conception Vessel 6) at the *hara*, some smaller, such as Crooked Pond (Liver 8).

It is a blisteringly hot summer day. You are walking across a field, your mouth dry with thirst, your head starting to throb from the sun. In the distance you see a wood. Getting closer, you see there is a fence around it, but it proves to be easy to jump over. Then you are in a leafy grove, cool and refreshingly dark. You keep walking to the center of the wood, and there, to your great delight, you see a pond, glistening and clear. A heavenly pond. You take off your clothes and jump in. You are suddenly immersed in another dimension, weightless, fluid, and cool.

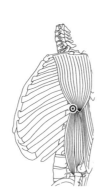

*Heavenly Palace*

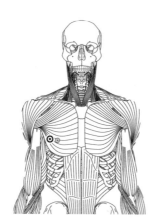

*Heavenly Pond HP1*

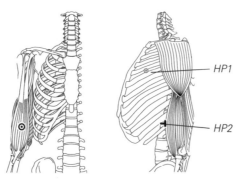

*Heavenly Spring HP2, anterior view (left) and lateral view with HP1 and HP2 (right)*

HP1

HP2

This point is capable of enhancing the transition from normal "sunlight" consciousness, to "water-being" or "oceanic" consciousness. It is located ½ inch (1.3 centimeter) immediately lateral to the nipple, on the pectoral muscle. Use this to begin easing the removal of the client's street armor, and to begin the process of opening his heart protector at its source. This will deepen heartfulness in the subsequent work. Apply posterior and medial pressure first, and once you are "hooked up" to the point, begin to move your energy and intention in a superior direction.

Heavenly Spring (Heart Protector 2) is used in women, rather than Heavenly Pond, because of the proximity of breast tissue. Heavenly Spring is located halfway down the anterior face of the biceps muscle, about three Acupuncture Chinese Inches[2] inferior to the axillary crease line.

■ Heaven Rushing Out,
Conception Vessel 22, Cervical 7

This point's name is also translated as Celestial Chimney. It is on the conception vessel, which, strictly speaking, is not a meridian but a vessel, that is, a major conduit of energy, like a major river of the body. It can handle more energy flow than the smaller tributaries that are the meridians.

Heaven Rushing Out is relevant when the spiritual self is not being supported by physical action – a lack of outer alignment to the inner. A keynote symptom is heart pain, that radiates to the back. The heart has to do with sense of destiny and purpose, so heart pain, combined with a lack of alignment to purpose, is an indication for our employing window work. Heaven Rushing Out is intimately concerned with emotional and spiritual expression – it is a throat soul point. In acupuncture it is used in the treatment of aphonia (loss of speech).

This point is located immediately inferior to the "glossy surface" of the Adam's apple, at its juncture with the cricoid cartilage. It is located just inferior to the thyroid gland, where the tissue "feel" changes from fatty to gristly, and it may be found as far inferior as the center of the suprasternal notch in the anterior midline. For finger contact, the point is located on the superior surface of the cricoid. Place your free hand under the neck, so that you have a "sending" finger on Heaven Rushing Out and a receiving, or "mother," hand under the neck (everything returns to the Great Mother). Your intention is to continue to take the neck "off" the rest of the body. First use a gentle posterior pressure with your cricoid finger, then move superiorly with your intention. You are encouraging the champagne to come up out of the bottle.

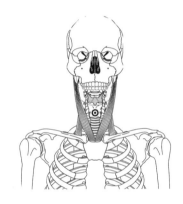

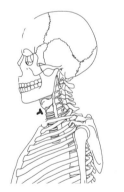

*Heaven Rushing Out CV22, anterior and lateral views*

Copyright © 1995 Nielsen/Garbett

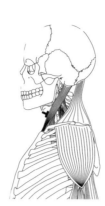
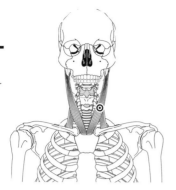

*People Welcome ST9, anterior and lateral views*

■ People Welcome, Stomach 9, Cervical 6

This point is also called Human Welcome (which slightly alters its meaning to me) and Man's Progress, which gives it another interpretation altogether. At Heaven Rushing Out, energy is leaving the body. At People Welcome, energy – people – is being welcomed in. Imagine a candlelit house deep in the forest at dusk. The doors are open. You are welcome to come in.

This is a very sedating point – of blood, of energy – and work here tends to make a person more receptive. This point is traditionally used to reduce blood pressure. We might choose to work with this point when the client "asks" for something related to sensing a need for support and nurturance from other people. It is on the stomach meridian; the stomach has to do with being fed. Opening this window allows the client to let nurturing energy in. In acupuncture, over-sedation here is regarded as able to cause a loss of consciousness, or even death, so treat this point with great care when using finger pressure and intention.

People Welcome is level with the cricoid cartilage, at the anterior border of the sternocleidomastoid. It is immediately anterior to the body of the sixth cervical vertebra. When you are at the correct location your fingertips will pick up the pulsation of the common carotid artery. Use this point gently, and only apply pressure to one side at a time.

■ Heavenly Pillar, Urinary Bladder 10, Atlanto-Occipital Joint

The name of this point is also translated as Celestial Pillar. It is one of the "sea of chi" points – in other words, not just a pond of energy, but a much larger resource. "Pillar" gives the feeling of being supported, being in touch with who we are and the world around us. We are also in touch with our inner strength when our pillar points are working optimally. The energy that transits and is located at these points has to do with will, ambition, and inner fortitude, rather like some of the energetics embodied in the field of the mandible.

Heavenly Pillar dysfunction may manifest as a deep sadness or anxiety, related to a lack of inner strength or will. The client is sad because he cannot summon the strength of will to break through his inertia and despondency. Somehow he knows that something is amiss, and that in normal times he could "shake himself out of it." This awareness of dysfunction coupled with the inability to do anything effective about it is, as we have seen, a hallmark of the need for "window" work.

Samson brought down the temple by pushing apart the pillars. The Heavenly Pillars support our temple, the head. The cords of semispinalis capitus

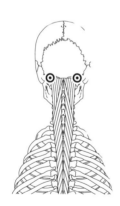
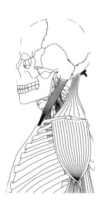

*Heavenly Pillar UB10, posterior and lateral views*

represent the pillars. This point is located at the lateral borders of the muscle as it inserts into the occiput.

Heavenly Pillar is ½ inch (1.3 centimeter) lateral to Wind Palace (Governor Vessel 16), and very slightly superior to it. It is a major hypnagogic point. Apply an anterior and superior-directed delicate pressure and intention. The subtle combination of angle, pressure, and intention determines its effectiveness. Normalization of this point is vital in furthering the release of the head from the neck. It is an important "trigger point" for release of rectus capitus posterior minor, and for working with muscle contraction headaches.

■ Support And Rush Out,
Large Intestine 18, Cervical 5

This point is also known as Protuberance Assistant. Use it when the client feels a lack of support in his life, or feels out of touch with his inner strength. The point is all about connecting heaven and earth, and being able to bring both into the world. Gentle pressure here helps free the head's connectedness to the body. Support the head, letting it know that it is being taken care of, and allow tension to rush out. It is a quietly euphoric technique.

Support and Rush Out is located on the middle part of the sternocleidomastoid, in the middle of the muscle belly, at the precise level of the fifth cervical vertebra. Locate this point by taking contact midway between the clavicular attachment of the muscle and the mastoid tip. Looked at from the front, this is just where the horizontal, sloping plane of the shoulder changes into the vertical plane of the neck.

■ Heavenly Window,
Small Intestine 16, Cervical 4

This point, also known as Celestial Window, is used to open a "window to heaven," especially in those who need help in perceiving how to change a negative behavior pattern into a productive and harmonious one.

This point is halfway between the last point (Support and Rush Out) and the mastoid tip. In other words, it is located halfway up the sternocleidomastoid (see Point Location, above). It is lateral to the spinal cord itself, at the level of the fourth cervical vertebra, exactly in the middle of the neck as seen laterally. Compared with the location of Support and Rush Out, Heavenly Window is one vertebra more superior. This is a place where most bodyworkers' fingertips go instinctively while doing neck work.

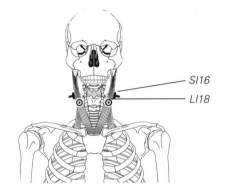

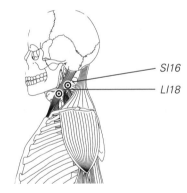

*Support and Rush Out LI18, and Heavenly Window SI16, anterior and lateral views*

Copyright © 1995 Nielsen/Garbett

257

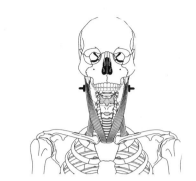

*Heavenly Appearance SI17, anterior view*

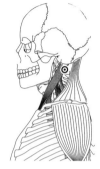
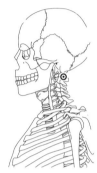

*Heavenly Appearance SI17, lateral view showing muscle attachment (left) and bony contact (right)*

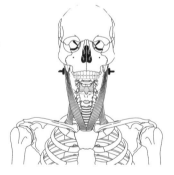
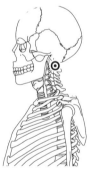

*Heavenly Window TW16, anterior and lateral views*

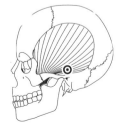
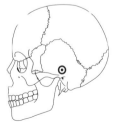

*Ear Gate TW21, lateral view with temporalis (left) and bony contact (right)*

■ Heavenly Appearance, Small Intestine 17, Cervical 2

The name is also translated as Celestial Countenance. This point can be used to produce a strong movement of energy from the head downward into the body. As such it is very useful in spiritual emergencies when the client is too much in his "heaven," and has lost all contact with the earth, and needs to be brought down as a matter of urgency. When this point is dysfunctional it can result in so much energy leaving the head that deafness or tinnitus can ensue. Use this point when the client has symptoms of hearing or energy deficit in the head, or in the "heavenly" aspects of his spiritual life, and also when he senses that something is not connected in his life. It would also be indicated when life actions are not in accord with beliefs, and when the client can see this but has no control over the pattern. This would apply to all addictions, once they are conscious.

The point is located halfway between Small Intestine 16 and the earlobe, on the lateral face of the sternocleidomastoid muscle. It is at the level of the body of axis (the second cervical vertebra). Use slow, deep pressure in a medial, then superior, direction, fingertips just anterior to the bulging lateral mass of the transverse process of axis.

■ Heavenly Window, Triple Warmer 16, Cervical 1

This has the same name in English as Small Intestine 16, but it is expressed in Chinese with different characters: there is more than one way of looking into heaven.

Triple Warmer 16 is located immediately inferior to the mastoid tips. Press an index or middle finger gently medially at the tip of mastoid and you will feel the lateral mass of the atlas (first cervical vertebra). One you have the right location, use thumb-pad contact and direct your intention and pressure medially. You are operating at the immediate level of foramen magnum, and the medulla oblongata and Wind Palace (see above). Calming work here may be helpful in anxiety, and to soothe the ruffled heart in heart palpitations. Triple Warmer 16 is used when there is too much heat in the body.

■ Ear Gate, Triple Warmer 21, Zygomatic Arch

This is not a traditional window point, but one that I have found useful in inducing specific states of consciousness. "Gates" are ways in, in this case to discrete pea-sized aggranulations of gray matter called the mammillary bodies, which help regulate and fine-tune our sense of well-being. Energetic contact with these deep structures helps induce inner illumination and content.

The mammillary bodies are located just anterior to the red nucleus, and posterior to the pituitary stalk, inferior to the hypothalamus, and anterior to the pons. Their access point, Ear Gate, is located just where the auricle of the ear merges with the superior aspect of the temporal portion of the zygomatic arch. The point is immediately superior to the temporal portion of the zygomatic arch, and is best located with the client's mouth open.

Once you have the exact location, use your middle fingers as energy transmitters, pointing them directly at each other, toward the very center of the brain. Once your middle fingers have located the "gate" and you can feel your energy begin to penetrate inside the client's head, begin to access your own energy field using a power breath or *chi kung* technique. Focus your projected energy, like a rainbow or laser beam, on the mammillary bodies, lighting them up. (For further information, see Chapter 25, The Temporals.)

■ Wind Palace, Governor Vessel 16, Atlanto-Occipital Joint

There are many subcategories of spiritual energy in Chinese medicine, and "wind" is sometimes included among them. However, it is safer to say that wind relates to energetic movement in the body. This energetic movement eddies up the spinal canal and vertebral column, the domain of the earth, to arrive at its "palace" – the highest physical home of the spirit. As the palace guards (muscle contraction and atlanto-occipital compression) step aside, Wind Palace opens up, and wind energy can expand through the potential stricture of the foramen magnum into the "heaven" of the expanded space of the cranium. Wind Palace is where we connect heaven and earth, and therefore it is an important transition place, one of the most important in the whole dreambody.

Sometimes, as in nature, wind gets out of control, which can manifest as muscle spasms or whole-body convulsions. Wind Palace connects directly to the brain, and if there is too much wind in the brain, there can be convulsions, epilepsy, or palsy.

*Wei chi*[3] is the defensive energy of the body, said to exist just outside and inside the surface of the skin, which aids in combating colds and chills. At a metaphysical level, *wei chi* has to do with energetic protection, such as the kind that bodyworkers need in order not to hang on to "other people's stuff." Wind Palace is a very good point for strengthening the *wei chi*. It is also a "sea of marrow" point – a place where we can access the very deepest level of energy in the body.

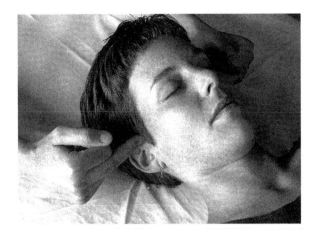
*Ear Gate, directed energy to mammillary bodies*

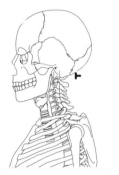
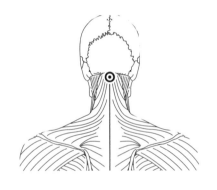
*Wind Palace GV16, posterior view with muscle attachments (left) and lateral view showing bony contact (below)*

Copyright © 1995 Nielsen/Garbett

Wind Palace is located on the midline, ⅓ inch (8 millimeters) inferior to the inion, in the gap between the occiput and the superior aspect of the atlas. Place your nondominant hand in a cupping contact on the frontal, and the middle finger of your dominant hand into contact with Wind Palace. Now bring the client's head into slight backward-bending and introduce slight traction to bring about a gental transition into hypnagogic consciousness. Gently drive your Wind Palace middle finger towards the falx, and the center line of your nondominant "mother" hand.

Be sensitive to the cranial wave and alert for the unfolding of unwinding patterns. This is a good technique to facilitate the gentle unwinding of the head from the neck, and is also effective to stop nosebleeds (when you would bend the head further into backward-bending). It may help in frontal headaches as well, where you hold the head in neutral position or in very slight forward-bending and deepen the pressure you are applying with your thumb until you sense release at the falx, occiput, and atlas.

■ Middle Of Man,
Governor Vessel 26, Cervical 1

Middle of Man is located at the apex of the curve of the anterior nasal spine. Take a fingertip contact with the middle finger of your dominant hand, making sure you are just anterior to bone contact. Span the greater wings of the sphenoid with the thumb and middle finger of your other hand, resting the metacarpophalangeal joint at glabella with a meaningful physical and energetic contact. Direct energy in to the hypothalamus from Middle of Man, which is the cerebral center of identity, and the central initiator of wakefulness. Meet that line of energy with a transverse line directed medially from each greater wing. Finally bring in a vector of energy from your glabella contact to the hypothalamus. This technique helps people to "come home" to the place where a deeper level of identity resides. It is deeply stabilizing. (See also Chapter 42, Cardinal Eight Protocol.)

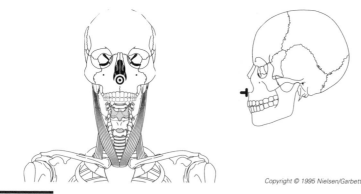

Copyright © 1995 Nielsen/Garbett

**Above:**
*Middle of Man GV26, anterior and lateral views*

**Right:**
*Middle of Man coupled with sphenoid contact*

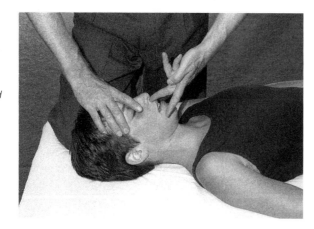

■ Broken Bowl, Stomach 12, Mid-Clavicle
This is the place you go to mend the broken bowl – to bring disparate parts back into a harmonious whole, to achieve the return of the Holy Vessel. Broken Bowl is an integration point for many energy pathways, and a good completion and balancing point for all of the window points. It is the supreme balancer.

This point is located midway between the acromion tip and the sternoclavicular joint, and lies just posterior to the superior ridge of the clavicle. It is best reached from the head end of the table and contacted bilaterally, using both of your thumbtips in contact with the points, with your fingers on the anterior face of the clavicles, providing gentle opposition to your thumbs.

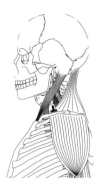
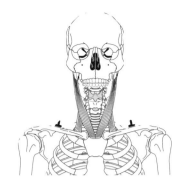

*Broken Bowl ST12, anterior and lateral views*

■ Hundred Meeting Places,
Governor Vessel 20, Vertex

This point is also known as Hundred Convergences. It is sahasrara, the crown soul, and is located at vertex. Working on the basis of opposites, attention to the field at Hundred Meeting Places is good for hemorrhoids and to treat clients who experience pain in sexual intercourse. It often assists in the treatment of sacral pain, and may be helpful in lumbago.

Locate Hundred Meeting Places by taking a line of sight directly superior from the ear canal aperture to the top of the head. This gives you vertex. Feel for the slight depression, or change of tissue tone, at the suture. As the crown soul, this point has perhaps the most widespread capabilities of any single point in acupuncture, craniosacral work, and energy work. You can easily reach any part of the body from here. It is especially good for transmitting energy down the "Red Road" of the spinal cord. To do this, find the suture with fingernails or thumbnails, and apply pressure in an inferior direction, sending energy down to the tip of the coccyx, and even to the soles of the feet. It is important to visualize the spinal canal, and permeate it with your energy, which you project in a warm, tender, ever-moving inferior direction.

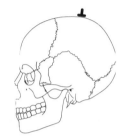
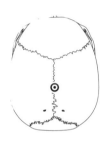

*Hundred Meeting Places, lateral and superior views*

Copyright © 1995 Nielsen/Garbett

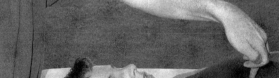
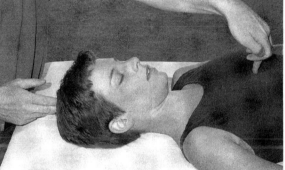

*Hundred Meeting Places and optional contact with heart*

# Glossary

**Ancestor Spirits** A Native American description for intelligent forms of non-corporeal energy, related to the subject through ancestral lineage, or through clan or tribal association. Information from ancestor spirits may be accessible in altered states of consciousness, at times of great need, or in moments of danger. The concept of resourcing ancestor spirit wisdom has some similarities to the concept of "guides." Access to such wisdom may also be facilitated by ancestor spirit ceremonies, which may also help access nonhabitual neurological pathways to the right cerebral cortex, or to little understood subcortical areas.

**Archaic Wound** When a physical, emotional or spiritual trauma is too severe to integrate into conscious memory at the time of the incident, the dreambody stores it away for future assimilation, or release. Also known as a "psychotic corner," "energy cyst," and an "area of condensed experience, or "COEX."

**Asterion** Asterion is located at the intersection of the posterior superior margin of the petrous portion of the temporal bone with the lambdoid suture. It literally means "little star," for its fanciful resemblance to the emanations of three starbursts of light.

**Bindu** An accessory soul-center, Bindu is the Hindu name for the energy point on the sagittal suture just posterior to the vertex of the head, where the spirit is said to leave the body at the moment of death, to join the soul. Some people sense this occurring; it is called witnessing the gyre.

**Blueprint Level** The operations level, or level where patterns of movement are formulated. The deepest level of the physical dimension of the dreambody.

**Bodhisatva** A Buddhist term for one who has attained their enlightenment but decides to postpone their union with *Nirvana* (approximately "heaven") until they have helped all other sentient beings to attain enlightenment.

**Borderline Heads** A head which appears normal until either stressed, or touched innocuously and exceedingly lightly in craniosacral work, when it suddenly (and often alarmingly) exhibits symptoms such as migraine or vertigo. This means that the head, while appearing normal, has in fact at least one underlying lesion pattern or archaic wound that needs only the smallest of inputs to tip it over the edge into symptom manifestation.

**Bramacharya** Literally celibacy, but inferring a spiritual choice in the search for a passionate connection with God.

**Bregma** A landmark located at the intersection of the coronal and sagittal sutures, some two inches (five centimeters) anterior to the crown of the head.

**Chakra** An area of condensed non-neurological energy, or chi, associated with specific states of consciousness, feelings, archetypes and shadows, polarities and colors. There are seven chakras in the Hindu system, seven in the ancient Egyptian, nine in the Sufi, and three principal ones, the *dantian*, in the Taoist. The Egyptians called the chakras "souls," a nomenclature I prefer to use.

**Chi**  Human non-neurological energy, present throughout the body and also flowing along the energy channels known in acupuncture as meridians and vessels. Synonymous with the Anglo-Saxon "life force," the Hindu *prana*, and the Japanese *ki*.

**Chi Kung**  The transmission of chi through space or through physical contact from healer to client, often accomplished with specific postures, mudras, use of the eyes, and breathing patterns. Requires years of disciplined training to master. Synonymous with *kime*.

**Chu'a Ka**  An ancient Mongolian warrior practice, a form of deep penetrating muscle massage done the day before battle to clear the body of any muscular or fascial restrictions; ideally also performed the day after battle, to exorcise residual trauma and tension.

**Clear The Confusion**  A psychic healing technique designed to clear the energetic space between the hemispheres of the brain, and to unwind tension in the falx cerebri.

**Compression Head**  A condition where there is no cranial wave, or a severely degraded wave, at the sphenobasilar joint, which usually means there is no cranial wave anywhere in the cranium, except in the mandible. This condition almost always is the result of severe trauma, including birth trauma. The atlanto-occipital joint is also usually compressed as well.

**Consciousness**  The presence of a meta-communicator, or "knower," distinct from instinctual process. Consciousness is that part of our being that can individuate from emotions or archetypal behavior, and do something of its own choosing instead.

**Contact High**  The transfer of specific states of consciousness through touch, or through physical proximity, as in *shaktipat*.

**Continuum**  An exquisitely fine movement-meditation discipline developed by Emily Conrad D'aoud. It is particularly effective in helping those with movement difficulties, spinal injury, or neurological impairment. It is also a very powerful tool for inner work.

**Core Link**  William Sutherland's name for the connection made by the spinal dura between the foramen magnum of the occiput and the second segment of the sacrum.

**Coronal Plane**  The lateromedial anatomical plane, running from one side of the body to the other. Similar, but not identical, to the plane of the coronal suture.

**Covert Awareness**  Coined by a Swiss psychologist at the turn of the century, covert awareness refers to noncortical ways of knowing and remembering. Similar, but not identical, to intuition.

**Cranial Wave (rhythm, pulse)**  The most discrete of the three motion patterns – breath, heartbeat and cranial wave – found in the human body. The cranial wave seems to have its source in involuntary muscle contractions that take place throughout the body in a tidal, ocean swell-like motion (the muscle contractions are themselves triggered by the fluctuant field, with the spiritual heart as its center. This involuntary motion is transmitted to the spinal cord and brain via the spinal nerves, the bones of the cranial base, and the mediastinum. Its normal range lies within 8 to 14 cycles per minute. It may be analogous to Traube-Hering waves (see below). The cranial wave is also called the cranial rhythm or cranial pulse.

**Domes and bowls, domed and bowled structures**  The dreambody can be considered as having a total of seven interrelated domes and bowls within it. It has four domed (cupola-shaped) structures – the calvarium, or top of the head; the tentorium cerebelli, the apex of the lungs, and the muscular portion of the respiratory diaphragm. It has three bowled (open upward, slightly cone-shaped) structures – the perineum, the central tendon of the respiratory diaphragm, and the cranial base.

**Dreambody**  A term coined by Arnold Mindell. As used in this book, dreambody denotes the sum of mind, body and spirit that is understood in most Western cultures to encompass the whole human being. We see the dreambody working perfectly when the spirit (or "psyche") communicates a body situation or need to the mind through dreams (see The Dream of the Sphenoid in Chapter 1, Visionary Craniosacral Work, and the section on C.G. Jung in Chapter 4, Vignettes in the History of Healing). The mind, body and spirit are not simply interconnected, they *are* one: dreambody means the totality.

***Encephalization Quotient*** The ratio between cerebral cortex surface area and body size; the higher this ratio is, the more intelligent the being. Humans have the highest "encephalization quotient" (E.Q.) of any land mammal; dolphins have the highest of any aquatic creature.

***Energy*** Human energy is called *chi* in China, *ki* in Japan, and *prana* in India. It is non-neurological force that travels along, but is not limited to, conduits known in acupuncture as energy vessels or meridians, and in Yoga as *nadis*. This energy *is* the spirit. Chi is transferable to another person through intention or through physical contact.

***Endosteal Dura*** The outer of the two layers of dura mater within the cranial cavity. It feels like a soft fingernail, and looks like prosciutto. It is firmly attached to the inside of the cranial bones, where it acts as periosteum, and to the inner (meningeal) layer of the dura mater.

***Energetic Loading*** Parts of the body have particular energies or emotions attached to them, or "loaded" into them. Thus the sphenoid is energetically imprinted with perception, and the energy of the inner eye; the liver with joyful assimilation or with angry biliousness, the legs with delight in movement, and so on.

***Epigamic Differentiation*** The evolutionary development of stimulating systems that are specific to one other individual (that is, systems that create pair-bonding). More commonly known as "falling in love." It encompasses two things. First, the hominid becomes an individual, distinct in behavior, appearance and scent from any other, and, because this individual is so distinctive, he attracts only a few potential mates. Second, it refers to the bonding of two such differentiated mates to each other, forming a monogamous pair bond. Thus human males fall in love, and care, protect and have sexual intimacy with that other; male baboons fall in sex, and mate with any female baboon who happens to be in estrus. Epigamic differentiation is thought to be a major reason for our development as a dominant species.

***Eyes Of A Dead Person*** This phrase, "to look at the world with the eyes of a dead person" originates in psychic perception work. It refers to the necessity to look at others, or events, as if you were dead. This means letting go of excitement, entanglements, performance anxiety, fear, the need to impress or be approved of, and competitiveness. It means seeing from selfless consciousness.

***Field*** The human energy field is invested in the body and also extends beyond it. It is composed of the following:

■ The piezoelectric field: This is created by tension or compression upon calcium crystals embedded in bone cells, which change their polarity depending upon the forces acting upon them. (See piezoelectric charge, below.) Sensitive fingers can discern changes in this field.

■ The meridian energy field: This encompasses all the non-neurological chi flowing within the meridians and energy vessels of the human body. It can be measured by changes in microelectrical resistance at acupuncture points. Local condensations of this field are called "chakras," or soul centers. I call this field, which is accessible to consciousness, "the spirit."

■ The extended human energy field, or aura: This is that part of the meridian energy field which extends beyond the body, and is visible to children, psychics, and those who have the gift of the inner eye.

■ The millivolt field: This is that part of the human electrical field that is measurable by electrocardiographs that pick up the discharge of the sinoatrial node (the heart's pacemaker). It can be detected throughout the body.

■ The neurological field: This is detectable by finely calibrated instruments that pick up the electrochemical energy that travels along the nerves, and is also detectable as changes in electrical activity in the human cortex.

■ The fluctuant field: This is the sum of the five fields mentioned above. The fluctuant field permeates and extends beyond the body, and seems to be the trigger for cranial wave formation. It gives off exceedingly faint radio waves. It is referred to in this book simply as "the field."

***Glabella*** An anatomical landmark on the cranium located between the eyebrows at the place commonly referred to as the "third eye." In acupuncture it is the point known as GV24.5. It has no name.

***Glamour*** This is an archaic English term that refers to an altered state of consciousness where non-normal abilities, such as inner-eye or inner-ear perception open up. It is synonymous to Shunryu Suzuki's "larger me." It is frequently mentioned in Marion Zimmer Bradley's Arthurian novel *The Mists of Avalon*.

***Guides*** A spirit guide is a non-corporeal form of energy that may be accessed to gather information or wisdom not ordinarily available to the subject. There may or may not be a family, or clan, relationship to the subject. The guide(s) may or may not have lived on this planet. Also known as "guardian angels." (See "Ancestor Spirits," above). Guides are further broken down into inner and outer guides. Inner guides are part of your own archetypal resource material; outer guides are sources external to you.

***Homeostatic Threat*** Homeostasis is the ability of a system to regulate its internal metabolism; homeostatic threat refers to a situation when a healer is moving into disequilibrium because she is giving out more energy than she has coming in. Give of the water (energy) overflowing from the brim of your well; never dip your bucket down the well, into your energy reserves, because then you are entering homeostatic threat. You are likely to become first flat, then dull, and finally to sicken.

***Hundred Meeting Places*** An acupuncture point, known technically as Governor Vessel 20, located at vertex, the intersection of the coronal and sagittal sutures. It is the crown soul, sahasrara, in the Hindu chakra system.

***Hyparxis*** A term used by ancient Greek philosophers to denote the necessity of understanding the world using both of what we would now call the right and the left hemispheres, as well as the intuitive heart – perception of the all and everything from a place of unity.

***Inner Eye Reading*** An intuitive assessment of another person's soul and dreambody based upon inner-eye perception – that is, based upon seeing beneath the surface appearance of things, into a deeper reality.

***Intuition*** The paranormal ability to sense that which is not apparent, spoken, or visible. Intuition encompasses clairvoyance, sensing another's deepest inner feelings, and gaining insight into what really troubles another. It includes the ability to sense what another person really needs to first heal, and then to find fulfillment.

***Intuitive Heart*** The words intuitive heart, spiritual heart and heavenly heart all refer to aspects of the heart as the energetic center of the body and the field, the most important of the seven souls according to the ancient Egyptian understanding.

■ Intuitive Heart refers to the part of the heart that feels, instinctively, or through empathy, what troubles everyone.

■ Spiritual Heart is that part of the heart that aspires to unconditional love, and loves selflessly.

■ Heavenly Heart is concerned with internal (often euphoric) processes, not necessarily with sensing others, or with giving love. Heavenly Heart is the center of meditative processes such as the "circulation of the light" described in the ancient Chinese text *The Secret of The Golden Flower.*

***Ki and Kime*** *Ki* is the Japanese word for *chi. Kime* refers to the projection of energy across space or through touch, and is thus synonymous to Chi Kung.

***Lambda*** An anatomical landmark on the head, where both lambdoid sutures meet the posterior limit of the sagittal suture. From the word for the Greek letter "L," whose shape lambda mimics. In acupuncture this is the location of Strength Divider (Governor Vessel 18).

***Larger Me*** See Glamour.

***Lateral Thinking*** A phrase coined by Edward De Bono to denote the ability to solve problems by thinking in nonhabitual ways, such as correcting complaints that a lift system works too slowly by installing full length mirrors in the lobbies rather than the traditional problem solving route of re-writing the lift operating systems.

***Lesion Pattern*** A lesion is a fault: a cut on your skin is a skin lesion. A lesion in craniosacral work usually refers to an aberrant position, movement, piezoelectric charge or energetic "feel" in a cranial bone, or a pair of articulating bone structures. Most cranial lesion patterns are described according to faulty movements or positions, or both, at the sphenobasilar joint. (See Compression Head, above.)

***Liquid-Electric Motion Pattern*** One of three models that seek to explain the way that cranial bones behave, this model posits a fully floating spherical axis for each cranial bone, which is additionally influenced, as a quantum field, by the energetic presence of the healer. See also Similar Motion Model and Opposite Motion Model, and Chapter 19, Quantum Cranial: The Liquid-Electric Model.

***Lordosis*** The anterior convexity, or forward curvature, of the lumbar spine. It is usually used to connote an abnormal degree of anterior convexity; however, a mild anterior convexity is healthy and normal.

***Love, specifically unconditional love*** A non-neurological form of energy, whose communication through eye contact, speech, song, or touch constitutes the single most powerful healing force (both of self and other), known to mankind.

***"The Mechanism"*** Sutherland called the sum total of cranial bones, brain and cerebrospinal fluid, sacrum, the membrane system within the head and the spinal dura (see Core Link above), and the way they all move together and interact, The Mechanism.

***Meningeal Dura*** The inner of the two layers of dura within the cranial cavity. The meningeal dura forms the sickle-shaped reinforcing and supporting struts known as the falx cerebri and cerebelli, and the tentorium cerebelli. It approximates the arachnoid meningeal tissue via the subdural space.

***Midline Bones*** The occiput, sphenoid, frontal, vomer, ethmoid and mandible are all midline – that is, central and single – bones. The remaining cranial bones are all paired.

***Mudra*** A hand position that both externalizes and evokes a specific state of consciousness. Mudras find their origins in Yoga, Jainism, Buddhism and classical Indian dance. From the sanskrit meaning "a sign."

***Nasion*** An anatomical landmark located in the median or midline of the skull, where the nasal bones articulate with the frontal. Nasion is about ½ inch (1.3 centimeter) inferior to glabella.

***Neurocranium*** That part of the skull that encloses the brain.

***Opposite Motion Patterns*** One of three phases of cranial bone motion patterns. In opposite motion pattern movement cranial bones move alternately, that is, when one parietal bone flexes, its twin extends.

***"The Other"*** A poetic word form to describe nonordinary consciousness, especially when being guided by the use of intuitive heart, inner-eye and inner-ear information to arrive at decisions, or diagnoses.

***Paired Bones*** All cranial bones of which there are two on each side of the head, such as the zygomae or parietals.

***Pattern-Setters*** Some bones or muscles act as "pattern-setters," that is, they help to determine the behavior of adjacent or distant structures, by virtue of location or connections, and pass on aspects of their specific static position, cranial wave motion and energetic loading to other bones. Thus the sphenoid is a pattern-setter for the whole neurocranium; each lateral pterygoid muscle is a pattern-setter for the sphenoid and the mandible; the sacrum, connected to it by the core link, is a pattern-setter for the occiput, and so on.

***Piezoelectricity*** When a bone is compressed or placed under tension, the nonconducting inorganic crystals that make up 70 percent of the bone register a minute electrical charge, known as the piezoelectric polarity. Compression produces a negative piezoelectrical polarity in the bone, tension a positive one. The bone cells responsible for shaping bones after a fracture use these piezoelectric changes to either lay down (osteoclasts) or remove (osteoblasts) bone cells. Sensitive fingers can feel the change of piezoelectricity in a cranial bone and therefore deduce if it is under compression or tension, using this information to fine tune their treatment.

***Prana*** Synonymous with *chi*. *Prana* is energy present throughout the body, traveling along "nadis" (synonymous with meridians) and polarized into male energy *(pingala)* and female *(ida)*. When pingala and ida meet at the base of the spine they form the beginning of the double-helix energy form of the *kundalini,* which is the aspiring spiritual energy of the human being. Yogis learn to direct their prana at will, often attaining mastery over their autonomic nervous system.

***Prana Yama*** The yoga practice of using prescribed respiratory exercises to bring about changes in consciousness, physiology, or both. The best known example consists of closing one nostril while breathing in through the other, and alternating the nostril closure from one side to the other.

***Process, Process Oriented Psychology ("POP")*** Born out of the genius of Arnold Mindell, a Jungian psychotherapist based in Portland, Oregon, this is a body-oriented psychotherapy. Some of Mindell's techniques and insights are used in my unwinding work.

***Psyche*** An archetypal aspect of the spirit, imbued with psychological weight. The psyche is composed of three aspects – mythos, eros and logos, each with its own gifts and needs. Named after the comely heroine of a Greek myth, as recounted by Apuleius.

*Pterion*  An anatomical reference on the head, pterion is located at the temple where the greater wing of sphenoid, frontal, temporal and parietal bones approximate or touch each other. It is thus a meeting of four bones, whose specific architecture differs from person to person.

*Reciprocal Tension Membrane*  William Sutherland and Harold Magoun agreed upon this nomenclature to describe a system of slightly elasticated membranes within the neurocranium, consisting of the falx and tentorium, two spatially distinct but physiologically continuous parts composed of meningeal dura.

*Right Thinking*  This denotes the ability to think a choice through, considering all its possible ramifications, and arrive at a course of action that will create the most appropriate result, and the greatest possible common good. It is the opposite of slipshod, selfish thinking.

*Sagittal Plane, or anteroposterior plane*  A plane running from front to back through the middle of the body, identical to the plane of the sagittal suture.

*Secondary Signals*  Gestures, postural shifts, or changes of expression that often contradict, or give deeper information about, the client's primary message, or signal. Thus the person says "I'd love to meet you Saturday," but unconsciously scratches himself behind his left ear as he says so – a secondary signal that may give the deeper meaning "I'm confused about the prospect of meeting you Saturday." Secondary signals are useful keys in visionary craniosacral work that help the practitioner gauge what is really going on with the client.

*Self*  Self with a capital "S" refers to the higher self, or individuated and conscious Self.

*Self-splinting*  The muscles that move a joint (or cover a visceral area) go into a protective hypertonicity when the joint, bone or area is dislocated, broken or injured, to prevent further movement which might cause further internal injury. Thus one psoas muscle typically goes into a hypertonic spasm in lumbar intervertebral disc injury to prevent the disc rupturing any further. It is wise to address the cause of its self-splinting, and not just the "tight muscle." Reducing the disc rupture by craniosacral work results in a spontaneous normalization of the psoas muscle. It also works both ways. Sometimes releasing the psoas with deep tissue work will allow the vertebra to normalize its position, thus reducing the disc rupture.

*Shaktipat*  A Hindu term for the transmission of energy from guru to disciple, or healer to client, through touch, eye-to-eye contact, or through intermediary devices, such as when the guru touches the disciple through the delightful intermediary of a peacock feather.

*Shear*  A term from physics, "shear" refers to a break or displacement occurring along an internal plane in response to a force applied to the structure parallel to the plane. Shear is used to describe the movement or displacement that occurs in two sphenoid lesion patterns, vertical strain and lateral strain, in both of which cases a force applied to the outside of the head causes a displacement along the internal plane of the sphenobasilar joint.

*Similar Motion Patterns*  One of three phases of cranial bone motion patterns. In this model, each paired cranial bone moves into flexion, or extension, at the same time. Thus when one parietal bone flexes, so does the other, and they diverge, or hinge, at the sagittal suture as they do so.

*Soul*  Soul refers to that part of the dreambody that resides outside the body, and is connected to our seventh soul, Sahasrara. It holds within its ovoid boundaries the accumulated wisdom, aspiration and spiritual identity of the individual. The spirit joins the soul twenty to forty minutes after death.

*Souls, as in "Seven Souls"*  (See Chakras, above.) The Egyptians called the chakras "souls," a nomenclature I prefer to use because it is more meaningful to Western consciousness, as well as being more poetic.

*Soul Center*  See "Chakra" above.

*Soul State*  A nomenclature I use to describe an out-of-body technique where one deliberately moves from ordinary, body-centered consciousness to that of being at one with one's soul. This is done in inner-eye diagnosis the better to sense another being's totality. The same phenomena is reported in (involuntary) near-death experiences as "seeing my body lying there as if looking down from the ceiling." Soul state is typically above the right or left shoulder (for most people, it is above and slightly in front of the right shoulder).

*Special Three*  This refers to the three most important bones of the cranium in visionary craniosacral work – the sphenoid, temporals, and the mandible.

***Speed Reducers*** Four cranial bones (the ethmoid, palatines, vomer, and zygomae) act as "speed reducers." Each bone reduces the amplitude of the cranial wave coming in on one side of itself before the wave formations reach bones on another side. Speed reducer bones do this through sutural sliding, and/or through malleability, and via osseous plasticity. Thus the zygomae reduces the "speed" (more accurately, the amplitude) of the cranial wave reaching it from the sphenoid before transmitting it to the maxillae.

***Spirit*** The field of the body. The moment this field collapses, we begin to move into the experience of death; there is no more electrical energy to cause the heart to contract, no more neurological energy to allow the brain to be alive. It takes twenty to forty minutes for the field and the spirit to close down completely, and for the spirit to leave the body and merge with the soul. During this time there is still a cranial wave in the body, which is triggered by the meridian field. It gradually disappears as the chi ebbs away.

***Spiritual Heart*** See Intuitive Heart, above.

***Still Point*** A spontaneous or induced cessation of the cranial wave formations. A still point is usually a moment of rest, sometimes is euphoric, and may last from a few seconds to as long as a minute. Still points are times when the cranial wave formations reorganize, optimally when the soma sheds a dysfunctional cranial wave pattern, and establishes a better one. The still point ends as the new pattern emerges.

***Still Point Breathing*** A meditative practice of inducing the cessation of the breath at the end of the out-breath and/or the end of the in-breath. This is done to facilitate specific states of consciousness, such as deep stillness or moving into a glamour. It also occurs spontaneously.

***Sutherland*** William Garner Sutherland D.O., 1873–1954, American osteopath, intuitive and deductive genius, the founder of cranial osteopathy.

***Traube-Hering waves*** These are sometimes called "third order waves," that is, a third motion present in the body distinct from respiration and heartbeat. Traube observed these waves of changing arterial pressure in animals whose thorax was opened and diaphragm was paralyzed. Traube noted that certain much longer wavelike variations occur during sleep. These sleeping waves are probably cranial wave formations. Russian investigators have found third order waves partly responsible for the same type of cerebrospinal fluctuations reported by Sutherland.

***Vector*** Movement of thrust or intention along a specified angle; used in cranial work when we "vector" energy or pressure along an exact angle designed to reach a target tissue, such as the pineal gland, or a specific target suture such as the one between the lesser wing of the sphenoid and the frontal bone, a suture that we cannot touch directly.

***Viscerocranium*** That part of the cranial bone structure that does not enclose the brain, such as the zygomae, maxillae and mandible. It denotes the face.

***Visionary Touch*** A nonhabitual way of touching that harnesses the deep perception of underlying structures and combines it with the transmission of energy to those structures. Simultaneously the healer focuses her awareness ("listening") on the information held in, or broadcast by, those target structures.

***Voice Dialogue*** A variation on Gestalt therapy pioneered by Hal Stone and Sidra Winkelman, Voice Dialogue turns on the dramatization or externalization of normally dormant "sub-personalities," or archetypal representations within us. Thus the frightened child within us is given his "time in court" to speak of his fears; the dutiful daughter gets consulted about her loyalty issues, and so on. Bringing these archetypes to consciousness helps in the understanding of complex life situations and interpersonal difficulties.

***Wind Palace*** This is an acupuncture point, Governor Vessel 16, located in the dorsal midline of the atlanto-occipital joint. "Wind" in traditional Chinese medicine refers to the spirit and its movements throughout the body; "palace" to a lofty location for the spirit, a place we do not visit often, where entry is normally barred by guards. I consider it the beginning of the channel of the inner eye.

# Notes

## Chapter 16   An Anatomical Guided Tour through the Cranial Field

1. Itzak Bentov, *Stalking the Wild Pendulum*, p. 110, Dutton, 1977.)

2. Robert Ornstein, *The Evolution of Consciousness*, p. 40, Prentice Hall, 1991.

3. David Michael and Ernest Retzlaff, "A Preliminary Study of Cranial Bone Movement in the Squirrel Monkey," pp. 886–9, *Journal of the American Osteopathic Association*, Vol. 74, 5/75

4. Lyons Pertucelli, *Medicine: An Illustrated History*, p. 431, Abradale, 1987

5. Frank Netter, *The Musculoskeletal System, Part 1*, p. 187, Ciba Geigy, 1987

6. "The Bones of Chile's Dead Tell their Tales," p. B1 & B11, *New York Times*, 1/14/95

7. Malcolm W. Browne, "Computers Help Chilean Dead Tell Their Tales," p. B1 & B11, *New York Times*, 1/14/92

8. Kenneth A.R.Kennedy, "Morphological Variations in Ulnar Supinator Crests and Fossae as Identifying Markers of Occupational Stress," *Journal of Forensic Science*, 10/83

9. John Noble Wilford, "Skeletons Record the Burden of Work: Skeletons Offer Clues to Owners' Occupations" p. 15, *New York Times*, 10/27/87

10. John Noble Wilford, "It's All in the Bones," *San Francisco Chronicle*, 12/13/87

11. Kenneth A.R. Kennedy and M. Yasar Iscan, *Reconstruction of Life from the Skeleton*, Alan R. Liss Inc., 1989

12. Werner Platzer, *Locomotor System*, pp. 52–53, Thieme, 1986

13. Harrison Fryette, *Principles of Osteopathic Technic* [sic], p. 73, Academy of Applied Osteopathy, 1954

14. Alan Stoddard, *Principles of Osteopathic Technique*, pp 69–74, Hutchinson Medical, London, 1969

15. Angus Cathie, *Growth and Nutrition of the Body with Special Reference to the Head*, Academy of Applied Osteopathy Yearbook, 1962

16. Henry Gee, "When Head-Butting is a Way of Life," *Nature-Times News Service*, London, 5/28/89

17. Sandra Blakeslee, "Evolution of Tabby Cat Mapped in Brain Study," pp. B5 & B8 *New York Times*, 1/12/93

18. For more information see "The Ageing Mind Proves Capable of Lifelong Growth," *New York Times*, 2/21/84

19. Werner Platzer, *Locomotor System*, pp. 22, Thieme, 1986

20. Ernest Retzlaff *et al.*, "The Structures of Cranial Bone Sutures," *Journal of the American Osteopathic Association*, Vol. 75, pp. 607–8, 2/76

21. Harold I. Magoun, *Osteopathy in the Cranial Field*, pp. 12–13, The Cranial Academy, 1976

22. N. Giblin and A. Alley, "Studies in Skull Growth: Coronal Suture Fixation," *Anatomical Record*, Vol. 88, No. 2, 2/44

23. R.S. Stowe *et al.*, *Measurement of Bone Torsion in Vivo Via Biostereoroentgenography*, Thirteenth International Congress for Photogrammetry, Helsinki, 7/76

24. David Michael and Ernest Retzlaff, "A Preliminary Study of Cranial Bone Movement in the Squirrel Monkey," pp. 886–9, *Journal of the American Osteopathic Association*, Vol. 74, 5/75

25. Harold Schmeck Jr, "Scientist Sheds Light on Bone and Enamel Growth," p. B6, *New York Times*, 7/19/88

26. Forrest Nielsen, *Biochemical and Physiologic Consequences of Boron Deprivation in Humans*, pp. 59–63, Environmental Health Perspectives, 11/7/94

27. James B. Wyngaarden and Lloyd H. Smith Jr., *Textbook of Medicine*, p. 1322, Saunders, 1982

28. Harold M. Schmeck Jr, "Scientist Sheds Light on Bone and Enamel Growth," p. B6, *New York Times*, 7/19/95

29. James Wyngaarden and Lloyd H. Smith Jr, *Textbook of Medicine*, p. 1323, Saunders, 1982

30. Robert O. Becker and Gary Selden, *The Body Electric*, pp. 60–65, Quill, 1985

31. Frank Netter, *The Musculoskeletal System, Part 1*, p. 188, Ciba-Geigy, 1987

32. Robert M. Poole, "The Incredible Machine," p. 129, *National Geographic*, 1986

33. "Skylab" was inhabited in 1973 and 1974 for a total of 84 days

34. Frank Netter, *The Musculoskeletal System, Part 1*, p. 186, Ciba Geigy, 1987

35. Associated Press, "439 Days in Space," (Valery Polyakov, 439 days ending March 1995), *New York Times* 3/23/95

36. *Guiness Book of Records*, "Space Records," traveled 98.1 million miles, returned 2/5/87, Bantam, 1989

37. Peter Rambaut and James Johnston, "Prolonged Weightlessness and Calcium Loss in Man," *Acta Astronautica*, Vol. 6, pp. 1113–1122,

38. William J. Broad, "New Attack Planned on Ills of Space Travel," pp. B5, B9, *New York Times*, 7/11/95

39. Stephen Crane, "Metabolic Bone Disease," in Harrison's *Principles of Internal Medicine*, p. 2028, McGraw Hill, 1974

40. Jennifer Steinhauser "Teen-Age Girls Talk Back on Exercise," *New York Times*, 1/4/95

41. "Theory on Calcium and Bone Loss is Disputed," *New York Times*, 1/22/87

42. Frank Netter, *The Musculoskeletal System, Part 1*, p. 186, Ciba Geigy, 1987

43. Belinda Lees *et al.*, "Differences in proximal femur bone density over two centuries," *The Lancet*, Vol. 341, 3/13/93

44. *Discover*, p. 13, 8/93

45. Frank Netter, *The Musculosketal System*, Vol. 1, p. 227, Ciba Geigy, 1987

46. Associated Press, "Gymnastics May Toughen Women's Bones," *New York Times*, 11/25/94

47. Reuters, "Walking a Mile a day Helps Delay Bone Loss," p. B9, *New York Times*, 12/7/94

48. William Sutherland, pp. 144–145, *Collected Writings of William Garner Sutherland D.O., D. Sc. (Hon)* ed. by Adah S. Sutherland and Anne L. Wales, Sutherland Teaching Foundation, 1967

49. John Dobbing and Jean Sands, "Vulnerability of Developing Brain, IX, The Effect of Nutritional Growth Retardation on the Timing of the Brain Growth Spurt," *Biology of the Neonate* 19, 1971

50. J.J. Pritchard *et al.*, "The Structure and Development of Cranial and Facial Sutures," Part 1, pp. 73–86, *Journal of Anatomy*, 1/56

51. Elizabeth Rosenthal, "A High-Tech View of the Sinuses Offers Answers to Chronic Problems," p. B7, *New York Times*, 6/19/91

52. Vanio Vannini, *Atlante Del Corpo Umano*, p. 66, Fabri Editori, (Milan) 1982

53. Harold I. Magoun, *Osteopathy in the Cranial Field*, pp. 183, 189, The Cranial Academy, 1976

54. Ada S. Sutherland and Anne L. Wales, *Collected Writings of William Garner Sutherland*, pp. 89–91, The Sutherland Cranial Teaching Academy, 1967

55. Harold I. Magoun, *Osteopathy in the Cranial Field*, p. 181, The Cranial Academy, 1976

56. Denis Brookes, *Lectures on Cranial Osteopathy*, p. 68, Thorsons, 1981

### *Chapter 17    Reciprocal Tension Membrane*

1. William G. Sutherland, *The Reciprocal Tension Membrane*, audio recording of a lecture given in 1953

2. William G. Sutherland, *The Cranial Bowl*, p. 46, The Cranial Academy, 1948

3. Ernest W. Retzlaff *et al.*, "The Structures of Cranial Bone Sutures," *Journal of the American Osteopathic Society*, Vol. 75, pp. 607–8, 2/76

4. William Sutherland, *The Cranial Bowl*, pp. 56–57, The Cranial Academy, 1948

5. Jack Worsley, *The Meridians of Chi Energy: Point Reference Guide*, p. 5, The College of Traditional Chinese Acupuncture, (England), 1979

6. William Sutherland, *Collected Writings of William Garner Sutherland D.O., D. Sc. (Hon)* pp. 90–91, ed. by Adah S. Sutherland and Anne L. Wales, Sutherland Teaching Foundation, 1967

7. Harold I. Magoun, *Osteopathy in the Cranial Field*, p. 70, The Cranial Academy, 1976

8. William G. Sutherland quoting from Still's *Philosophy of Osteopathy* in Harold I. Magoun, *Osteopathy in the Cranial Field*, p. v, The Cranial Academy, 1976

9. Vernon B. Mountcastle, *Medical Physiology*, pp. 1121–1122, C.V. Mosby Company, 1974

10. Gary W. Goldstein and A. Loris Betz, "The Blood Brain Barrier," *Scientific American*, 9/86

11. Harold K. Kimelberg and Michael D. Norenberg, "Astrocytes," pp. 66–76, *Scientific American*, 4/89

12. Vernon B. Mountcastle, *Medical Physiology*, pp. 1116–1118, C.V. Mosby Company, 1974

13. Frank H. Netter, *The Nervous System*, p. 44, Ciba Geigy, 1967

14. Vernon B. Mountcastle, *Medical Physiology*, p. 1118, C.V. Mosby Company, 1974

15. Vernon B. Mountcastle, *Medical Physiology*, pp. 1116–1118, C.V. Mosby Company, 1974

16. Arthur C. Guyton, *Basic Neuroscience*, p. 36, W.B. Saunders, 1987

17. Frank Netter, *The Nervous System*, pp. 102 & 108, Ciba Geigy, 1967

18. Zvi Karni and John Upledger *et al.*, "Examination of the Cranial Rhythm in Long-Standing Coma and Chronic Neurological Cases," p. 275, *Craniosacral Therapy*, Eastland Press, 1983

19. Reynold Spector and Conrad E. Johanson, "The Mammalian Choroid Plexus," p. 70, *Scientific American*, 11/89

20. Reynold Spector and Conrad E. Johanson, "The Mammalian Choroid Plexus," p. 70, *Scientific American*, 11/89

21. John E. Upledger and Jon D. Vredevoogd, *Craniosacral Therapy*, p. 14, Eastland Press, 1983

22. Vernon B. Mountcastle, *Medical Physiology*, p. 1118, C.V. Mosby Company, 1974

23. John H. Moyer et al, "Effect of Increased Jugular Pressure on Cerebral Hemodynamics," *Journal of Applied Physiology* 7, 11/54

24. Harold I. Magoun, "Whiplash Injury: A Greater Lesion Complex," *The Journal of the American Osteopathic Association*, Vol.63, 2/64

25. Israeli Shin Bet security service agents use a form of torture known politely as "shaking." This consists of prolonged and extremely violent oscillation of the suspects shoulders, done in such a way that it quickly leads to uncontrollable large-amplitude, high velocity cranial movements, reminiscent of the movements that occur momentarily in whiplash injury. "Shaking" results in the same kind of spinal pain as whiplash injury does, and has led to the suspect's death on at least one occasion. See Barton Gellman, "Israelis Break A Code of Silence: Interrogation Practices Get a Rare Public Airing," p. 2, *International Herald Tribune*, 10/23/95

26. Similar phenomena occur in schizophrenia: See Harold I. Magoun, *Osteopathy in the Cranial Field*, pp. 315–317, The Cranial Academy, 1976

27. Daniel Goleman, "Probing the Enigma of Multiple Personality," p. 1, 27, *New York Times* 6/28/88

## Chapter 18   The Stomatognathic System

1. John C. Pierrakos, "Anatomy of Evil," p. 89, from *Meeting the Shadow*, ed. by Connie Zweig and Jeremiah Abrams, Tarcher, 1991

2. Wilhelm Reich, *Ether, God and Devil*, p. 292, Doubleday, 1973

3. Stanley Kelleman, *Emotional Anatomy*, pp. 96–102, Center Press, 1985

4. A.C. Fonder, *The Dental Physician*, pp. 127, 267, Medical Dental Arts, 1985

5. C.M. Guzay, *The Quadrant Theorum*, Doctors Dental Service, 1980

6. Stephen D. Blood, "The craniosacral mechanism and the temporomandibular joint," *Journal of the American Osteopathic Association*, Vol. 86, 8/86

7. Guzay and Fonder describe the base of the dens as the precise source of mandibular motion. This may be so. However, the atlanto-occipital and atlantoaxial joints are so intertwined – energetically, mechanically, neurologically and through dural attachments – that the different motions involved in aggression, chewing, and stress spread motion throughout the suboccipital area. Wherever it can, the body spreads mechanical loads. This area is no exception. in the liquid-electric model, the mandible's spherical axis of motion is at the atlanto-occipital joint, formed by an imaginary sphere that rests at the base of the dens.

8. A.C. Fonder, *Basal Facts*, p. 142 Vol. 5, No. 4

9. S.L. Washburn, "The Relation of the Temporal Muscle to the Form of the Skull," *Anatomical Record*, Vol. 99, 11/47

10. Yochanan Rywerant, *The Feldenkrais Method: Teaching By Handling*, Harper and Row, 1983

11. Steve Jones *et al.*, *The Cambridge Encyclopedia of Human Evolution*, pp. 72–73, Cambridge University Press, 1994

12. C. Loring Brace *et al.*, "Gradual Change in Human Tooth Size in the Pleistocene and Post-Pleistocene," pp. 705–720, *Evolution*, Vol. 41, No. 4, 1987

13. C. Loring Brace *et al.*, "Gradual Change in Human Tooth Size in the Pleistocene and Post-Pleistocene," pp. 705–720, *Evolution*, Vol. 41, No. 4, 1987

14. Robert Burns, *Address to the Toothache*, ed. J. A. Mackay, *Robert Burns: The Complete Poetical Works*, Alloway Publishing, 1993

15. Harold I. Magoun, "Dental Equilibrium and Osteopathy," *The Journal of the American Osteopathic Association*, Vol. 74, 6/75

16. Melvin Henningsen, *Living Osteology of Interest to the Dentist*, Part 1, Dental Digest 63, 10/57

17. A.C. Fonder, *The Dental Physician*, p. 105, Medical Dental Arts, 1985

18. Ernest G. Baker, "Alteration in Width of Maxillary Arch and Its Relation to Sutural Movement of Cranial Bones," *Journal of the American Osteopathic Association*, Vol. 70, No. 6, 2/71

19. John Upledger and Zvi Karni, "Mechanical Electrical Patterns During Craniosacral Osteopathic Diagnosis and Treatment," pp. 782–91, *Journal of the American Osteopathic Association*, Vol. 78, 7/79

20. Adah S. Sutherland and Anne L. Wales, *Collected Writings of William Garner Sutherland*, pp. 90–91, Sutherland Cranial Teaching Foundation, 1967

21. See Chapter 11, The Seven Souls

22. Robert E. Ornstein, *The Mind Field*, pp. 21–35, Viking, 1976

23. Elizabeth Deuress, *The Seen and the Unseen*, pp. 101–117, Smith Barnes, 1924

24. Aelred C. Fonder, *The Dental Physician*, p. 94, Medical Dental Arts, 1985

25. Hans Selye, "The Nature of Stress," pp. 131–150 of A.C. Fonder's *The Dental Distress Syndrome*, Medical Dental Arts, 1993

26. Lisa Seachrist, "Mimicking the Brain: Using computers to investigate neurological disorders," pp. 62–63, *Science News*, Vol. 148, 7/22/95

27. A.C. Fonder, *The Dental Distress Syndrome*, pp. 12–25, Medical Dental Arts, 1993

28. Casey M. Guzay, "Efficiency in Occlusal Function," pp. 93–125 in *The Dental Distress Syndrome*, by Aelred C. Fonder, Medical Dental Arts, 1993

29. Edna M. Lay, "The Osteopathic Management of Temporomandibular Joint Dysfunction," from *Clinical Management of Head, Neck and TMJ Pain*, ed. Harold Gelb, W.B. Saunders, 1985

30. A.C. Fonder, *The Dental Physician*, pp. 148–151, Medical Dental Arts, 1985

31. See Chapter 24, The Sphenoid

32. I. Krejci and F. Lutz, *Zahnfarbene Adhasive Restaurationen im Seitenzahnbereich*, University of Zurich, 1994

33. I. Krejci *et al.*, *In-vitro-testverfahren Zur Evaluation Dentaler Restaurationsysteme*, University of Zurich, 1994 (Chewing simulator proves the need for ceramic inlays both above and below)

34. Bruce Ingersoll and Rose Gutfeld, "Medical Mess: Implants in Jaw Joint Fail, Leaving Patients in Pain and Disfigured," *Wall Street Journal*, p. 1, 8/31/93

35. Stanley Kelleman, *Emotional Anatomy*, pp. 92–93, Center Press, 1985

36. William G. Sutherland, *The Cranial Bowl*, p. 119–124, The Cranial Academy, 1948

37. Cupped: imagine a teacup's saucer, open superiorly; domed, imagine a cupola. For more information on the body's cupped and domed structures, see Chapter 9, Diagnosis

38. Meyer Silverman, "Effect of Skull Distortion on Occlusal Equilibrium," *Journal of Prosthetic Dentistry*, 4/73

39. Harold I. Magoun, "Dental Equilibrium and Osteopathy," *The Journal of the American Osteopathic Association*, Vol. 74, 6/75

40. David Denton, *Craniopathy and Dentistry*, privately published in Los Angeles, 1979

41. Stephen D. Blood, "The craniosacral mechanism and the temporomandibular joint," *Journal of the American Osteopathic Association*, Vol. 86, 8/86

42. Aelred C. Fonder, *The Dental Physician*, pp. 93–95, Medical Dental Arts, 1985

43. Ernest G. Baker, "Alteration in Width of Maxillary Arch and Its Relation to Sutural Movement of Cranial Bones," *Journal of the American Osteopathic Association*, Vol. 70, No. 6, 2/71

44. S.L. Washburn, "The Relation of the Temporal Muscle to the Form of the Skull," *Anatomical Record*, Vol. 99, 11/47

45. Ernest W. Retzlaff *et al.*, "Temporalis muscle Action in Parietotemporal Suture Compression," *The Journal of the American Osteopathic Association*, Vol. 78, 10/78

46. Alexander Lowen, *The Betrayal of the Body*, pp. 62–70, Macmillan, 1967

47. See Chapter 11, The Seven Souls, on Vishuddha

### Chapter 19   Quantum Cranial

1. Richard P. Feynman, *What Do You Care What Other People Think*, p. 136, Bantam, 1989

2. Arnold Mindell, *City Shadows*, p. 52, Routledge, Keagan, Paul, 1988

3. See Chapter 4, *Vignettes in the History of Healing*, p. 60

4. William Sutherland, *The Cranial Bowl*, p. 54, Free Press Company, 1948

5. Frank Netter, *The Central Nervous System*, p. 110, Ciba Geigy, 1967

6. Johannes Setekleiv, *Spontaneous Rhythmic Activity in Smooth Muscles*, Norske Legeforening, 1964, Neurological Laboratory, Anatomical Institute, University of Oslo, Norway.

7. Nephi Cottam, *The Story of Craniopathy*, privately published, 1936

8. Harold I. Magoun, *Osteopathy in the Cranial Field*, The Cranial Academy, 1966

9. William Sutherland, *Collected Writings of William Garner Sutherland*, ed. Adah S. Sutherland and Anne L. Wales, Sutherland Cranial Teaching Foundation, 1967

10. Viola Frymann, "A Study of the Rhythmic Motions of the Living Cranium," pp. 928–945, *Journal of the American Osteopathic Association*, Vol. 70, 5/71

11. R.H. Woods and J.M Woods describe it as the "Sutherland wave," in "A Physical Finding Related to Psychiatric Disorders," *Journal of the American Osteopathic Association*, Vol. 60, pp. 988–993, 8/61

12. Marion Woodman, from "Addiction and Sacred Emptiness," (audiotape) care of Inner City Books, Box 1271, Station Q, Toronto, Canada M4T2P4.

13. William Sutherland, *Collected Writings of William Garner Sutherland*, pp. 201–205, ed. Adah S. Sutherland and Anne L. Wales, Sutherland Cranial Teaching Foundation, 1967

14. Viola M. Frymann, "A Study of Rhythmic Motions of the Living Cranium," p. 928–945, *Journal of the American Osteopathic Association*, Vol. 70, 5/71

15. Zvi Karni, John Upledger *et al.*, "Examination of the Cranial Rhythm in Long-Standing Coma and Chronic Neurological Cases," pp. 607–608, *The Journal of the American Osteopathic Association*, Vol. 75, 2/76

16. Rudolf Steiner, *Life Between Death and Rebirth*, pp. 82–83, Anthroposophic Press, 1968

17. Jacques Lusseyran, *And There Was Light*, pp. 24–25, Parabola Books, 1987

18. John E. Upledger and Zvi Karni, "Mechanical Electrical Patterns During Craniosacral Osteopathic Diagnosis and Treatment," p. 782–91, *Journal of the American Osteopathic Association*, Vol. 78, 7/79

19. Richard E. Kappler, "Osteopathy in the Cranial Field," pp. 13–18, *The Osteopathic Physician*, 2/79

20. H. Somberg, "The Relation of the Spinal Subarachnoid and Perineural Spaces," *Journal of Neuropathy and Experimental Neurology*, 4/47

21. Ralph F. Erlinghausen, *The Circulation of the Cerebrospinal Fluid through the Connective Tissue System*, Academy of Applied Osteopathy Yearbook, 1969.

22. Yuri Moskalenko, *Cerebral Pulsation in the Closed Cranial Cavity*, Izv Akad Nauk USSR, Vol. 620, No. 4, 9/61

23. John Upledger and Jon Vredevoogd, *Craniosacral Therapy*, "Examination of the Cranial Rhythm in Long-Standing Coma and Chronic Neurological Cases," p. 275, Eastland Press, 1983

24. Melvin Morse, *Transformed By the Light*, p. 56, Ballantine, 1992

25. Sogyal Rinpoche, *Tibetan Book of Living and Dying*, p. 330, Harper Collins, 1992

26. Ian Wilson, *The After Death Experience: The Physics of the Non-Physical*, William Morrow, 1987

27. Kenneth Ring, *Life at Death: A Scientific Investigation of the Near-Death Experience*, Coward, McCann and Geoghegan, 1980

28. Raymond A. Moody, *Life after Life*, p. 42, Stackpole Books, 1976

28. Denis Brookes, *Lectures on Cranial Osteopathy: A Manual for Practitioners and Students*, p. 57, Thorsons, 1981 (See also Ian Wilson, *The After Death Experience: The Physics of the Non-Physical*, p. 168, William Morrow, 1987)

29. Viola Frymann, "A Study of Rhythmic Motions of the Living Cranium," p. 928–945, *Journal of the American Osteopathic Association*, Vol. 70, 5/71

30. See also Dexter G. Girton *et al.*, "Observation of Very Slow Potential Oscillations in Human Scalp Recordings," pp. 561–568, *Electroencephalography and Clinical Neurophysiology*, Elsevier Scientific Publishing House, Amsterdam, 1973

31. Cary Baynes, *The I-Ching*, p. 655, Princeton University Press, 1990

32. David K. Michael and Ernest K. Retzlaff, "A Preliminary Study of Cranial Bone Motion in the Squirrel Monkey," p. 886–889, *Journal of the American Osteopathic Association*, Vol. 74, 5/75

33. F. Bruce Lamb, *Wizard of the Upper Amazon*, p. 169, Houghton Mifflin, 1974

34. John C. Pierrakos, p. 89 of *Meeting the Shadow*, ed. Connie Zweig and Jeremiah Abrams, Tarcher, 1991

35. See Chapter 11, Dialoguing the Seven Souls.

36. Dong Shaoming, "Some Like It Hot: The Chinese Idea of the Dantian," pp. 6–7, *Heaven Earth*, Vol. 1, 1/92

37. Robert Bly, *The Kabir Book*, p. 6, Beacon Press, 1977

38. See Chapter 8, Waiting for the Mandala

39. For further information on the other four brain patterns see Michael Hutchison, *Megbrain*, pp. 86–87, Ballantine, 1987

40. N.A. Aladzhalov *et al.*, *The Ultralow Frequency Spectrum of Electrical Phenomenon in the Brain*, translated from Doklady Akademii Nauk USSR, Vol. 197, No. 4, 4/71

41. Gay Gaer Luce, *Biological Rhythms in Psychiatry and Medicine*, p. 142, U.S. Department of Health, Education and Welfare, 1970

42. Edward T. Hall, "The Dance of Life," from the preamble of Doris Lessing's *Under My Skin*, Harper Collins, 1995

43. For more information, see the Wintreberg experiments on cartilaginous fish as mentioned in H. Laborit's *Stress and Cellular Function*, Lippincott, 1959

44. Marion Woodman, *The Ravaged Bridegroom: Masculinity in Women*, Inner City Books, 1990

45. R. H. Blyth, *Zen in English Literature and Oriental Classics*, p. 129, The Hokuseido Press (Tokyo) 1942

46. Deepak Chopra, from a lecture series entitled *Quantum Healing Workshop*, Mystic Fire Audio Tapes, 1990

47. Don Johnson, *The Protean Body*, p. 145, Harper and Row, 1977

48. Harold I. Magoun, *Osteopathy in the Cranial Field*, p. 226, The Cranial Academy, 1976

49. David K. Michael and Ernest K. Retzlaff, "A Preliminary Study of Cranial Bone Motion in the Squirrel Monkey," pp. 886–889, *Journal of the American Osteopathic Association*, Vol. 74, 5/75

50. Ernest W. Retzlaff *et al.*, "Nerve Fibers and Endings in Cranial Sutures," *The Journal of the American Osteopathic Association*, Vol. 77, 2/78

51. Frank Netter, *Musculoskeletal System*, p. 187–188, Ciba Geigy, 1987

52. John E. Upledger and Zvi Karni, "Mechanical Electrical Patterns During Craniosacral Osteopathic Diagnosis and Treatment," p. 782–91, *Journal of the American Osteopathic Association*, Vol. 78, 7/79

53. Deepak Chopra, from a lecture series entitled *Quantum Healing Workshop*, Mystic Fire Audio Tapes, 1990

54. Ram Dass, *The Yoga of Daily Life*, Dolphin Tapes, 1970

55. Fred L. Mitchell *et al.*, "Accuracy and Perceptual Decision Delay in Motion Perception," p. 149, *Journal of American Osteopathic Association*, Vol. 78, 10/78

56. Major Betrand DeJarnette, *Cranial Technique*, 1968, and *SacroOccipital Technique*, 1981, (both privately published in Nebraska City, NE).

57. Wilhelm Reich, *Ether, God and Devil*, p. 292, Doubleday, 1973

58. Margaret Attwood, *The Robber Bride*, p. 146, Doubleday, 1993

59. Alfred J. Zeigler, "Illness as Descent into the Body," from *Meeting the Shadow*, p. 95, ed. by Connie Zweig and Jeremiah Abrams, Tarcher, 1991

60. Jack Schwarz in *Healers on Healing*, edited by Richard Carlson, p. 18, St Matin's Press, 1989

61. Don Johnson, *The Protean Body*, p. 145, Harper Colophon, 1977

62. "... that which is clinically proved needs no other evidence." Sir James Padget

63. William Sutherland, *The Cranial Mechanism*, audio recording, 1953

64. Zvi Karni, John Upledger *et al.*, "Examination of the Cranial Rhythm in Long-Standing Coma and Chronic Neurological Cases," p. 275, *Craniosacral Therapy*, Upledger and Vredevoogd, Eastland Press, 1983

### Chapter 20   The Central Nervous System

1. Robert Ornstein and Richard F. Thompson, *The Amazing Brain*, p. 9, Houghton Mifflin, 1984

2. Roger Lewin, *In the Age of Mankind*, p. 179, Smithsonian Books, 1988

3. Donald Johanson and Maitland Edey, *Lucy*, p. 320–327, Simon and Shuster, 1981

4. Oliver Sacks, *Making Up the Mind*, New York Review of Books, pp. 44, 4/8/93

5. David B. Chamberlain, "The Outer Limits of Memory" p. 4, *Noetic Sciences Review*, Autumn 1990

6. Steve Jones *et al.*, *The Cambridge Encyclopedia of Human Evolution*, p. 108, Cambridge University Press, 1994

7. John Dobbing and Jean Sands, "Vulnerability of Developing Brain, IX, The Effect of Nutritional Growth Retardation on the Timing of the Brain Growth Spurt," *Biology of the Neonate* 19, 1971

8. Angus Cathie, "Growth and Nutrition of the Body with Special Reference to the Head," *Academy of Applied Osteopathy Yearbook*, 1962

9. Michael Hutchison, *Megbrain*, p. 47, Ballantine, 1987

10. Daniel Goleman, "Feeling Cheerfull?" p. B5 & B9, *New York Times*, 2/11/91

11. Harold I. Magoun, *Osteopathy in the Cranial Field*, p. 35, The Cranial Academy, 1976

12. Reynold Specter and Conrad E. Johanson, "The Mammalian Chroroid Plexus," pp. 68–74, *Scientific American*, 11/89

13. J. Robert McLintic, *Physiology of the Human Body*, p. 177, John Wiley & Sons, 1975

14. Frederick E. Jackson, *The Pathophysiology of Head Injuries*, pp. 67–93, Vol. 18, Clinical Symposium, 7/66

15. Dominance occurs by a kind of neuronal Darwinism: the fittest neuron gets to the target area first, establishing its preeminence. See Robert J. Cabelli *et al.*, "Inhibition of Ocular Dominance Column Formation By Infusion of NT-4/5 or BDNF," pp. 1662–1666, *Science*, Vol. 267, 3/17/95

16. Ronald E. Kalil, "Synapse Formation in the Developing Brain," pp. 76–85, *Scientific American*, 12/89

17. Steve Jones *et al.*, *The Cambridge Encyclopedia of Human Evolution*, pp. 107–108, Cambridge University Press, 1994

18. Daniel Goleman, "Feeling Cheerfull?" p. B5, B9, *New York Times*, 2/11/91

19. Daniel Goleman, "Mapping the Brain's Scratch Pad," p. 10, *International Herald Tribune*, 5/4/95

20. Robert E. Ornstein, *The Mind Field*, pp. 34–35, Viking, 1976

21. Melvin Morse M.D., *Transformed By the Light*, p. 156 & 211 Ballantine, 1992

22. Oliver Sacks, *Making Up the Mind*, New York Review of Books, p. 42, 4/8/93

23. Mitchell Glickstein, "The Discovery of the Visual Cortex," pp 118–127, *Scientific American*, 9/88

24. Harold I. Magoun, *Osteopathy in the Cranial Field*, p. 25, The Cranial Academy, 1976

25. Steve Jones *et al.*, *The Cambridge Encyclopedia of Human Evolution*, pp. 107–110, Cambridge University Press, 1994

26. Frank Netter, *The Nervous System*, p. 73, Ciba Geigy, 1967

27. Arthur C. Guyton, *Basic Neuroscience*, p. 12, W. B. Saunders and Co, 1987

28. Natalie Angier, "In a First, Scientists Grow a Brain Cell," p. B5, *New York Times*, 5/4/90

29. Sandra Blakeslee, "A Pathway that Carries the Signals of a Caress," p. B9, *New York Times*, 11/23/94

30. Charles Jennings, "New visions of the cortex," pp. 635–636, *Nature*, Vol. 375, 6/22/95

31. Sandra Blakeslee, "How the Brain Might Work: A New Theory of Consciousness," p. B7, *New York Times*, 3/21/95

32. Marcia Baringa, "Researchers Get a Sharper Image of the Human Brain," pp. 803–804, *Science*, Vol. 268, 5/12/95

33. M.I. Sereno *et al.*, "Borders of Multiple Visual Areas in Humans Revealed by Functional Magnetic Resonance Imaging," pp. 889–893, *Science*, Vol. 268, 5/12/95

34. Sandra Blakeslee, "Medical Movies: Watching the Brain at Work," *International Herald Tribune*, 6/3/93

35. Steve Jones *et al.*, *The Cambridge Encyclopedia of Human Evolution*, p. 121, Cambridge University Press, 1994

36. John Horgan, "Fractured Functions: Does the Brain have a Supreme Integrator?," pp. 36–37, *Scientific American*, 12/93

37. Philip J. Hilts, "Photos Show Mind Recalling a Word," p. 1, *New York Times*, 11/11/91

38. Sandra Blakeslee, "Brain Yields New Clues on Its Organization for Language," *New York Times*, 9/10/91

39. William K. Stevens, "Neanderthals Possessed Anatomy for Speaking," p. C22, *New York Times*, 4/27/89

40. Bruce Bower, "Talk of Ages: A Tiny Bone Rekindles Arguments Over the Roots of Speech and Language," pp. 24–26, *Science News*, Vol. 136, 7/8/89

41. Melvin Morse, *Transformed By the Light*, pp. 156, 211, Ballantine, 1992

42. Marcia Barinaga, "Remapping the Motor Cortex," pp. 1696–1698, *Science*, Vol. 268, 6/23/95

43. "Study May Explain How Eye Achieves Link with Brain," *New York Times*, 2/11/92

44. Arthur C. Guyton, *Basic Neuroscience*, p. 13, W.B. Saunders Company, 1987

45. Mitchell Glickstein, "The Discovery of the Visual Cortex," pp. 118–127, *Scientific American*, 9/88, and also 12/88, p. 58.

46. See the fascinating study by Francis Crick and Christof Koch, "Are we aware of neural activity in primary visual cortex?," pp. 121–123, *Nature*, Vol. 375, 5/11/95

47. Charles Jennings, "New visions of the cortex," pp. 635–636, *Nature*, Vol. 375, 6/22/95

48. Robert Ornstein and Richard F. Thompson, *The Amazing Brain*, p. 8, Houghton Mifflin Company, 1984

49. Marguerite Holloway, "Profile: Doreen Kimura plumbs male and female brains," pp.40–42, *Scientific American*, 10/90

50. Bennet A. Shaywitz *et al.*, "Sex differences in the functional organization of the brain for language," pp. 607–609, *Nature*, Vol. 373, 2/16/95

51. Ruben C. Gur *et al.*, "Sex Differences in Regional Cerebral Glucose Metabolism During a Resting State," pp. 528–531, *Science*, Vol. 267, 1/27/95

52. Sandra Blakeslee, "Evolution of Tabby Cat Mapped in Brain Study," pp. B5 & B8 *New York Times*, 1/12/93

53. Sandra Blakeslee, "New Way to Map Brain Helps Surgeons Cure Some Epilepsy," p. B9, *New York Times*," 10/25/88

54. Warren Leary, "New Wave of Drugs Expected to Improve Epilepsy Treatment," *New York Times*, p. B6, 11/30/93

55. Sandra Blakeslee, "How Surgery Can Counter Epilepsy," *International Herald Tribune*, 10/1/92

56. Robert E. Ornstein, *The Nature of Human Consciousness*, pp. 87–100

57. Daniel Goleman, "Brain Structure Differences Linked to Schizophrenia in Study of Twins," *New York Times*, 3/22/90

58. *Scientific American*, p. 40, 6/90,

59. Jane Brody, "Human Eye is Reported to Set Clock for the Body," *New York Times*, 1/5/95

60. William P. Gordon, *Sleep: A Guide for Professionals*, p. 16, Institute for Cortex research and Development, 1986

61. Arthur T. Winfree, "The Timing of Biological Clocks," *Scientific American Library*, 1987

62. Richard J. Wurtman and Judith J. Wurtman, "Carbohydrates and Depression," p. 68, *Scientific American*, 1/89

63. See the research on melatonin and sleep as published in *The Proceedings of the National Academy of Sciences*, 3/1/94

64. Jacob Liberman, *Light, Medicine of the Future*, Bear and Company, 1991

65. Mircea Eliade, *Patanjali and Yoga*, particularly pp. 50–59, Schoken Books, 1975

66. See *The Yoga Sutras of Patanjali*, Krishnamacharya Yoga Mandiram, Madras, India, 1985

67. John Allman and Leslie Brothers, "Faces, Fear and the Amygdala," pp. 613–614, *Nature*, Vol. 372, 12/15/94

68. Joseph E. LeDoux, "Emotion, Memory and the Brain," pp. 50–57, *Scientific American*, 6/94

69. John P. Angleton, ed. *The Amygdala: Neurobiological Aspects of Emotion, Memory and Mental Dysfunction*, Wiley Liss, 1992

70. Cheryl L. Grady *et al.*, "Age-Related Reductions in Human Recognition Memory Due to Impaired Encoding," pp. 218–221, *Science*, Vol. 269, 7/14/95

71. Joseph E. LeDoux, "Emotion, Memory and the Brain," pp. 53, *Scientific American*, 6/94. Larry Cahill et al, "The amygdala and emotional memory," pp. 295–296, *Nature*, Vol. 377. 9/28/95

72. Larry R. Squire and Stuart Zola-Morgan, "The Medial Temporal Lobe System," *Science*, p. 1380, 9/20/91

73. Philip J. Hilts, "A Brain Unit Seen as Index for Recalling Memories," pp. B5, *New York Times*, 9/24/91

74. Arthur C. Guyton, *Basic Neuroscience*, p. 22, W. B. Saunders and Company, 1987

75. William P. Gordon, *Sleep: A Guide for Health Professionals*, pp. 9–11, Institute for Cortex Research and Development, 1986

76. See Chapter 37, Headaches and Chapter 18, The Stomatognathic System

77. John P. Welsh *et al.*, "Dynamic organization of motor control within the olivocerebellar system," pp. 453–457, *Nature*, Vol. 374, 3/30/95 (Particularly interesting for its description of olivary organization of movements in rhythmic sequence by the entrainment of motor neuron firing patterns.)

78. David A. McCormick, "The cerebellar symphony," pp. 412–413, *Nature*, Vol. 374, 3/30/95

79. Harold K. Kimelberg and Michael D. Norenberg, "Astrocytes," pp. 66–76, *Scientific American*, 4/89

80. "Spinal Cord Injuries: New Optimism Blooms for Developing Treatments," p. 218, *Science*, Vol. 258, 10/9/92

### *Chapter 21    Technical Introduction*

1. Jane E. Brody, "Brain Tumors Increasing," p. 9, *International Herald Tribune*, 7/6/95

2. Florence Rush, *The Best Kept Secret: Sexual Abuse of Children*, pp. 4–5, 137–138, Prentice Hall, 1980. The author notes the comment that "incest ... is far more common than ever reported," (p. 138)

3. Ellen Bass and Laura Davis, *The Courage to Heal: A Guide for Women Survivors of Child Sexual Abuse*, p. 20, Harper and Row, 1988 (Authors estimate that 33% of young women and 14% of young men are sexually abused before age 18)

4. See also Diana Russell, *The Secret Trauma: Incest in the Lives of Girls and Women*, Basic Books, 1986

5. C.G. Jung, *The Secret of the Golden Flower*, p. 83, trans. Carey Baynes, Arkana, 1984

## Chapter 22    *The Sacrum*

1. Harrison H. Fryette, "Principles of Osteopathic Technic," p. 68, *Academy of Applied Osteopathy*, 1966

2. John Wernham, *Lectures On Osteopathy*, pp. 32–33, Maidstone College of Osteopathy, undated (circa 1993)

3. Alan Stoddard, *Manual of Osteopathic Practice*, p. 185, Hutchinson Medical Publications, 1969

4. James Cyriax, *Textbook of Orthopedic Medicine*, Vol. 1, pp. 360–361, Bailliere Tindall, 1984

5. D. Sashin, "A Critical Analysis of the Anatomy and the Pathologic Changes of the Sacro-Iliac Joint," p. 895, *Journal of Bone and Joint Surgery*, Vol. 12A, 1930

6. note: osteopathic physicians generally disagree, from clinical experience, with the orthopedic observation of fusion By fifty: See Harrison H. Fryette, *Principles of Osteopathic Technic*, pp. 69–75, Academy of Applied Osteopathy, 1966

7. C. Owen Lovejoy, "Evolution of Human Walking," pp. 118–125, *Scientific American*, 11/88

8. R. McNeill Alexander, "Human Locomotion," pp. 80–85 in *The Cambridge Encyclopedia of Human Evolution*, ed. Steve Jones *et al.*, Cambridge University Press, 1994

9. Alan Stoddard, *Manual of Osteopathic Practice*, pp. 184–185, Hutchinson Medical Publications, 1969

10. James Cyriax, *Textbook of Orthopedic Medicine*, Vol. 1, p. 360, Balliere Tindall, 1984

11. Harold I. Magoun, *Osteopathy in the Cranial Field*, p. 142, The Cranial Academy, 1967

12. James Cyriax, *Textbook of Orthopedic Medicine*, Vol. 1, pp. 360–361, Balliere Tindall, 1984

13. Harrison H. Fryette, *Principles of Osteopathic Technic*, p. 73, Academy of Applied Osteopathy, 1966

14. William Sutherland, *Collected Writings of William Garner Sutherland D.O., D. Sc. (Hon)*, pp. 90–91, 157–168, ed. by Adah S. Sutherland and Anne L. Wales, Sutherland Teaching Foundation, 1967

15. See Alan Watts, *Tao: The Watercourse Way*, Pantheon Books, 1975

16. John C. Pierrakos, *The Energy Field in Man and Nature*, Institute of Bio-energetic Analysis, undated

17. Jerry A. Johnson, *The Essence of Internal Martial Arts*, Vol. I, pp. 113–120, Ching Lien Healing Arts, 1994

18. William Sutherland, *Collected Writings of William Garner Sutherland D.O., D. Sc. (Hon)*, pp. 19–20, ed. by Adah S. Sutherland and Anne L. Wales, Sutherland Teaching Foundation, 1967

19. Adolf Guggenbuhl-Craig, "The Demonic Side of Sexuality," from *Meeting the Shadow*, pp. 98–99, ed. by Connie Zweig and Jeremiah Abrams, Tarcher, 1991

20. Alexander Lowen, *The Betrayal of the Body*, pp. 64–70, Macmillan, 1970

21. Edward T. Hall, "The Dance of Life," from the preamble of Doris Lessing's *Under My Skin*, Harper Collins, 1995

22. See Chapter 11, Dialoguing the Seven Souls, and Chapter 9, Diagnosis provide more information and questions on the soul centers

23. H. Vincent Langley, *Essential Treatments in Manipulative Therapy*, p. 12, Castle Carey Press (England), 1963

24. See the watercolor by Tennessee Dixon entitled *Pluto and Persephone*

25. Glynn Isaac and Richard E.F. Leakey, "Human Ancestors," p. 59, *Scientific American*, 1979

26. C. Owen Lovejoy, "The Evolution of Human Walking," p. 118, *Scientific American*, 11/88

27. John Napier, "The Antiquity of Human Walking," pp. 50–60 in "Human Ancestors," *Scientific American*, 1979

28. Gerda and Mona-Lisa Boysen, *Biodynamik Des Lebens*, p. 45, Synthesis Verlag, 1987

29. A. T. Still, "Osteopathy: Research and Practice," 1910, reprinted by Eastland Press, 1992

30. S.G. John Wernham, *Lectures on Osteopathy*, p. 28, Maidstone College of Osteopathy, undated, circa 1993

31. Jack Worsley, *The Meridians of Chi Energy: Point Reference Guide*, p. 5, The College of Traditional Chinese Acupuncture, U.K. 1979

32. In Japan, the pubis is sometimes referred to as "the secret bone"

## Chapter 23    *The Occiput*

1. C.B. Stringer, "Evolution of Early Humans," pp. 244–249, in *The Cambridge Encyclopedia of Human Evolution*, ed. Steve Jones *et al.*, Cambridge University Press, 1994

2. See Chapter 3, A History of Human Evolution

3. Denis Brookes, *Lectures on Cranial Osteopathy*, p. 13, Thorsons, 1981

4. William Sutherland, *Collected Writings of William Garner Sutherland D.O., D. Sc. (Hon)*, pp. 90–91, *Bent Twigs*, ed. by Adah S. Sutherland and Anne L. Wales, Sutherland Teaching Foundation, 1967

5. Harold I. Magoun, *Osteopathy in the Cranial Field*, p. 50, The Cranial Academy, 1976

6. William G. Sutherland, *The Cranial Bowl*, pp. 30–31, The Cranial Academy, 1948

7. L. Bolk, "On the Premature Obliteration of Sutures in the Human Skull," *American Journal of Anatomy*, Vol. 17, No. 4, 5/15/15

8. Viola Frymann, "Relation of Disturbances of Craniosacral Mechanisms to Symptomatology of the Newborn: Study of 1,250 Infants," *Journal of the American Osteopathic Association*, pp. 1059–1075, Vol. 65, 6/66

9. William Sutherland, *Collected Writings of William Garner Sutherland D.O., D. Sc. (Hon)*, pp. 144–145, *Bent Twigs*, ed. by Adah S. Sutherland and Anne L. Wales, Sutherland Teaching Foundation, 1967

10. *Oxford Dictionary of Quotations,* Third Edition, p. 150, Oxford University Press, 1985

11. See Chapter 7, Perception

12. Jack Worsley, *The Meridians of Chi Energy: Point Reference Guide,* p. 5, The College of Traditional Chinese Acupuncture, U.K. 1979

13. Frederick E. Jackson, "The Pathophysiology of Head Injuries," pp. 67–93, *Clinical Symposia,* July–December 1966

14. Meyer Silverman, "Effect of Skull Distortion on Occlusal Equilibrium," *Journal of Prosthetic Dentistry,* 4/73

15. Ada S. Sutherland, *With Thinking Fingers,* p. 88, The Cranial Academy, 1963

16. Stephen J. Blood, "The craniosacral mechanism and the temporomandibular joint," p. 87, *Journal of the American Osteopathic Association,* Vol. 86, 8/86

17. Edna M. Lay, "The Osteopathic Management of Temporomandibular Joint Dysfunction," from *Clinical Management of Head, Neck and TMJ Pain,* ed. Harold Gelb, W.B. Saunders, 1985

18. Harold I. Magoun, "Whiplash Injury: A Greater Lesion Complex," *The Journal of the American Osteopathic Association,* Vol. 63, 2/64

19. John H. Moyer *et al.,* "Effect of Increased Jugular Pressure on Cerebral Hemodynamics," *Journal of Applied Physiology 7,* 11/54

20. See Chapter 24, The Sphenoid

21. Lao Tzu, *Tao Te King,* Trans. Gia-Fu Feng and Jane English, Vintage, 1972

22. See Chapter 45, Windows to the Sky

## Chapter 24   The Sphenoid

1. Denis Brookes, *Lectures On Cranial Osteopathy,* p. 13, Thorsons, 1981

2. Harold I. Magoun, *Osteopathy in the Cranial Field,* p. 13, The Cranial Academy, 1976

3. Harold I. Magoun, *Osteopathy in the Cranial Field,* pp. 138–142, The Cranial Academy, 1976

4. Because of a last minute update, there is no footnote number 4.

5. L. Bolk, "On the Premature Obliteration of Sutures in the Human Skull," *American Journal of Anatomy,* Vol. 17, No. 4, 5/15/15

6. Frederick E. Jackson, "The Pathophysiology of Head Injuries," pp. 67–93, *Clinical Symposia,* July–December 1966

7. S.L. Washburn, "The Relation of the Temporal Muscle to the Form of the Skull," *Anatomical Record,* Vol. 99, 11/47

8. *The Anatomy of Sleep,* p. 66, Hoffman-LaRoche, 1966

9. Harold I. Magoun, "A Pertinent Approach to Pituitary Pathology," appearing in *The D.O.,* Vol. 11, 7/71

10. Olive M. Stretch, "The Pituitary and the Ageing Process in relation to the Cranial Concept," in *Lectures on Cranial Osteopathy* by Denis Brookes, Thorsons, 1981

11. H. Somberg, "The Relation of the Spinal Subarachnoid and Perineural Spaces," *Journal of Neuropathy and Experimental Neurology,* 4/47

12. Reynold Specter and Conrad E. Johanson, "The Mammalian Choroid Plexus," pp. 68–74, *Scientific American,* 11/89

13. John H. Moyer *et al.,* "Effect of Increased Jugular Pressure on Cerebral Hemodynamics," *Journal of Applied Physiology 7,* 11/54

14. Daniel Goleman, "Cool Smile, Warm Frown?" pp. B1–8, *New York Times,* 7/18/89

15. William P. Gordon, *Sleep: A Guide for Health Professionals,* pp. 25–26, Stanford University, 1986

16. Harold I. Magoun, *Osteopathy in the Cranial Field,* pp. 27, 30, The Cranial Academy, 1976

17. Barbara Ann Brennan, *Hands of Light: A Guide to Healing through the Human Energy Field,* p. 42–43, Bantam, 1987

18. Jacques Lusseyran, *And There Was Light,* pp. 19, 33, Parabola, 1987

19. *The Bible,* American Standard Version, Matthew 6, 22 and Luke 11, 34

20. "Interview with Master Jing Hui," *Heaven Earth,* p. 3, China Advocates, 1/92

21. Miyamoto Musashi, *A Book of Five Rings,* p. 54, Overlook Press, 1974

22. Mirabai *For Love of the Dark One,* p. 75, trans. Andrew Schelling, Shambala, 1993

23. Neal Karlen, "The Woodstock Notion," *New York Times,* p. A13, 8/5/94

24. Willard Johnson, *Riding the Ox Home,* p. 29, Beacon Press, 1982

25. Oliver Sacks, *The Man Who Mistook His Wife for A Hat,* Summit Books, 1985

26. *The Anatomy of Sleep,* p. 72, Hoffman-LaRoche, describing Professor A.C. Aitken of Edinburgh University, 1966

27. Jacob Liberman, *Light, Medicine of the Future,* p. 124, Bear & Co, 1991

28. William P. Gordon, *Sleep: A Guide for Health Professionals,* p. 16, Stanford University, 1986

29. Elisabeth Rosenthal, "Pulses of Light Give Astronauts New Rhythms," *New York Times,* 4/23/91

30. Elisabeth Rosenthal, "A High-Tech View of the Sinuses Offers Answer to Chronic Problems," p. B7, *New York Times,* 6/19/91

31. Harold I. Magoun, *Osteopathy in the Cranial Field,* p. 122, 30, The Cranial Academy, 1976

32. John C. Pierrakos, "Anatomy of Evil," p. 89, from *Meeting the Shadow,* p. 83, ed. by Connie Zweig and Jeremiah Abrams, Tarcher, 1991

33. Yatri, *Unknown Man: The Emergence of a New Species,* p. 168–169, Simon and Schuster, 1988

34. T.R. Miles, *Dyslexia,* pp. 15–23, Granada Publishing, 1993

35. Wade Roush, "Arguing Over Why Johnny Can't Read," pp. 1896–1898, *Science,* Vol. 267, 3/31/95

36. Viola Frymann, "Learning Difficulties of Children Viewed in the Light of the Osteopathic Concept," *The Journal of the American Osteopathic Association,* Vol. 76, 9/76

37. Harold I. Magoun, *Osteopathy in the Cranial Field,* p. 291, The Cranial Academy, 1976

38. Gina Kolata, "Study Reports That Dyslexia Isn't Always Permanent," p. A15, *New York Times,* 1/16/92

39. Meyer Silverman, "Effect of Skull Distortion on Occlusal Equilibrium," *Journal of Prosthetic Dentistry,* 4/73

40. Stephen J. Blood, "The craniosacral mechanism and the temporomandibular joint," p. 87, *Journal of the American Osteopathic Association,* Vol. 86, 8/86

41. Aelred C. Fonder, *The Dental Distress Syndrome,* p. 22, Medical Dental Arts, 1993

42. Peter R. Brotchie *et al.,* "Head position signals used by parietal neurons to encode location of visual stimuli," pp. 232–235, *Nature,* Vol. 375, 5/18/95

43. Alfred J. Zeigler, "Illness as Descent into the Body," from *Meeting the Shadow,* p. 95, ed. by Connie Zweig and Jeremiah Abrams, Tarcher, 1991

44. John E. Upledger, "The Relationship of Craniosacral Examination Findings in Grade School Children with Developmental Problems," *The Journal of the American Osteopathic Association,* Vol. 77, 6/78

45. Edgar D. Mitchell, *Psychic Exploration,* p. 295, Putnam, 1974

46. Margaret Attwood, *The Robber Bride,* p. 146, Doubleday, 1993

47. Viola Frymann, "Relation of Disturbances of Craniosacral Mechanisms to Symptomatology of the Newborn: Study of 1,250 Infants," *Journal of the American Osteopathic Association,* pp. 1059–1075, Vol. 65, 6/66

48. H. Somberg, "The Relation of the Spinal Subarachnoid and Perineural Spaces," *Journal of Neuropathy and Experimental Neurology,* 4/47

49. Harold I. Magoun, "Whiplash Injury: A Greater Lesion Complex," *The Journal of the American Osteopathic Association,* Vol. 63, 2/64

## Chapter 25   The Temporals

1. Denis Brookes, *Lectures On Cranial Osteopathy,* p. 90, Thorsons, 1981

2. Harold I. Magoun, *Osteopathy in the Cranial Field,* p. 149, The Cranial Academy, 1976

3. In California, the same condition is known as "North Ear" or "Surfer's Ear," and is more prevalent in the windward ear.

4. Kenneth A.R. Kennedy, "Morphological Variations in "Ulnar Supinator Crests and Fossae as Identifying Markers of Occupational Stress," *Journal of Forensic Science,* 10/83

5. Kenneth A.R. Kennedy and M. Yasar Iscan, *Reconstruction of Life from the Skeleton,* Alan R. Liss Inc., 1989

6. *The Bible,* Revised Standard Version, Exodus 3:5

7. Robert Fulghum, *All I Really Need To Know I Learned In Kindergarten,* pp. 6–7, Villard Books, 1990

8. Milan Kundera, *The Unbearbale Lightness of Being,* Faber and Faber, 1984

9. Milton Erickson, *Healing In Hypnosis,* Irvington, 1989

10. Stanley Kelleman, *Emotional Anatomy,* pp. 90–99, Center Press, 1985

11. Harold I. Magoun, "Whiplash Injury: A Greater Lesion Complex," *The Journal of the American Osteopathic Association,* Vol. 63, 2/64

12. Denis Brookes, *Lectures On Cranial Osteopathy,* p. 91, Thorsons, 1981

13. Seymour Diamond and Jose Medina, "Headaches," pp. 12–20, *Clinical Symposia,* Vol. 41, No. 1, Ciba Geigy, 1989

14. Harold I. Magoun *Osteopathy in the Cranial Field,* pp. 269, 308–310, The Cranial Academy, 1976

15. See Richard Rhodes, "The General and World War III," p. 47, *New Yorker,* 6/19/95, for a famous example of adaptation to Bell's Palsy

16. Linda Pezzano, "Touch Healed My Paralysis," pp. 66–68, *Natural Health,* March–April 1995.

17. Valerie A. Fildes, *Breasts, Bottles and Babies: A History of Infant Feeding,* Edinburgh University Press, distributed by Columbia University Press

18. Jessie R. Thomson, *Natural and Healthy Childhood,* pp. 22–24, 28–29, Bloomfield Books, 1986

19. Denis Brookes, *Lectures On Cranial Osteopathy,* p. 119, Thorsons, 1981

20. Aelred C. Fonder, *The Dental Distress Syndrome,* p. 85, Medical Dental Arts, 1993

21. Aelred C. Fonder, *The Dental Physician,* pp. 183–199, Medical Dental Arts, 1985

22. Aelred C. Fonder, *Hearing Loss and Its Relation to Malocclusion of the Teeth,* privately published in Rock Falls, IL, 1957

23. See Chapter 45, Windows To The Sky

24. See version of this technique demonstrated by William Sutherland and described by Harold I. Magoun in *Osteopathy in the Cranial Field,* pp. 155–156, The Cranial Academy, 1976

25. William Sutherland, *Collected Writings of William Garner Sutherland D.O., D. Sc. (Hon),* pp. 990–91, ed. by Adah S. Sutherland and Anne L. Wales, Sutherland Teaching Foundation, 1967

26. William G. Sutherland, *The Cranial Bowl,* pp. 54–55, Free Press Co, 1948

27. Jack Worsley, *The Meridians of Chi Energy: Point Reference Guide,* p. 6, The College of Traditional Chinese Acupuncture, U.K. 1979

28. See The Four-Chambered Heart Meditation, in Chapter 2, The Mind is Like a Sword

29. F. M. Alexander, *The Use of the Self,* Gollanz, 1985

30. W. Barlow, *The Alexander Principle,* Gollanz, 1973

### Chapter 26   The Parietals

1. See Chapter 11, Dialoguing the Seven Souls
2. S.L. Washburn, "The Relation of the Temporal Muscle to the Form of the Skull," *Anatomical Record*, Vol. 99, 11/47
3. John Noble Wilford, "Fossil Findings Fan Debate on Human Origins," p. B10, *New York Times*, 2/14/89
4. Ada Sutherland, *As the Twig is Bent*, p. 9, undated, circa 1960
5. "Skullduggery: Pundits ponder perforated prehistoric pates from Peru," p. 34, *Scientific American*, 6/90
6. David K. Michael and Ernest W. Retzlaff, "A Preliminary Study of Cranial Bone Movement in the Squirrel Monkey," *Journal of the American Osteopathic Association*, Vol. 74, pp. 886–889, 5/75
7. Zvi Karni and John Upledger et al: found a parietal bone amplitude of 10–25 microns with dial gauges, and one to one and a half millimeters with digital palpation. See "Examination of the Cranial Rhythm in Long-Standing Coma and Chronic Neurologic Cases," Appendix B of Upledger's *Craniosacral Therapy*, Eastland Press, 1983
8. Joseph Campbell, *Oriental Mythology: The Masks of God*, p. 198, Arkana, 1991
9. Beautifully narrated in Joseph Campbell's *Transformational Myths*, audio recordings by Mythology Limited, 1989
10. See the serpents hovering above the crown, from an illustration dating back to 2,000 B.C., on p. 170 of Joseph Campbell's *Oriental Mythology: The Masks of God*, Arkana, 1991. (The same motif was repeated in Bertolucci's 1994 film, "Little Buddha")
11. Jack Worsley, *The Meridians of Chi Energy: Point Reference Guide*, p. 5, The College of Traditional Chinese Acupuncture, U.K. 1979
12. R.H. Blyth, *Zen in English Literature and Oriental Classics*, p. 26, Hokuseido Press (Tokyo), 1942
13. Melvin Morse, *Transformed By the Light*, p. 156, Ballantine, 1992
14. Yatri, *Unknown Man: The Birth of a New Species*, p. 86, Simon and Schuster, 1988
15. Jerry A. Johnson, *The Essence of Internal Martial Arts*, Vol. II, p. 113–124, Ching Lien Healing Arts, 1984

### Chapter 27   The Frontal

1. L. Bolk, "On the Premature Obliteration of Sutures in the Human Skull," *American Journal of Anatomy*, Vol. 17, No. 4, 5/15/15
2. Harold I. Magoun, *Osteopathy in the Cranial Field*, pp. 5, 165, The Cranial Academy, 1976
3. Elizabeth Culotta, "New Finds Rekindle Debate Over Anthropoid Origins," p. 1851, *Science*, Vol. 268, 6/30/95
4. Elwyn L. Simons, "Skulls and Anterior Teeth of Catopithecus (Primates:Anthropoidea) from the Eocene and Anthropoid Origins," p. 1885, *Science*, Vol. 268, 6/30/95

5. Sperm whales regularly dive to more than 3,300 feet (1,000 meters) and stay down for up to one hour. Source: American Cetacean Society, P.O. Box 1391, San Pedro, CA 90733
6. Lawrence K. Altman, "Ingenuity and a Miraculous Recovery," p. B5, *New York Times*, 7/26/88
7. Edward Rothstein, "Distinguishing the Grandiose from the Charming," p. B1, *New York Times*, 2/11/92
8. Tim Hilchey, "Skull and Air Sacs Tune Dolphin Sonar," *New York Times*, 11/10/92
9. Denis Brookes, *Lectures on Cranial Osteopathy*, p. 68, Thorsons, 1981
10. William G. Sutherland, *The Cranial Bowl*, pp. 36–38, The Cranial Academy, 1948
11. Elisabeth Rosenthal, "A High-Tech View of the Sinuses Offers Answer to Chronic Problems," p. B7, *New York Times*, 6/19/91
12. See Chapter 10, "Working with the Inner Eye"
13. William G. Sutherland, *The Cranial Bowl*, p. 35, The Cranial Academy, 1948
14. Daniel Goleman, "Mapping the Brain's Scratch Pad," p. 10, *International Herald Tribune*, 5/4/95
15. John H. Moyer *et al.*, "Effect of Increased Jugular Pressure on Cerebral Hemodynamics," *Journal of Applied Physiology 7*, 11/54

### Chapter 28   The Ethmoid

1. Barry Holstun Lopez, *Of Wolves and Men*, p. 48–50, Charles Scribner's Sons, 1978
2. "Protein That Helps the Nose to Smell," *New York Times*, 8/2/88
3. Natalie Angier, "Powerhouse of Senses, Smell, at Last Gets Its Due," p. B5 & B8, *New York Times*, 2/14/95
4. Sandra Blakeslee, "Human Nose May Hold An Additional Organ for A Real Sixth Sense," p. B6, *New York Times*, 9/7/93

### Chapter 29   The Vomer

1. Vanio Vannini, *Atlante Del Corpo Umano*, p. 66, Gruppo Editoriale Fabri, (Turin) 1989
2. Dong Shaoming, "The Chinese Idea of the Dantian," p. 7, *Heaven Earth*, Vol. 1, No. 3, China Advocates, 1/92
3. Wojciech Tarnowski, in a lecture given 11/90 to the Cranial Association in England, notes a dental colleague whose wife's torus totally disappeared after cranial treatment
4. Harold I. Magoun, *Osteopathy in the Cranial Field*, p. 122, The Cranial Academy, 1976

### Chapter 30   The Zygomae

1. Frank Netter, *Atlas of Human Anatomy*, plate 94 (no page number), Ciba Geigy, 1992
2. Sheridan Morley, "Recalling Dietrich: Better in Real Life," p. 12, *International Herald Tribune*, 5/9/92

### Chapter 31   The Maxillae

1. J.J. Pritchard *et al.,* "The Structure and Development of Cranial and Facial Sutures," Part 1, pp. 73–86, *Journal of Anatomy,* 1/56
2. Stephen J. Blood, "The craniosacral mechanism and the temporomandibular joint," p. 87, *Journal of the American Osteopathic Association,* Vol. 86, 8/86
3. Edna M. Lay, "The Osteopathic Management of Temporomandibular Joint Dysfunction," from *Clinical Management of Head, Neck and TMJ Pain,* ed. Harold Gelb, W.B. Saunders, 1985
4. Aelred C. Fonder, *The Dental Distress Syndrome,* pp. 10–25, Medical Dental Arts, 1993
5. William Sutherland, *Collected Writings of William Garner Sutherland D.O., D. Sc. (Hon),* pp. 41–43, ed. by Adah S. Sutherland and Anne L. Wales, Sutherland Teaching Foundation, 1967
6. Kabir, *The Kabir Book,* trans. Robert Bly, p. 6, Beacon Press, 1977
7. Lao Tzu, *Tao Te Ching,* chapter 56, trans. Gia-Fu Feng and Jane English, Vintage Books, 1972
8. See Chapter 3, A History of Human Evolution
9. Aelred C. Fonder, *The Dental Physician,* pp. 273–304, Medical Dental Arts, 1985
10. William G. Sutherland, *The Cranial Bowl,* pp. 119–124, The Cranial Academy, 1948
11. Ernest G. Baker, "Alteration in Width of Maxillary Arch and Its Relation to Sutural Movement of Cranial Bones," *Journal of the American Osteopathic Association,* Vol. 70, No. 6, 2/71
12. Stephen J. Blood, "The craniosacral mechanism and the temporomandibular joint," p. 87, *Journal of the American Osteopathic Association,* Vol. 86, 8/86
13. Harold I. Magoun, *Osteopathy in the Cranial Field,* pp. 122, The Cranial Academy, 1976
14. See Chapter 18, The Stomatognathic System
15. Harold I. Magoun, *Osteopathy in the Cranial Field,* p. 282–283, The Cranial Academy, 1976

### Chapter 32   The Palatines

1. William Sutherland, *Collected Writings of William Garner Sutherland D.O., D. Sc. (Hon)* pp. 101–114, ed. by Adah S. Sutherland and Anne L. Wales, Sutherland Teaching Foundation, 1967
2. Vanio Vannini, *Atlante Del Corpo Umano,* p. 66, Fabbri Editori, (Turin) 1989

### Chapter 33   The Auditory Tubes

1. Robert M. Poole, *The Incredible Machine,* p. 287–290, National Geographic Society, 1986
2. Michael D. Levitt, Veterans Affairs Medical Center, suggests that 79 percent of Native Americans, 75 percent of African Americans, 51 percent of Hispanics and 21 percent of Whites are milk-intolerant. Associated Press, *Japan Times,* p. 20, 7/7/95
3. Warren E. Leary, "Study Doubts Milk-Intolerance Impact," p. B9, *New York Times,* 7/12/95
4. Jane E. Brody, "New Appreciation of Sinus Infections in Children and What Steps Should Be Taken," p. B6, *New York Times,* 12/28/89
5. Valerie A. Fildes, *Breasts, Bottles and Babies,* Edinburgh University Press, distributed by Columbia University Press, c. 1988
6. Harold I. Magoun, *Osteopathy in the Cranial Field,* p. 215, The Cranial Academy, 1976
7. See Harold I. Magoun's *Osteopathy in the Cranial Field,* p. 155, for alternate approaches to this technique, and a photograph of William G. Sutherland applying it.
8. Miyamoto Musashi, *A Book of Five Rings,* pp. 45–46, The Overlook Press, 1974

### Chapter 34   The Mandible

1. C.B. Stringer, "Evolution of Early Humans," p. 249, *The Cambridge Encyclopedia of Human Evolution,* ed. Steve Jones, Cambridge University Press, 1994
2. See Chapter 3, A History of Human Evolution
3. Stanley Kelleman, *Emotional Anatomy,* pp. 90–99, Center Press, 1985
4. S.L Washburn, "The Relation of the Temporal Muscle to the Form of the Skull," *Anatomical Record,* Vol. 99, 11/47
5. Marcia Barinaga, "Remapping the Motor Cortex," pp. 1696–1698, *Science,* Vol. 268, 6/23/95
6. S.D. Smith, *Atlas of Temporomandibular Orthopedics,* Medical College of Philadelphia, 1982
7. Aelred C. Fonder, *The Dental Physician,* pp. 97–100, Medical Dental Arts, 1985
8. See also *Basal Facts,* p. 142 Vol. 5, No. 48
9. Aelred C. Fonder, *The Dental Distress Syndrome,* pp. 12–13, Medical Dental Arts, 1993
10. Stephen J. Blood, "The craniosacral mechanism and the temporomandibular joint," p. 87, *Journal of the American Osteopathic Association,* Vol. 86, 8/86
11. However, the lack of a symphisis does allow greater biting force to be exerted on a chosen side. See Christopher Dean, "Jaws and Teeth," p. 56, *The Cambridge Encyclopedia of Human Evolution,* ed. Steve Jones *et al.,* Cambridge University Press, 1994
12. Harold I. Magoun, "Dental Equilibrium and Osteopathy," *The Journal of the American Osteopathic Association,* Vol. 74, 6/75
13. See Chapter 18, The Stomatognathic System, for more information
14. See Chapter 31, Maxillae and Chapter 11, Dialoguing the Seven Souls
15. Erika L. Rosenberg, "Facing the Facts," pp. 569–570, *Nature,* 2/16/95
16. Alan J. Fridlund, *Human Facial Expression: An Evolutionary View,* Academic Press, 1994
17. Hans Selye, "The Nature of Stress," appearing in pp. 131–150, *The Dental Distress Syndrome,* by Aelred C. Fonder, Medical Dental Arts, 1993

18. John C. Pierrakos, in *Meeting the Shadow*, p. 89, ed. by Connie Zweig and Jeremiah Abrams, Tarcher, 1991

19. Adolf Guggenbuhl-Craig, "The Demonic Side of Sexuality," from *Meeting the Shadow*, pp. 98–99, ed. by Connie Zweig and Jeremiah Abrams, Tarcher, 1991

20. Alexander Lowen, *The Betrayal of the Body*, p. 268, Collier, 1967

21. Fritz Perls, *Ego, Hunger and Aggression*, Gestalt Journal Press, 1992

22. Frederick E. Jackson, "The Pathophysiology of Head Injuries," pp. 67–93, *Clinical Symposia*, July–December 1966

23. Stanley Kelleman, *Emotional Anatomy*, pp. 90–99, Center Press, 1985

24. Stephen D. Blood, "The craniosacral mechanism and the temporomandibular joint," *Journal of the American Osteopathic Association*, Vol. 86, 8/86

25. Keith Mason, *Medicine for the 21st Century*, p. 102, Element, 1992

26. Donald J. Dalessio, ed., *Wolff's Headache and Other Head Pain*, 4th edition, Oxford University Press (New York), 1980

27. Seymour Diamond and Jose Medina, "Headaches," pp. 2–4, *Clinical Symposium*, Vol. 41, No. 1, 1989

28. H. Vincent Langley, *Essential Treatment in Manipulative Therapy*, p. 12, Castle Cary Press, (England) 1963

### Chapter 35  Craniosacral Work with Infants

1. Hugo Lagercrantz and Theodore A. Slotkin, "The Stress of Being Born," see photograph on p. 107, *Scientific American*, 6/86

2. Adah S. Sutherland, *As the Twig Is Bent*, The Cranial Academy, undated (c. 1960)

3. Anthony DeCasper, "Recognition of Language May Begin in the Womb," University of North Carolina, after research with women in their 32d week of pregnancy. Newborn babies, given the choice of hearing speech or heart beat out of either ear, chose to listen to heartbeat with their left ear, and speech with their right. *New York Times*, c. 8/13/91

4. See Chapter 3, "A History of Human Evolution"

5. Steven Pinker, *The Language Instinct*, Morrow, 1994

6. C. Owen Lovejoy, "Evolution of Human Walking," p. 125, *Scientific American*, 11/88

7. Robert G. Tague and C. Owen Lovejoy, "The Obstetric Pelvis of A.L. 288–1 (Lucy)," *Journal of Human Evolution*, Vol. 15, pp. 237–255, 5/86

8. Hugo Lagercrantz and Theodore A. Slotkin, "The Stress of Being Born," pp. 100–107, *Scientific American*, 6/86

9. In *Osteopathy in the Cranial Field*, p. 226, Magoun cites uterine contractions as capable of exerting an overpressure of from 4.5 to 26.5 pounds per square inch (.25 to 1.30 Bar)

10. In Frymann's "Relation of Disturbances of Craniosacral Mechanisms to Symptomatology of the Newborn, Study of 1,250 Infants," she documents finding less than 12% of newborn babies to have healthy heads. See pp. 1059–1075, *The Journal of the American Osteopathic Association*, Vol. 65, 6/66

11. Harold I. Magoun, *Osteopathy in the Cranial Field*, p. 143, The Cranial Academy, 1976

12. Beryl Arbuckle, "The Cranial Aspect of Emergencies of the Newborn," pp. 507–511, *The Journal of the American Osteopathic Association*, Vol. 47, 5/48

13. Viola M. Frymann, "The Trauma of Birth," pp. 197–205, *Osteopathic Annals*, 5/76

14. Edith E. Dovesmith, "The Growing Skull and the Injured Child," pp. 34–39, *American Association of Osteopaths Yearbook*, 1967

15. John Dobbing and Jean Sands, "Vulnerability of Developing Brain, IX, The Effect of Nutritional Growth Retardation on the Timing of the Brain Growth Spurt," *Biology of the Neonate 19*, 1971

16. Viola Frymann, "Learning Difficulties of Children Viewed in the Light of the Osteopathic Concept," *The Journal of the American Osteopathic Association*, Vol. 76, 9/76

17. Meyer Silverman, "Effect of Skull Distortion on Occlusal Equilibrium," *Journal of Prosthetic Dentistry*, 4/73

18. Denis Brookes, in *Lectures on Cranial Osteopathy* on p. 127, describes this delightfully as "taking a turn around the room." Thorsons, 1981

19. Joseph E. LeDoux, "Emotion, Memory and the Brain," pp. 50–57, *Scientific American*, 6/94

20. Jessie R. Thomson, *A Natural and Healthy Childhood*, pp. 57–60, Bloomfield Books, 1986

21. Stanley Greenspan *et al.*, *Diagnostic Classification of Mental Health and Developmental Disorders of Infancy and Early Childhood*, 1994, available through telephoning 1 800 899 4301

22. Daniel Goleman, "A Psychiatric Manual for the Smallest Children," *New York Times*, 1/4/95

23. David B. Chamberlain, "The Outer Limits of Memory," pp. 4–13, *Noetic Sciences Review*, Autumn 1990

24. B. Bower, "Conscious memories may emerge in infants," p. 86, *Science News*, Vol. 148, 8/5/95

25. John Horgan, "Brain Storm," p. 24, *Scientific American*, 11/94

### Chapter 36  Bad Backs

1. See Chapter 3, A History of Human Evolution

2. B.A. Wood, "Evolution of Australopithecines," p. 237, *The Cambridge Encyclopedia of Human Evolution*, ed. Steve Jones *et al.*, Cambridge University Press, 1994

3. G.H. Brundtland *et al.*, "Height, Weight and Menarche of Oslo Schoolchildren During the Last 60 Years," *Annals of Human Biology*, Vol. 7, pp. 307–322, 1980

4. As of June 1995, the height of Tokyo grade school desks has been raised five times since 1945

5. Frank Netter, *Musculoskeletal System, Part 1,* p. 125, Ciba Geigy, 1987

6. Ruthy Alon, *Mindful Spontaneity,* p. 297, Prism Press, 1990

7. Alan Stoddard, *Manual of Osteopathic Practice,* p. 6, Hutchinson Medical, (London) 1969

8. C. Owen Lovejoy, "Evolution of Human Walking," *Scientific American,* 11/88, p. 121

9. Stanley Keleman, *Emotional Anatomy,* p. 99, Center Press, 1985

10. John C. Pierrakos, "Anatomy of Evil," p. 89, from *Meeting the Shadow,* p. 83, ed. by Connie Zweig and Jeremiah Abrams, Tarcher, 1991

11. D.H. Lawrence, "Healing," from *Selected Poems,* p. 114, Viking, 1959

12. A.L. Cochrane, *Working Group on Back Pain,* p. 7, Her Majesty's Stationary Office, London, 1979

13. Stanley J. Bigos, *Acute Low Back Pain in Adults,* p. 1, U.S. Department of Health and Human Services, 1994

14. R.T. Benn and P.H.N. Wood, *Pain in the Back,* pp. 14, 121

15. C.V. Burton, *Lumbosacral Arachnoiditis,* pp. 3, 24

16. Michael Winerip, "It's Always Good to Take An X-Ray. But Necessary?" p. B8, *New York Times,* 3/2/94

17. John G. Fleagle, "Primate locomotion and posture," pp. 75–79, *The Cambridge Encyclopedia of Human Evolution,* ed. Steve Jones *et al.,* Cambridge University Press, 1994

18. A. Nachemson, "Measurement of Intradiscal Pressure," p. 1, *Acta Orthop. Scand.,* Suppl. 43, 1960

19. J. Puschel, "Water Content of Normal And Degenerated Intervertebral Discs," *Beitr. Path. Anat,* Vol. 84, No. 123, 1930

20. R. Wasse, *Philosophical Transactions,* (London), Innys, 1724

21. H. Somberg, "The Relation of the Spinal Subarachnoid and Perineural Spaces," *Journal of Neuropathy and Experimental Neurology,* 4/47

22. Ralph F. Erlinghausen, "The Circulation of the Cerebrospinal Fluid through the Connective Tissue System," *Academy of Applied Osteopathy Yearbook,* 1969.

23. A. Nachemson, "Review of Mechanics of the Lumbar Disc," pp. 14 & 129, *Rheum. Rehab,* 1975

24. William G. Sutherland, *Collected Writings of William Garner Sutherland D.O., D. Sc. (Hon)* pp. 17–20, ed. by Adah S. Sutherland and Anne L. Wales, Sutherland Teaching Foundation, 1967

25. James Cyriax, *Textbook of Orthopedic Medicine,* Vol. 1, pp. 235–236

26. K.L. Kelsey, "Epidemiological Study of Acute Lumbar Intervertebral Discs," p. 144, *Rheumat. Rehab.,* Vol. 14, 1975

27. Alan Stoddard, *Manual of Osteopathic Practice,* p. 59, Hutchinson Medical, London, 1969

28. John Wernham, *Lectures on Osteopathic Technique,* p. 111, Maidstone College of Osteopathy, undated, c. 1993

29. Yochanan Rywerant, *The Feldenkrais Method: Teaching By Handling,* Harper and Row, 1983

30. Moshe Feldenkrais, *Awareness through Movement,* Harper Collins, 1990

31. Emily Conrad-Da'oud, *Life on Land,* Tilbury Press, forthcoming in 1996

32. M.A. Edgar and S. Nundy, "Innervation of the Spinal Dura Mater," p. 530, *Neural. Neurosurg. Psychiat.,* Vol. 29, 1966

33. J.S. Collis, *Lumbar Discography,* Charles C. Thomas, 1963

34. James Cyriax, *Textbook of Orthopedic Medicine,* Vol. 1, p. 229, Balliere Tindall (England), 1984

35. James Cyriax, *Textbook of Orthopedic Medicine,* Vol. 1, p. 331, Balliere Tindall (England), 1984

36. James Cyriax, *Textbook of Orthopedic Medicine,* Vol. 1, p. 329, Balliere Tindall (England), 1984

37. Alan Stoddard, *Manual of Osteopathic Practice,* pp. 65–72, Hutchinson Medical, London, 1969

38. Alan Stoddard, *Manual of Osteopathic Practice,* p. 148, Hutchinson Medical, London, 1969

39. James Cyriax, *Textbook of Orthopedic Medicine,* Vol. 2, p. 4, Balliere Tindall (England), 1982

40. M.I.V. Jayson *et al., Intervertebral Discs: Nuclear Morphology and Bursting Pressures,* p. 308, Ann. Rheum. Dis., 1973

41. Vasily Aleksayev holds the world record in the snatch at five-hundred sixty-two pounds (255 kilos)

42. Harrison Fryette, *Principles of Osteopathic Technic (sic),* p. 117, Academy of Applied Osteopathy, 1966

43. Harrison Fryette, *Lectures on Osteopathic Technique,* p. 24, Academy of Applied Osteopathy, 1966

44. For more information on this topic, see Martin Rush, *Decoding the Secret Language of Your Body,* Simon and Schuster, 1995

45. Alec Milne, *Back Pain and Psychosomatic Stress,* lecture at the Kingston Clinic, Edinburgh, 1971 (See *Psychosomatic Stress: Asthma and Allergy,* by the same author, Kingston, 1986)

46. Alfred J. Zeigler, "Illness as Descent into the Body," from *Meeting the Shadow,* p. 95, ed. by Connie Zweig and Jeremiah Abrams, Tarcher, 1991

47. For more information see the guidelines on the treatment of prostatic enlargement by John D. McConnell *et al.,* published in 1994 by the Federal Agency for Health Care Policy and Research. (For information call 800 358 9295)

48. A. Magora, "Relations Between Low-Back Pain and Occupation," p. 12, *Industrial Med. Surg.,* Vol. 41, 1972

49. See John Wernham, *Lectures on Osteopathic Technique,* pp. 65–67 with the emphasis on the "wedge" of the sacrum. The mechanics of car seats accentuate the "wedge's" compression into the coxal bones. Maidstone College of Osteopathy, c.1993 (undated)

50. Sandra Blakeslee, "A Pathway That Carries the Signals of a Caress," p. B9, *New York Times*, 11/23/94

51. Alexander Lowen, *Love and Orgasm*, Macmillan, 1965

52. Adolf Guggenbuhl-Craig, "The Demonic Side of Sexuality," from *Meeting the Shadow*, pp. 98–99, ed. by Connie Zweig and Jeremiah Abrams, Tarcher, 1991

53. See Chapter 11, The Seven Souls, on Swadisthana, and Chapter 34 The Mandible

54. R.D. Laing, *The Divided Self*, pp. 66–77, Pantheon, 1962

55. Stanley Keleman, *Emotional Anatomy*, p. 70, Center Press, 1985

56. Stanley Keleman, *Emotional Anatomy*, p. 126, Center Press, 1985

57. Alex Gray, *Sacred Mirrors*, see the chapter entitled "Progress of the Soul," Inner Traditions International, 1990

58. Reynold Spector, "Vitamin Homeostasis in the Central Nervous System," pp. 1393–1398, *New England Journal of Medicine*, 6/16/77

59. M.F.K. Fisher, *The Gastronomical Me*, North Point Press, F, S & G, 1989

60. Alan Stoddard, *Manual of Osteopathic Practice*, p. 81, Hutchinson Medical, London, 1969

61. *The Anatomy of Sleep*, p. 30, Hoffman-LaRoche, 1966, no author accredited

62. Alex Beam of *The Boston Globe*, "Napping: It's Not Just for Kids Anymore," *The Monterey Herald*, p. 1D, 3/3/95.)

63. Daniel Goleman, "Feeling Sleepy? An Urge to Nap is Built In," p. B9, *New York Times*, 9/12/89

64. *The Anatomy of Sleep*, p. 63, Hoffman-LaRoche, 1966

65. "Astronauts Grow Too Tall," *New York Times*, 7/12/94

66. Gretel Erlich, *The Solace of Open Spaces*, p. 130, Penguin Books, 1985

67. Anthony Storr, *Solitude*, p. 36, Ballantine Books, 1988

68. Alec Milne, *Insight and Shamanism*, lecture in November 1993, Carmel, California

69. Stanley Keleman, *Emotional Anatomy*, p. 69, Center Press, 1985

70. Ruthy Alon, *Mindful Spontaneity*, p. 299, Prism Press, 1990

71. Alex Gray, *Sacred Mirrors*, pp. 54–55, Inner Traditions International, 1990

72. John Wernham, *Lectures on Osteopathy*, p. 6, Maidstone College of Osteopathy, 1992

73. K.L. Kelsey, "Epidemiological Study of Acute Lumbar Intervertebral Discs," p. 144, *Rheum. Rehab.*, Vol. 14, 1975

74. Harrison Fryette, *Principles of Osteopathic Technic*, pp. 77, 123, Academy of Applied Osteopathy, 1966

75. Stanley J. Bigos *et al.*, *Acute Low Back Problems in Adults*, U.S. Government Printing Office, 1994

76. Hank Herman, "Back Pain: Signal That Should Not Be Ignored," p. B10, *New York Times*, 2/11/91

77. The body also does its own limiting through muscle splinting and tissue "blocking," particularly when a disc rupture is involved

78. Alan Stoddard, *Manual of Osteopathic Practice*, p. 128, 149, Hutchinson Medical, London, 1969

79. Hank Herman, "Some Sports Aren't a Pain in the Back," p. B10, *New York Times*, 2/11/91

80. For further information, see James Cyriax, *Textbook of Orthopedic Medicine*, Vol. 1, pp. 332–336

81. C.N. Shealy, "The Role of Spinal Facets in Back and Sciatic Pain," *American Association for the Study of Headache*

82. James Cyriax, *Textbook of Orthopedic Medicine*, Vol. 1, pp. 332, Balliere Tindall, 1984

83. John Wernham, *Lectures in Osteopathy*, p. 9, Maidstone College of Osteopathy, c. 1992 (undated)

84. Edward De Bono, *De Bono's Thinking Course*, Facts on File, 1986

85. Edward De Bono, *Master Thinkers Handbook*, International Center for Creative Thinking, 1990

86. Harrison Fryette, *Principles of Osteopathic Treatment*, p. 105, Academy of Applied Osteopathy, 1966

87. Alan Stoddard, *Manual of Osteopathic Practice*, p. 149, Hutchinson Medical, London, 1969

88. James Cyriax, *Textbook of Orthopedic Medicine*, Vol. 1, p. 235, Balliere Tindall (London) 1984

89. Miyamoto Musashi, *A Book of Five Rings*, pp. 53–54, Overlook Press, 1974

90. For in-depth coverage, see Jerry A. Johnson, *The Essence of Internal Martial Arts*, Vols. I and II, Ching Lien Healing Arts, 1994

91. Peter Ralston, *The Principles of Effortless Power*, pp. viii–xviii, North Atlantic Books, 1989

92. F. Matthias Alexander, *The Use of the Self*, Gollancz, 1984

93. W. Barlow, *The Alexander Principle*, Gollancz, 1973

94. See Elaine Louie, "The Fit Commandment: Health Is Next to Godliness," p. B2, *New York Times*, 7/12/95

### Chapter 37 Headaches

1. Seymour Diamond and Jose L. Medina, "Headaches," p. 2, *Clinical Symposia*, Vol. 41, No. 1, Ciba Geigy, 1989

2. Kins Loree, "Headache Pain," *Massage and Bodywork Quarterly*, Summer 1994, pp. 38–41

3. Seymour Diamond and Jose L. Medina, "Headaches," Vol. 41, No. 1, p. 12, *Clinical Symposia*, Ciba Geigy, 1989

4. Denis Brookes wisely points out that "anti-social tendencies" can ensue from frontal bone impaction, which may lead to frontal and/or orbital headache, and "because the behavior centers in the frontal lobe are directly beneath this field." See his *Lectures on Cranial Osteopathy*, p. 88, Thorsons, 1981

5. This may be a serious development: See note regarding brain tumors at end of chapter

6. Jane E. Brody, "Brain Tumors Increasing," p. 9, *International Herald Tribune*, 7/6/95

7. John Upledger and Jon D. Vredevoogd, *Management of Autogenic Headache*, pp. 232–241, Osteopathic Annals, No. 6, 6/79

8. Frank H. Netter, *The Nervous System*, p. 164, Ciba Geigy, 1967

9. Steve Jones *et al.*, *The Cambridge Encyclopedia of Human Evolution*, p. 196, Cambridge University Press, 1994

10. Seymour Diamond and Jose L. Medina, "Headaches," pp. 14–15, *Clinical Symposia*, Vol. 41, No. 1, Ciba Geigy, 1989

11. Elisabeth Rosenthal, "Drug Shows Promise in Treating Migraines," *New York Times*, 6/5/94

12. William G. Sutherland, *The Cranial Bowl*, pp. 115–116, The Cranial Academy, 1948

13. Oliver Sacks, *Migraine*, University of California Press, 1992

14. George W. Thorn *et al.*, "Principles of Internal Medicine," p. 23, *Harrison's Principles of Internal Medicine*, McGraw Hill, 1950

15. Kins Loree, "Headache Pain," *Massage and Bodywork Quarterly*, Summer 1994, pp. 38

16. See Chapter 3, A History of Human Evolution, and Chapter 20, The Central Nervous System

17. John Horgan, "Brain Storm: Controlling chaos could help treat epilepsy," p. 24, *Scientific American*, 11/94

18. "Mystifying Headaches," p. 80, *The Economist*, 3/2/91

19. Stuart L. Brown, *Animals at Play*, pp. 2–35, National Geographic Society, Vol. 186, No. 6, 12/84

20. Seymour Diamond and Jose L. Medina, "Headaches," Vol. 41, No. 1, p. 4, *Clinical Symposia*, Ciba Geigy, 1989

21. Revenge, or "retaliatory aggression," however, does play a part in society, both ours and that of other primates. See T.H. Clutton-Brock and G.A. Parker, "Punishment in animal societies," pp. 209–216, *Nature*, Vol. 373, 1/19/95

22. Harold I. Magoun, *Osteopathy in the Cranial Field*, pp. 276–277, The Cranial Academy, 1976

23. George W. Thorn *et al.*, "Principles of Internal Medicine," p. 20, *Harrison's Principles of Internal Medicine*, McGraw Hill, 1950

24. Seymour Diamond and Jose L. Medina, "Headaches," Vol. 41, No. 1, p. 5, *Clinical Symposia*, Ciba Geigy, 1989

25. George W. Thorn *et al.*, "Principles of Internal Medicine," p. 21, *Harrison's Principles of Internal Medicine*, McGraw Hill, 1950

26. Jane E. Brody, "Migraine" p. B8, *New York Times*, 1/8/92

27. Michael Moskowitz, cited in Jennifer Allen's "Oh My Aching Head," p. 72, *Life*, 2/94

28. Seymour Diamond and Jose L. Medina, "Headaches," Vol. 41, No. 1, pp. 4, *Clinical Symposia*, Ciba Geigy, 1989

29. See the computer simulation of exactly this phenomena in Lisa Seachrist's "Mimicking the Brain: Using computers to investigate neurological disorders," pp. 62–63, *Science News*, Vol. 148, 7/22/95

30. Courtney Childs and Bruce Doneux, Counselors working with the U.S. Army "Light Infantry" at Fort Ord, California

31. Harold I. Magoun found that the greater wing was usually elevated on the affected side. See his *Osteopathy in the Cranial Field*, p. 120, The Cranial Academy, 1976

32. William Sutherland, *Collected Writings of William Garner Sutherland D.O., D. Sc. (Hon)*, pp. 86–88, ed. by Adah S. Sutherland and Anne L. Wales, Sutherland Teaching Foundation, 1967

33. James Cyriax, *Textbook of Orthopedic Medicine*, Vol. I, p. 75, Balliere Tindall, 1982

34. Seymour Diamond and Jose L. Medina, "Headaches," Vol. 41, No. 1, p. 19, *Clinical Symposia*, Ciba Geigy, 1989

35. Cohen et al, "Electroencephalographic Laterality Changes During Human Sexual Orgasm," pp. 189–199, *Archives of Sexual Behaviour*, Vol. 5, No. 3, 1976

36. *The Anatomy of Sleep*, p. 29, Hoffman-LaRoche, 1966, author unacknowledged

37. George W. Thorn et al, "Principles of Internal Medicine," pp. 24–25, *Harrisons Principles of Internal Medicine*, McGraw Hill, 1950

### Chapter 38 Brain Tumors

1. Natalie Angier, "Cellular Phone Scare Discounted," pp. B5–B6, *New York Times*, 2/2/93

2. Jane E. Brody, "Brain Tumors Increasing," p. 9, *International Herald Tribune*, 7/6/95

3. Natalie Angier, "Rising Incidence of Brain Tumors," p. B7, *New York Times*, 7/31/90

4. Stanley I. Rapoport and Devra Lee Davis, *Journal of the National Cancer Institute*, 1990

5. Robert O. Becker and Gary Selden, *The Body Electric*, pp. 60–67, Quill, 1985

6. Yang Jwing-Ming, *Chinese Qigong Massage*, pp. 6–17, YMAA Publication Center, 1992

7. Jane E. Brody, "Possible Links Are Being Explored Between Babies' Health and Fathers' Habits and Working Conditions," p. 15, *New York Times*, 12/25/91

8. Birgitta Floderus, National Institute of Occupational Health, Sweden

9. Samuel Milham Jr., *The American Journal of Epidemiology*, 1988

10. Judy Makin, Carleton University, Ottowa

11. See the series of articles by Paul Brodeur entitled "Annals of Radiation (Cancer and Power Lines)," *The New Yorker*, 1990

12. John C. Pierrakos, *The Energy Field in Man and Nature*, Institute of Bio-energetic Analysis, undated

13. Maria Feychting and Anders Ahlbom, Karolinska Institute, Stockholm
14. Robert O. Becker and Gary Selden, *The Body Electric*, pp. 278–329
15. Yuri Kholodov, "Subliminal Stress," on small-gauss fields affecting brain, appearing in Robert O. Becker and Gary Selden, *The Body Electric*, pp. 276–277, Quill, 1985
16. *International Herald Tribune*, 5/15/95
17. See also: Jeffrey D. Saffer and Sarah J. Thurston, "Cancer Risk and Electromagnetic Fields," p. 22, *Nature*, Vol. 375, 5/4/95
18. *New York Times*, 11/29/93
19. See Chapter 19, The Liquid Electric Model
20. See also Holger Kalweit, *Shamans, Healers and Medicine Men*, p. 230: "... as the Hopi say, the human being speaks with God." Shambala, 1987
21. Larry Dosey, *Healing Words: The Power of Prayer and the Practice of Medicine,* Harper Collins, 1993
22. Holger Kalweit, *Shamans, Healers and Medicine Men*, pp. 162–174, Shambala, 1987
23. See Chapter 45, Windows to the Sky

## Chapter 45   *Windows to the Sky*

1. *Scientific American*, p. 81, 5/91
2. An "Acupuncture Chinese Inch," is measured as the distance between the greatest divergence points of the two creases formed on the client's index finger when it is bent at right angles at the first and second phalangeal joints.
3. Jerry A. Johnson, *The Essence of Internal Martial Arts*, Vol. I, p. 302, Ching Lien Healing Arts, 1994

# Bibliography

**Articles, Books, Research Papers,
Audio Tapes and Film**

Jeanne Achterberg, *Imagery in Healing: Shamanism and Modern Medicine*, Shambala, 1985

Jeanne Achterberg and G. Frank Lewis, *Imagery
and Disease*, Institute for Personality and
Ability Testing Inc, Illinois, 1984

*Acute Low Back Problems in Adults: Assessment
and Treatment*, U. S. Department of Health
and Human Services, 1994

N. A. Aladzhalov et al, *The Ultralow Frequency
Spectrum of Electrical Phenomenon in the
Brain*, translated from Doklady Akademii
Nauk USSR, Vol. 197, No. 4, 4/71

F. Matthias Alexander, *Constructive Conscious
Control of the Individual*, Gollanz, 1987

R. McNeill Alexander, "Human Locomotion,"
pp. 80–85 in *The Cambridge Encyclopaedia
of Human Evolution*, ed. Steve Jones et al,
Cambride University Press, 1994

Ruthy Alon, *Mindful Spontaneity*, Prism Press,
1990

*The Anatomy of Sleep*, Hoffman-LaRoche, 1966

W. French Anderson, *Gene Engineering*, Omni,
Vol. 13, No. 10, 7/91

John P. Angleton, ed. *The Amygdala:
Neurobiological Aspects of Emotion, Memory
and Mental Dysfunction*, Wiley Liss, 1992

Lucius Apuleius, *The Tale of Cupid & Psyche*,
Shambala Centaur Editions, 1992

Beryl Arbuckle," The Cranial Aspect of
Emergencies of the Newborn," pp. 507–511,
*The Journal of the American Osteopathic
Association*, Vol. 47, 5/48

Angeles Arrien, *The Four-Fold Way*, Harper Collins,
1993

Angeles Arrien, *Signs of Life*, Arcus, 1992

Angeles Arrien, *The Tarot Handbook*, Arcus Books,
1987

W.H. Auden, *Epistle To A Godson and Other
Poems*, Random House, 1972

F.G. Bailey, *The Prevalence of Deceit*, Cornell
University Press, 1991

Ernest G. Baker, "Alteration in Width of Maxillary
Arch and Its Relation to Sutural Movement of
Cranial Bones," *Journal of the American
Osteopathic Association*, Vol. 70, No. 6, 2/71

R. Robin Baker and Mark A. Bellis, *Human Sperm
Competition: Copulation, Masturbation and
Infidelity*, Chapman and Hall, 1994

Betty F. Balcombe, *As I See It*, Piatkus Books, 1994

Betty F. Balcombe, *The Energy Connection*, Piatkus
Books, 1993

Michael Balter, "Did Homo Erectus Tame Fire
First?" p. 1570, *Science*, Vol. 268, 6/16/95

Jean-Claud Baral, *Visceral Manipulation*, Eastland
Press, 1988

Marcia Barinaga, "Anthropologists Overturn Old
Ideas About New Developments,"
pp. 364–365, *Science*, Vol. 268, 4/21/95

Marcia Barinaga, "The Brain Remaps its Own
Contours," *Science*, Vol. 258, 10/92

Marcia Barinaga, "Remapping the Motor Cortex,"
pp. 1696–1698, *Science*, Vol. 268, 6/23/95

W. Barlow, *The Alexander Principle*, Gollancz,
1973

Ellen Bass and Laura Davis, *The Courage to Heal: A Guide for Women Survivors of Child Sexual Abuse,* Harper and Row, 1988

Cary Baynes translation of the Wilhelm edition of the I-Ching, Princeton University Press, 1990

E.A. Bennet, *C.G.Jung,* 1961

Rollin E. Becker, "Diagnostic Touch: Its Principles and Application," pp. 165–177, *Academy of Aplied Osteopathy Yearbook,* 1965

Robert O. Becker and Gary Selden, *The Body Electric,"* Quill, 1985

Michael J. Benton, "Diversification and extinction in the history of life," p. 52, *Science,* Vol. 269, 4/7/95

Itzak Bentov, *Stalking the Wild Pendulum,* Dutton, 1977

The Bible, Standard Version and Revised Standard Version

Stanley J. Bigos, *Acute Low-Back Pain in Adults,* U.S. Department of Health and Human Services, 1994

Stephen J. Blood, "The Craniosacral Mechanism and the Temporomandibular Joint," pp. 516–519, *The Journal of the American Osteopathic Association,* Vol. 86, No. 8, 8/86

Robert Bly, *The Kabir Book,* Beacon Press, 1977

R. H. Blyth, *Zen in English Literature and Oriental Classics,* The Hokuseido Press (Tokyo) 1942

L. Bolk, "On the Premature Obliteration of Sutures in the Human Skull," *American Journal of Anatomy,* Vol. 17, No. 4, 5/15/15

M. Bolte and C.J. Hogan, "Conflict over the age of the Universe," pp. 399–402, *Nature,* Vol. 376, 8/3/95

Edward de Bono, *Parallel Thinking: From Socratic to de Bono Thinking,* Viking, 1993

Edward De Bono, *Master Thinkers Handbook,* International Center for Creative Thinking, 1990

Bruce Bower, "Conscious memories may emerge in infants," p. 86, *Science News,* Vol. 148, 8/5/95

Bruce Bower, "Talk of Ages: A Tiny Bone Rekindles Arguements Over the Roots of Speech and Language," pp. 24–26, *Science News,* Vol. 136, 7/8/89

Gerda and Mona-Lisa Boysen, *Biodynamic Des Lebens,* Synthesis Verlag, 1987

C. Loring Brace et al, "Gradual Change in Human Tooth Size in the Pleistocene and Post-Pleistocene," pp. 705–720, *Evolution,* Vol. 41, No. 4, 1987

Barbara Ann Brennan, *Hands of Light: A Guide To Healing Through the Human Energy Field,* Bantam, 1987

Barbara Ann Brennan, *Light Emerging: The Journey of Personal Healing,* Bantam, 1993

M. Brodrick and A.A. Morton, *Concise Dictionary of Egyptian Archeology,* p. 94, Methuen, 1922

Denis Brookes, *Lectures On Cranial Osteopathy,* Thorsons, 1981

Peter R. Brotchie et al, "Head position signals used by parietal neurons to encode location of visual stimuli," pp. 232–235, *Nature,* Vol. 375, 5/18/95

Stuart L. Brown, "Animals at Play," pp. 2–35, *Magazine of the National Geographic Society,* Vol. 186, No. 6, 12/84

Norman O. Brown, *Love's Body,* Random House, 1966

G.H. Brundtland et al, "Height, Weight and Menarche of Oslo Schoolchildren During the last 60 Years," *Annals of Human Biology,* Vol. 7, pp. 307–322, 1980

Gautama the Buddha, *The Dhammapada: The Sayings of the Buddha,* trans. Thomas Byron, Random House, 1976

E.A. Wallis Budge, *The Gods of the Egyptians,* Vols. 1 and 2, Dover, 1969

E.A. Wallis Budge, *From Fetish To God In Ancient Egypt,* Dover, 1988

James F.T. Bugenthal *Intimate Journeys,* Jossey-Bass, 1990

Vern L. Bullough, *Science in the Bedroom: A History of Sex Research,* Basic Books, 1995

Margaret Bunson, *The Encyclopaedia of Ancient Egypt,* Facts on File, 1991

Robert Burns, *Robert Burns: The Complete Poetical Works,* ed. J. A. Mackay, Alloway Publishing, 1993

Maxwell Cade and Nona Coxhead, *The Awakened Mind,* Delacorte Press, 1979

Joseph Cambell, *The Masks of God: Creative Mythology,* Penguin, 1976

Joseph Campbell, *Oriental Mythology: The Masks of God,* Arkana, 1991

Fritzjof Capra, *The Tao of Physics,* Shambala, 1975

Richard Carlson, ed., *Healers on Healing,* St. Martin's Press, 1989

Robert Carroll, "Between fish and amphibian," pp. 389–390, *Nature,* Vol. 373, 2/2/95

Angus Cathie, "Growth and Nutrition of the Body with Special Reference to the Head," *Academy of Applied Osteopathy Yearbook*, 1962

David B. Chamberlain, "The Outer Limits of Memory," *Noetic Sciences Review*, Autumn 1990

Bruce Chatwin, *Songlines*, Jonathan Cape, 1987

Deepak Chopra, *Ageless Body, Timeless Mind*, Harmony Books, 1993

Cohen et al, "Electroencephalographic Laterality Changes During Human Sexual Orgasm," pp. 189–199, *Archives of Sexual Behavior*, Vol. 5, No. 3, 1976

A.L. Cochrane, *Working Group On Back Pain*, Her Majesty's Stationary Office, London, 1979

Joel E. Cohen, "Population Growth and Earth's Human carrying Capacity," pp. 341–346, *Science*, Vol. 269, 7/21/95

Elizabeth Collins, "Unadvertised Receptivity," pp. 24 & 26, *Scientific American*, 11/87

Emily Conrad-Da'oud, *Life on Land*, Tilbury Press, forthcoming in 1996

Robert H. Coombs, *Inside Doctoring*, Praeger, 1986

Paulo Coelho, *The Alchemist*, Harper Collins, 1993

Alan Cowey and Peter Stoerig, "Blindsight in monkeys," pp. 247–249, *Nature*, Vol. 373, 11/19/95

Thomas Cleary, *Zen Master Keizan*, North Point Press, 1990

T.H. Clutton-Brock and G.A. Parker, "Punishment in animal societies," pp. 209–216, *Nature*, Vol. 373, 1/19/95

Paul Colinvaux, *Why Big Fierce Animals Are Rare*, Princeton University Press, 1978

Robert H. Coombs, *Inside Doctoring*, Praeger, 1986

Calvin Cottam, "Cranial Manipulation Roots," Part 1, *Digest of Chiropractic Economics*, Vol. 23, No. 4, Jan/Feb 1981

Nephi Cottam, *The Story of Craniopathy*, Privately Published, 1936

Ted Crail, *Apetalk and Whalespeak*, J.P. Tarcher, 1981

Francis Crick and Christof Koch, "Are we aware of neural activity in primary visual cortex?," pp. 121–123, *Nature*, Vol. 375, 5/11/95

Elizabeth Culotta, "Birth Tale Gets a New Twist," p. 365, *Science*, Vol. 268, 4/21/95

e.e. cummings, *Collected Poems* Harcourt Brace and Co, New York, 1926

James Cyriax, *Textbook of Orthopaedic Medicine*, Vols I and II, Balliere Tindall, 1984

Donald J. Dalessio, ed., *Wolff's Headache and Other Head Pain*, 4th edition, Oxford University Press (New York), 1980

Major Betrand DeJarnette, *Cranial Technique – 1968*, privately published in Nebraska City, Nebraska, 1968

Major Betrand DeJarnette, *Sacro Occipital Technique – 1981*, privately published in Nebraska – City, Nebraska, 1968

Arthur Deikman, *The Observing Self: Mysticism and Psychotherapy* Beacon Press, 1982

Robin Dennell, "In search of Neanderthals," p. 397, *Nature*, Vol. 376, 8/3/95

David Denton, *Craniopathy and Dentistry*, privately published in Los Angeles, 1979

Taisen Deshimaru, *The Way to the Martial Arts*, E. P. Dutton, 1982

Elizabeth Deuress, *The Seen and the Unseen*, Smith Barnes, U.K., 1924

Seymour Diamond and Jose Medina, "Headaches," *Clinical Symposium*, Vol. 41, No. 1, 1989

Annie Dillard, *Teaching a Stone To Talk*, Harper Collins, 1982

John Dobbing and Jean Sands, "Vulnerability of Developing Brain, IX, The Effect of Nutritional Growth Retardation on the Timing of the Brain Growth Spurt," *Biology of the Neonate* 19, 1971

Larry Dossey, "The Light of Health, the Shadow of Illness," from *Meeting the Shadow*, p. 93, ed. by Connie Zweig and Jeremiah Abrams, Tarcher, 1991

Larry Dossey, *Healing Words: the Power of Prayer and the Practice of Medicine*, Harper Collins, 1993

Karlfried Graf Von Durkheim, *Hara: The Vital Center of Man*, George Allen and Unwin, 1985

Albert Einstein, *Einstein: A Portrait*, compiled by Mark Winokur, Pomegranite Art Books, 1984

Mircea Eliade, *Shamanism*, Princeton University Press, Bollingen, 1974

Mircea Eliade, *Patanjali and Yoga*, Schoken Books, 1975

Henri Ellenberger, "Psychiatry from Ancient to Modern Times," in *The American Handbook of Psychiatry*, Vol. 1, ed. S. Arieti, Basic Books, New York, 1974

Frederick T. Elworthy, *The Evil Eye*, Citadel, copyrighted in 1895 (no recent publication date found)

Gretel Ehrlich, *The Solace of Open Spaces*, Penguin Books, 1985

Ralph F. Erlinghausen, "The Circulation of the Cerebrospinal Fluid Through the Connective Tissue System," *Academy of Applied Osteopathy Yearbook*, 1969.

B. d'Espignat, "The Quantum Theory and Reality," *Scientific American*, pp. 158–181, 11/89:

Clarissa Pinkola Estes, *Women Who Dance With Wolves*, Ballantine Books, 1992

W. Y. Evans-Wentz, *The Tibetan Book of the Dead*, Oxford University Press, 1960

Moshe Feldenkrais, *Awareness through Movement*, Harper Collins, 1990

Richard P. Feynman, *What Do You Care What Other People Think*, Bantam, 1989

Joshua Fischman, "Human Origins," pp. 37–40, *Discover*, 1/95

Joshua Fischman, "Painted Puzzles Line the walls of an Ancient Cave," p. 614, *Science*, Vol. 267, 2/3/95

Aelred C. Fonder, *The Dental Physician*, Medical Dental Arts, 1985

Aelred C. Fonder, *The Dental Distress Synndrome*, Medical Dental Arts, 1994

Richard Feely, *Clinical Cranial Osteopathy*, Cranial Academy, 1975

Richard P. Feynman, *Surely You're Joking, Mr Feynman: Adventures of a Curious Character*, Vintage, 1985

Francesca Freemantle and Chogyam Trungpa, *The Tibetan Book of the Dead*, Shambala, 1975

Philip Freund, *Myths of Creation*, Transatlantic Arts, 1975

Viola Frymann, "Relation of Disturbances of Craniosacral Mechanisms to Symptomatology of the Newborn: Study of 1,250 Infants," *Journal of the American Osteopathic Association*, pp. 1059–1075, Vol. 65, 6/66

Viola Frymann, "Learning Difficulties of Children Viewed in the Light of the Osteopathic Concept," *The Journal of the American Osteopathic Association*, Vol. 76, 9/76

Viola Frymann, "A Study of the Rhythmic Motions of the Living Cranium," pp. 928–945, *Journal of the American Osteopathic Association*, Vol. 70, 5/71

Joseph T. Fuhrmann, *Rasputin: A Life*, Praeger, 1990

Robert Fulghum, *All I Really Need to Know I Learned in Kindergarten*, pp. 6–7, Villard Books, 1990

Jack Gaines, *Fritz Perls: Here and Now*, Integrated Press, 1979

Albert M. Galaburda et al, "Cerebral Lateralization," pp. 428–456, *Archives of Neurology*, Vol. 42, 5/85

Alain Gehin, *Atlas of Manipulative Techniques*, Eastland Press, 1985

N. Giblin and A. Alley, "Studies in Skull Growth: Coronal Suture Fixation," *Anatomical Record*, Vol. 88, No. 2, 2/44

Dexter G. Girton et al, "Observation of Very Slow Potential Oscillations in Human Scalp Recordings," pp. 561–568, *Electroencephalography and Clinical Neurophysiology*, Elsevier Scientific Publishing House, Amsterdam, 1973

Mitchell Glickstein, "The Discovery of the Visual Cortex," pp. 118–127, *Scientific American*, 9/88

Gary W. Goldstein and A. Loris Betz, "The Blood Brain Barrier," *Scientific American*, 9/86

Jane Goodall, *In The Shadow of Man*, Houghton Mifflin, 1971

William P. Gordon, *Sleep: A Guide For Professionals*, Institute for Cortex research and Development, 1986

Cheryl L. Grady et al, "Age-Related Reductions in Human Recognition Memory Due to Impaired Encoding," pp. 218–221, *Science*, Vol. 269, 7/14/95

Alex Gray, *Sacred Mirrors*, Inner Traditions, 1990

Phillip E. Greenman, "Roentgen Findings in the Craniosacral Mechanism," *The Journal of the American Osteopathic Association*, Vol.70, 9/70

Wolfgang Gretschmer, "Meditative Techniques in Psychotherapy," pp. 224–234 of *Altered States of Consciousness*, ed. Charles T. Tart, Doubleday Anchor, 1969

John Gribbin, *Schrodinger's Kittens and the Search for Reality*, Little, Brown, 1995

Donald Griffin, *The Question of Animal Awareness*, 1970

John A. Grim, *The Shaman*, University of Oklahoma Press, 1983

Stanislav Grof, *LSD Psychotherapy*, Hunter House, 1980

Stanislov Grof, *Spiritual Emergency Network*, Tarcher Putnam, 1989

Adolf Guggenbuhl-Craig, "The Demonic Side of Sexuality," from *Meeting the Shadow*, pp. 98–99, ed. by Connie Zweig and Jeremiah Abrams, Tarcher, 1991

Arthur Guirdham, *The Cathars and Reincarnation*, Neville Spearman, 1970

Arthur Guirdham, *We Are One Another*, C.W. Daniel, 1991

Ruben C. Gur et al, "Sex Differences in Regional Cerebral Glucose Metabolism During a Resting State," pp. 528–531, *Science*, Vol. 267, 1/27/95

Arthur C. Guyton, *Basic Neuroscience*, W. B. Saunders and Company, 1987

Edward T. Hall, *The Dance of Life: The Other Dimension of Time*, Anchor, 1989

Dora Jane Hamblin, *The Emergence of Man*, Time-Life Books, 1973

Chester L. Handy, "History of Cranial Osteopathy," pp. 269–272, *Journal of the American Osteopathic Association*, Vol. 47, 1/48

Barbara Hannah, *Jung, His Life and Work*, Perigree Books, 1976

Michael Harner, *The Way of the Shaman*, Harper Collins 1980

T. R. Harrison, *Principles of Internal Medicine* McGraw Hill, 1977

William Hart, *Vipassana Meditation as taught by S.N. Goenka*, Harper and Row, 1987

John Heider, *The Tao of Leadership*, Humanics, 1985

Werner von Heisenberg, *Physics and Philosophy: the Revolution in Modern Science*, Harper, 1958

Melvin Henningsen, "Living Osteology of Interest to the Dentist," Part 1 and 2, *Dental Digest* 63, 10/57 and 11/57

Eugen Herrigel, *Zen in the Art of Archery*, Pantheon Books, 1964

A.R. Hildebrand et al, "Size and structure of the Chicxulub crater revealed by horizontal gravity gradients and cenotes," pp. 415–417, *Nature*, Vol. 376, 8/3/95

J. Allan Hobson, *The Dreaming Brain*, Basic Books, 1989

Herbert Hoffman, *Icons of Immortality*, forthcoming in 1996

John Horgan, "Fractured Functions: Does the brain have a supreme integrator?" pp. 36–37, *Scientific American*, 12/93

John Horgan, "Brain Storm," p. 24, *Scientific American*, 11/94

John M. Howell, "Early Farming In Northwestern Europe" pp. 118–124, *Scientific American*, 11/87

Jing Hui, "Chinese Patriarch: The Life and Teaching of China's Great Buddhist Monk Xu Yun," published in *Heaven Earth*, China Advocates, Vol. 1 No. 3, 1/92

Glyn W. Humphreys, "Acting without 'seeing,'" *Nature*, Vol. 374, pp. 763–764, 4/27/95

Michael Hutchison, *Megabrain*, Ballantine, 1986

Sandra Ingerman, *Soul Retrieval*, Harper Collins, 1991

Jennifer Isaacs, *Autralian Dreaming*, Lansdowne, 1980

Frederick E. Jackson, "The Pathophysiology of Head Injuries," *Clinical Symposia*, July–December 1966

Arthur Janov, *The Primal Scream*, Putnam, 1970

Charles Jennings, "New visions of the cortex," pp. 635–636, *Nature*, Vol. 375, 6/22/95

Conrad E. Johanson, "Potential for Pharmocological Manipulation of the Blood-Cerebrospinal Fluid Barrier," appearing in *Implications of the Blood-Brain Barrier and its Manipulation*, Vol. 1, edited by Edward A. Neuwelt, Plenum Press, 1989.

Donald Johanson and James Shreeve, *Lucy's Child: The Discovery of A Human Ancestor*, Early Man Publications, 1989

Donald Johanson, *Lucy: The Beginnings of Mankind*, Simon & Shuster, 1981

Donald Johanson and Leon Johanson, *Ancestors: In Search of Human Origins*, Villard, 1994

Alex de Jonge, *The Life and Times of Grigarii Rasputin*, Coward, McCann and Geoghegan, 1982

Steve Jones et al, *The Cambridge Encyclopaedia of Human Evolution*, Cambridge University Press, 1994

Don Hanlon Johnson, *The Protean Body*, Harper and Row, 1977

Don Hanlon Johnson, *Body, Spirit and Democracy*, North Atlantic Books, 1994

Jerry A. Johnson, *The Essence of Internal Martial Arts*," Vols. 1 and II, Ching Lien Healing Arts, 1994

W. Brugh Joy, *Joy's Way*, Tarcher, 1982

C.G. Jung, *Modern Man In Search of A Soul*, translated by W.S. Dell and Cary Baynes, Harcourt, Brace and Company, 1933

C.G. Jung, *Four Archetypes: Mother/Rebirth/Spirit/Trickster*, Princeton University Press, 1992

C.G. Jung, *Man and His Symbols*, Aldus Books, London, 1964

C.G. Jung, *Collected Works*, translated by R.F.C. Hull, Bollingen Series XX, Princton University Press, 1980

Franz Kafka, *The Great Wall of China: Stories and Reflections*, Schocken Books, 1970

Holger Kalweit, *Shamans, Healers and Medicine Men*, Shambala, 1987

Richard E. Kappler, "Osteopathy in the Cranial Field," pp. 13–18, *The Osteopathic Physician*, 2/79

Ted J. Kaptchuk, *The Web That Has No Weaver: Understanding Chinese Medicine*, Congdon and Weed, 1983

Zvi Karni, John Upledger et al, "Examination of the Cranial Rhythm in Long-Standing Coma and Chronic Neurological cases," pp. 275–281 of *Craniosacral Therapy*, Upledger and Vredevoogd, Eastland Press, 1983

Akira Kasamatsu and Tomio Hirai, "An Electrocephalographic Study on the Zen Meditation," in Charles T. Tart, *Altered States of Consciousness*, Doubleday Anchor, 1969

Stanley Kelleman, *Emotional Anatomy*, Center Press, 1985

Kenneth A.R. Kennedy, "Morphological Variations in Ulnar Supinator Crests and Fossae as Identifying Markers of Occupational Stress," *Journal of Forensic Science*, 10/83

Kenneth A.R. Kennedy and M. Yasar Iscan, *Reconstruction of Life from the Skeleton*, Alan R. Liss Inc., 1989

Richard A. Kerr, "Did Darwin Get it All Right?" pp. 1421–1422, *Science*, Vol. 267, 3/10/95

Richard A. Kerr, "Timing Evolution's Early Bursts," pp. 33–34, Science, Vol. 267, 1/6/95

Harold K. Kimelberg and Michael D. Norenberg, "Astrocytes," pp. 66–76, *Scientific American*, 4/89

Jeffrey Kluger, "Magna Cum Laud Critters," pp. 18–22, *Discover*, 2/95

Samuel Noah Kramer, *Great Ages of Man: Cradle of Civilization*, Time-Life, 1967

I. Krejci and F. Lutz, *Zahnfarbene Adhasive Restaurationen im Seitenzahnbereich*, University of Zürich, 1994

I. Krejci et al, *In-vitro-testverfahren Zur Evaluation Dentaler Restaurationsysteme*, University of Zürich, 1994

Elisabeth Kubler-Ross, *Death: The Final Stage of Growth*, Simon and Schuster, 1975

H. Laborit, *Stress and Cellular Function*, Lippincott, 1959

Hugo Lagercranrtz and Thodore A. Slotkin, "The Stress of Being Born," *Scientific American*, pp. 100–107, 6/86

R.D. Laing, *The Divided Self*, Pantheon, 1962

F. Bruce Lamb, *Wizard of the Upper Amazon*, Houghton Mifflin, 1971

H. Vincent Langley, *Essential Treatments in Manipulative Therapy*, Castle Cary Press Somerset, (England) 1963

Edward O. Laumann et al, *The Social Organization of Sexuality: Sexual Practices in the United States*, University of Chicago Press, 1995

Robert Lawlor, *Voices of the First Day*, Inner Traditions, 1991

D. H. Lawrence, *Selected Poems*, New Directions Books, 1947

Edna M. Lay, "The Osteopathic Management of Temporomandibular Joint Dysfunction," from *Clinical Management of Head, Neck and TMJ Pain and Dysfunction*, ed Harold Gelb, W.B. Saunders, 1985

Richard Leakey, *Origins: The Emergence and Evolution of Our Species and Its Possible Future*, E.P. Dutton, 1982

Richard Leakey and Roger Lewin, *Origins Reconsidered*, E.P. Dutton, 1977

Joseph E. LeDoux, "Emotion, Memory and the Brain," pp. 50–57, *Scientific American*, 6/94

Richard B. Lee and Irven De Vore, *Kalahari Hunter-Gatherers*, Harvard University Press, 1976,

Belinda Lees et al, "Differences in proximal femur bone density over two centuries," *The Lancet*, Vol. 341, 3/93

Anthony J. Legge and Peter A. Rowley-Conwy, "Gazelle Killing In Stone Age Syria," pp. 88–95, *Scientific American*, 8/87

Frederick Lehrman, *The Sacred Ladscape*, Celestial Arts, 1988

Steven Levine, *A Gradual Awakening*, Anchor, 1979

Roger Lewin, *In the Age of Mankind*, Smithsonian Books, 1988

Jacob Liberman, *Light, Medicine of the Future*, Bear and Company, 1991

Andrei Linde, "The Self-Reproducing Inflationary Universe," pp. 48–55, *Scientific American*, 11/94

J. Little and B. Thompson, "Descriptive Epidemiology," in *Twinning and Twins*, MacGilvray et al, John Wiley, New York, 1988

Konrad Lorenz, *On Agression*, Bantam, 1966

C. Owen Lovejoy, "Evolution of Human Walking," pp. 121–131, *Scientific American*, 11/88

Alexander Lowen, *Love and Orgasm*, Macmillan, 1965

Alexander Lowen, *The Betrayal of the Body*, Collier, 1967

Alexander Lowen, *Bio-energetics*, Penguin, 1976

Gay Gaer Luce, *Biological Rhythms in Psychiatry and Medicine*, U.S. Department of Health, Education and Welfare, 1970

Jacques Lussyran, *And There Was Light*, Parabola, 1989

Norman Maclean, *A River Runs Through It and Other Stories*, The University of Chicago Press, 1976

Louis MacNeice, *Autumn Journal*, Faber and Faber Ltd., 1939

Thomas E. Mails, *The Plains Indians*, Bonanza Books, 1985

Shizuto Masunaga and Wataru Ohashi, *Zen Shiatsu: How to Harmonize Yin and Yang for Better Health*, Japan Publications (Tokyo) 1977

R.E.L. Masters and J. Houston, *The Varieties of Psychedelic Experience*," Holt, Rinehart, New York, 1966

David A. McCormick, "The cerebellar symphony," pp. 412–413, *Nature*, Vol. 374, 3/30/95

Alexander Marshack, "The Ecology and Brain of Two-handed Bipedalism: An Analytic, Cognitive and Evolutionary Assessment," in *Animal Cognition*, Lawrence Erlbaum Associates, 1984.

Keith Mason, *Medicine for the 21st Century*, Element, 1992

Kiiko Matsumoto and Stephen Birch, *Hara Diagnosis: Reflections on the Sea*, Paradigm Publications, 1988

Terence McKenna, *The Archaic Revival*, Harper, 1992

J. Robert McLintic, *Physiology of the Human Body*, John Wiley & Sons, 1975

David Michael and Ernest Retzlaff, "A Preliminary Study of Cranial Bone Movement in the Squirrel Monkey," pp. 886–9, *Journal of the American Osteopathic Association*, Vol. 74, 5/75

Stuart Miller, *Men and Friendship*, Gateway (England) 1986

A.A. Milne, *House At Pooh Corner*, Dell, 1923

Alec Milne *Psychosomatic Stress: Asthma and Allergy*, Kingston, (Scotland) 1962

Arnold Mindell, *Dreambody*, Sigo Press, 1982

Arnold Mindell, *City Shadows: Psychological Interventions in Psychiatry*, Routledge, 1988

Arnold Mindell *Working on Yourself Alone*, Arkana, 1990

Roberta DeLong Miller, *Psychic Massage*, Harper and Row, 1975

Herbert C. Miller, "Head Pain," pp. 135–142, the *Journal of the American Osteopathic Association*, Vol. 72, 10/72

Mira, *For Love of the Dark One*, trans. Andrew Schelling, Shambala, 1993

Edgar D. Mitchell, *Psychic Exploration*, Putnam, 1974

Fred L. Mitchell et al, "Accuracy and Perceptual Decision Delay in Motion Perception," p. 149, *Journal of American Osteopathic Association*, Vol. 78, 10/78

Stephen Mitchell, *The Enlightened Heart*, Harper and Row, 1989

Betty Clare Moffat, *Soulwork* Wildcat Canyon Press, 1994

Richard Monastrsky, "The Edicaran Enigma," pp. 28–30, *Science News*, Vol. 148, 7/8/95

Raymond A. Moody, *Life after Life*, Stackpole Books, 1976

Virginia Morell, " The Earliest Art Becomes Older – and More Common," pp. 1908 1909, *Science*, Vol. 267, 3/31/95

Melvin Morse, *Transformed By the Light*, Ballantine Books, 1992

Yuri Moskalenko, *Cerebral Pulsation in the Closed Cranial Cavity*, Izv Akad Nauk USSR, Vol. 620, No. 4, 9/61

Vernon B. Mountcastle, *Medical Physiology*, C.V. Mosby, 1974

John H. Moyer et al, "Effect of Increased Jugular Pressure on Cerebral Hemodynamics," *Journal of Applied Physiology* 7, 11/54

Max Muller, trans, *The Upanishads*, Part II, Dover (England) 1962

Miyamoto Musashi, *A Book of Five Rings*, Overlook Press, 1974

Charles Muses and Arthur M. Young, *Consciousness and Reality*, Outerbridge and Lazard, 1972

John Napier, *The Roots of Mankind*, London, 1971

National Institute of Mental Health Epidemiologic Catchment Area Study on Obsessive-Compulsive Disorders, 1988

Loil Neidhoefer, *Intuitive Koerperarbeit*, Transform, 1990

John G. Neihardt, *Black Elk Speaks*, Bison, 1932

Martin G. Netsky and S. Shulangshoti, *The Choroid Plexus in Health and Disease*, University Press of Virginia, 1975

Frank Netter, *The Musculoskeletal System*, Ciba-Geigy, 1987

Frank H. Netter, *The Nervous System*, Ciba-Geigy, 1967

Frank Netter, *Atlas of Human Anatomy*, Ciba-Geigy, 1989

Forrest Nielsen, "Biochemical and Physiologic Consequences of Boron Deprivation in Humans," pp. 59–63, *Environmental Health Perspectives*, 11/7/94

Robert M. Nideffer, *Ethics and Practice of Applied Sports Psychology*, Mouvement [sic] Publications, 1981

Tim O'Brien, *The Things They Carried*, Viking, 1991

Robert E. Ornstein, *The Mind Field*, Viking, 1976

Robert Ornstein and Richard F. Thompson, *The Amazing Brain*, Houghton Mifflin Company, 1984

Robert Ornstein, *The Evolution of Consciousness*, Prentis Hall, 1991

Frank A. Oski, *Don't Drink Your Milk: New Frightening Medical Facts about the World's Most Overrated Nutrient*, TEACH Services, Brushton, New York, 1992

Walter N. Pahnke and William A. Richards, "Implications of LSD and Experimental Mysticism," in *Altered States of Consciousness*, ed. Charles T. Tart, Doubleday Anchor, 1969

H. W. Parke and D. E. W. Wormell, *The Delphic Oracle*, Vol. 1 and 2, Blackwell, London, 1956

Carol Pearson, *The Hero Within*, Harper & Row, 1986

Fritz Perls, *Ego, Hunger and Aggression*, Gestalt Journal Press, 1992

Lyons Petrucelli, *Medicine: An Illustrated History*, Abradale Press/Harry N. Adams Inc, New York, 1987

John C. Pierrakos, "Anatomy of Evil," from *Meeting the Shadow*, ed. by Connie Zweig and Jeremiah Abrams, Tarcher, 1991

John C. Pierrakos, *The Energy Field in Man and Nature*, Institute of Bio-energetic Analysis, undated

Norman St Pierre, Richard Roppel, Ernest Retzlaff, "The Detection of Relative Movements of Cranial Bones," p. 289, *Journal of the American Osteopathic Association*, 12/76.

Stuart Piggot, *The Druids*, Thames and Hudson, 1985

Teresa Pijoan, *Healers on the Mountain*, August House, 1993

Steven Pinker, *The Language Instict*, Morrow, 1994

Werner Platzer, ed., *Locomotor System*, Thieme, 1986

Fred Plum and Jerome B. Posner, *The Diagnosis of Stupor and Coma*, 3rd edition, F.A.Davis Co, 1980

Robert M. Poole, *The Incredible Machine*, National Geographic Society, 1986

J.J. Pritchard et al, "The Structure and Development of Cranial and Facial Sutures," Part 1, pp 73–86, *Journal of Anatomy*, 1/56

W. Rahula, *What the Buddha Taught*, Grove Press, New York, 1959

Peter Ralston, *Cheng Hsin: The Principles of Efforless Power*, North Atlantic Books, 1989

Peter Rambaut and James Johnston, "Prolonged Weightlessness and Calcium Loss in Man," *Acta Astronautica*, Vol. 6, pp. 1113–1122,

Michael E. Rampino and Bruce M. Haggerty, " Mass Extinctions and Periodicity," pp. 617–618, *Science*, Vol. 269, 8/4/95

Wilhelm Reich, *Orgasmusreflex, Muskelhaltung und Korperausdruck*, Sexpol Verlag, 1937

Wilhelm Reich, *Willhelm Reich Uber Sigmund Freud*, Reich Archive 1954

Wilhelm Reich, *Ether, God and Devil*, Doubleday, 1973

Boyce Rensberger, "Bones of Our Ancestors," pp. 29–34, *Science*, 4/84

Ernest W. Retzlaff et al, "Nerve Fibers and Endings in Cranial Sutures," *The Journal of the American Osteopathic Association*, Vol. 77, 2/78

Ernest W. Retzlaff et al, "Temporalis Muscle Action in Parietotemporal Suture Compression," *The Journal of the American Osteopathic Association*, Vol. 78, 10/78

Ernest W. Retzlaff et al, "The Structures of Cranial Bone Sutures," *Journal of the American Osteopathic Society*, Vol. 75, pp. 607–8, 2/76

Rainer Maria Rilke, *Letters To A Young Poet*, Vintage Books, 1987

Kenneth Ring, *Life at Death: A Scientific Investigation of the Near-Death Experience*, Coward, McCann and Geoghegan, 1980

Sogyal Rinpoche, *The Tibetan Book of Living and Dying*, Harper Collins, 1992

Bryant Robey et al, "The Fertility Decline in Developing Countries," pp. 60–67, *Scientific American*, 12/93

Jelaluddin Rumi, *Open Secret*, trans. John Moyne and Coleman Barks, Threshold Books, 1984

Jelaluddin Rumi, *Unseen Rain*, trans. John Moyne and Coleman Barks, Threshold, 1986

Jelaluddin Rumi *We Are Three*, trans. Coleman Barks, Maypop Books, 1987

Jelaluddin Rumi, *Like This*, trans. Coleman Barks, Maypop, 1990

Peter Rutter, *Sex in the Forbidden Zone*, Fawcett Crest, 1989

Yochanan Rywerant, *The Feldenkrais Method: Teaching by Handling*, Harper and Row, 1983

Oliver Sacks, *The Man Who Mistook His Wife for a Hat*, Summit Books, 1985

Oliver Sacks, "Making Up the Mind," *New York Review of Books*, p. 42, 4/8/93

Oliver Sacks, *Migraine*, University of California Press, 1992

Oliver Sacks, "A Neurologist's Notebook: Prodigies," pp. 44–46, *The New Yorker*, 1/9/95

Jamie Sams and David Carson, *Medicine Cards*, Bear and Co, 1988

Lee Sannella, *The Kundalini Experience: Psychosis or Transcendence*, Integral Publishing, 1992

Bennet A. Shaywitz et al, "Sex differences in the functional organization of the brain for language," pp. 607–609, *Nature*, Vol. 373, 2/16/95

Steven Schumacher, *The Encyclopeadia of Eastern Philosophy and Religion*, Shambala, 1994

H.W. Schumann, *The Historical Buddha*, Arkana, London, 1989

Theodor Schwenk, *Sensitive Chaos*, Anthroposophic, 1990

Lisa Seachrist, "Mimicking the Brain: Using computers to investigate neurological disorders," pp. 62–63, *Science News*, Vol. 148, 7/22/95

*The Secret of the Golden Flower*, trans. from Chinese to German by Richard Wilhelm, trans. from German by Cary Baynes, Arkana, 1984

Hans Selye, *The Stress of Life*, p. 68, McGraw Hill, 1956

Hans Selye, "The Nature of Stress," pp. 131–150 of A.C. Fonder's *The Dental Distress Syndrome*, Medical Dental Arts, 1993

Richard Selzer, *Mortal Lessons*, Simon and Schuster, 1974

M.I. Sereno et al, "Borders of Multiple Visual Areas in Humnas Revealed by Functional Magnetic Resonance Imaging," pp. 889–893, *Science*, Vol. 268, 5/12/95

Johannes Setekleiv, *Spontaneous Rhythmic Activity in Smooth Muscles*, Norske Legeforening, 1964, Neurological Laboratory, Anatomical Institute, University of Oslo, Norway.

Bernie Siegel, *Love, Medicine and Miracles*, Harper Collins, 1990

Meyer Silverman, "Effect of Skull Distortion on Occlusal Equilibrium," *Journal of Prosthetic Dentistry*, 4/73

Marsha Sinetar, *Ordinary People as Monks and Mystics*, Paulist Press, 1986

Dong Shaoming, *Some Like It Hot: The Chinese Idea of the Dantian*, Heaven Earth, Vol. 1, 1/92

Shalila Sharamon and Bodo J Baginski, *Das Chakra Handbuch*, Windpferd, 1989

Marsha Sinetar, *Ordinary People as Monks and Mystics*, Paulist Press, 1986

S.D. Smith, *Atlas of Temporomandibular Orthopedics*, Medical College of Philadelphia, 1982

C. Snow-Harter and R. Marcus, "Exercise, Bone Mineral Density, and Osteoporosis," *Exercise and Sports Science Reviews*, ed. J. Holloszy, Williams and Wilkins, 1991

H. Somberg, "The Relation of the Spinal Subarachnoid and Perineural Spaces," *Journal of Neuropathy and Experimental Neurology*, 4/47

Reynold Specter and Conrad E. Johanson, "The Mammalian Chroroid Plexus," pp. 68–74, *Scientific American*, 11/89

Reynold Spector, "Micronutrient Homeostasis in Mammalian Brain and Cerebrospinal Fluid, *Journal of Neurochemsitry*, 1989.

"Spinal Cord Injuries: New Optimism Blooms for Developing Treatements," p. 218, *Science*, Vol. 258, 10/9/92

Larry R. Squire and Stuart Zola-Morgan, "The Medial Temporal Lobe System," *Science*, p. 1380, 9/20/91

Rudolf Steiner, *Life Between Death and Rebirth*, Anthroposophic Press, 1968

Suzanne K. Steinmetz, *The Cycle of Violence*, 1977

L. Le Shan, *The Medium, the Mystic and the Physicist*, Viking, 1974

"Skullduggery," p. 34, *Scientific American*, 6/90

Larry R. Squire and Stuart Zola-Morgan on the hippocampus, *Science*, 9/91

Andrew Taylor Still, *Philosophy of Osteopathy*, Edwards Brothers, Ann Arbor, Michigan, 1946

Andrew Taylor Still, *Osteopathy: Research and Practice*, 1910, reprinted by Eastland Press, 1992

Andrew Taylor Still, *Autobiography of Andrew T. Still, with a History of the Discovery & Development of the Science of Osteopathy*, 1897, reprinted by Ayer, 1972

Alan Stoddard, *Principles of Osteopathic Technique*, pp 69–74, Hutchinson Medical, London, 1969

Hal Stone and Sidra Winkelman, *Embracing Our Selves: The Voice Dialogue Manual*, Delos, 1983

Anthony Storr, *Human Agression*, Bantam, 1968

Anthony Storr, *Solitude*, Ballantine Books, 1989

Hyemeyohsts Storm, *Seven Arrows*, Ballantine, 1972

R. S. Stowe et al, *Measurement of Bone Torsion In Vivo Via Biostereoroentgenography*, Thirteenth International Congress for Photogrammetry, Helsinki, 7/76

Christopher Stringer and Clive Gamble, *In Search of the Neanderthal*, Thames and Hudson, 1993

Olive M. Stretch, "The Pituitary and the Ageing Process in realtion to the Cranial Concept," in *Lectures on Cranial Osteopathy* by Denis Brookes, Thorsons, 1981

Ada S. Sutherland, *With Thinking Fingers*, Cranial Academy, 1962

William G. Sutherland, *Collected Writings of William Garner Sutherland D.O., D. Sc. (Hon)* ed. by Adah S. Sutherland and Anne L. Wales, Sutherland Teaching Foundation, 1967

William G. Sutherland, *The Cranial Bowl*, Free Press, 1939

D.T. Suzuki, *Manual of Zen Buddhism*, Rider London, 1950

D.T. Suzuki, *Studies in Zen*, Dell, 1955

Shunryu Suzuki, *Zen Mind, Beginner's Mind*, Weatherhill, 1988

Thomas Szasz, *The Theology of Medicine*, Harper, 1977

Rabindranath Tagore, *Gitanjali* Macmillan, 1912

Reah Tannahill, *Sex in History*, Scraborough, 1980

Charles T. Tart, *Altered States of Consciousness*, Doubleday Anchor, 1969

Melicien Tettambel et al, "Recording of the Cranial Rhythmic Impulse," p. 149, *Journal of the American Osteopathic Association*, Vol. 78, 10/78

Edward J. Thomas, *The Life of Buddha*, Routledge (London) 1969

Jessie R. Thomson, *Natural and Healthy Childhood*, Bloomfield Books, 1927

Times Literary Supplement, *Two Faces of Jung*, 8/2/63

Nikolai Tolstoy, *The Quest for Merlin*, Little Brown, 1985

Steve Van Toller and George H. Dodd, *Perfumery: The Psychology and Biology of Fragrance*, 1989

E. Fuller Torrey, "Are Twins Really Identical," pp. 18–21, *Parabola*, Vol. XIX, No. 2, 5/94

Erik Trinkaus and Pat Shipman, *The Neandetals*, Alfred A. Knopf, 1993

Chuang Tzu, *Inner Chapters*, trans. Gia-Fu Feng and Jane English, Random House, 1974

Chuang Tzu, "Inner Chapters," trans. Stephen Mitchell, from *The Enlightened Heart*, Harper and Row, 1989

Lao Tzu, *Tao Te King*, trans. Gia-Fu Feng and Jane English, Vintage, 1972

*Understanding Acute Low Back Problems*, U. S. Department of Health and Human Services, 1994

John E. Upledger, "The Relationship of Craniosacral Examination Findings in Grade School Children with Developmental Problems," *The Journal of the American Osteopathic Association*, Vol. 77, 6/78

John E. Upledger et al, "Diagnosis and Treatment of Temporoparietal Suture Head Pain," *Osteopathic Medicine*, 7/78

John E. Upledger and Zvi Karni, "Mechanical Electrical Patterns During Craniosacral Osteopathic Diagnosis and Treatment," pp. 782–791, *Journal of the American Osteopathic Association*, Vol. 78, 7/79

John E. Upledger and Jon D. Vredevoogd, *Craniosacral Therapy*, Eastland Press, 1983

George E. Valliant, *Adaptation To Life*, Little, Brown, 1978

Vanio Vannini, *Atlante Del Corpo Umano*, Fabri Editori (Milan), 1982

Frances E. Vaughan, *Awakening Intuition*, Anchor Press, 1979

Alberto Viloldo and Stanley Krippner, *Healing States* Fireside, 1987

Anne L. Wales, "The Work of William Garner Sutherland, D.O., D.Sc. (Hon.)," *The Journal of the American Osteopathic Association*, Vol. 71, 1972

Alan Walker and Mark Teaford, "The Hunt For Proconsul," *Scientific American*, 1/89

Barbara Walker, *The Woman's Encyclopedia of Myths and Secrets*, Harper, 1983

Brian Browne Walker, trans., *I-Ching*, St Martin's Press, 1992

John Warfel, *The Head, Neck and Trunk*, Williams Wilkins, 1992

S.L. Washburn, "The Relation of the Temporal Muscle to the Form of the Skull," *Anatomical Record*, Vol. 99, 11/47

Alan Watts, *Tao: The Watercourse Way*, Pantheon Books, 1975

John P. Welsh et al, "Dynamic organization of motor control within the olivocerebellar system," pp. 453–457, *Nature*, Vol. 374, 3/30/95

John Wernham, *Lectures on Osteopathy*, Maidstone College of Osteopathy (England), circa 1993

M. Westcott, *Toward a Contemporary Psychology of Intuition*, Holt, Rinehart and Winston, New York, 1968

Ian Wilson, *The After Death Experience: The Physics of the Non-Physical*, William Morrow, 1987

Arthur T. Winfree, "The Timing of Biological Clocks," *Scientific American Library*, 1987

Jonathan Winson, "The Meaning of Dreams," pp. 86–96, *Scientific American*, 11/90

Marion Woodman, *The Ravaged Bridegroom: Masculinity in Women*, Inner City Books, 1990

R.H. Woods and J.M Woods, "A Physical Finding Related To Psychiatric Disorders," *Journal of the American Osteopathic Association*, Vol. 60, pp. 988–993, 8/61

Jack Worsley, *The Meridians of Chi Energy: Point Reference Guide*, The College of Traditional Chinese Acupuncture, U.K., 1979

Richard J. Wurtman and Judith J. Wurtman, "Carbohydrates and Depression," p. 68, *Scientific American*, 1/89

James B. Wyngaarden and Lloyd H. Smith Jr, *Textbook of Medicine*, Saunders, 1982

Yatri, *Unknown Man: The Mysterious Birth of a New Species*, Simon and Schuster, 1988

Shinzen Young, "Purpose and Method of Vipassana Meditation," *The Humanistic Psychologist*, Vol. 22, Spring 1994

Alfred J. Zeigler, "Illness as Descent into the Body," from *Meeting the Shadow*, p. 95, ed. by Connie Zweig and Jeremiah Abrams, Tarcher, 1991

Mark Zvelebil, "Postglacial Foraging in the Forests of Europe," pp. 104–106, *Scientific American*, 5/86

Zweig and Abrams, *Meeting the Shadow*, Tarcher, 1991

### Audio Tapes

Angeles Arrien, *The Story of Basque Mysticism*, Dolphin Tapes, 1982

Robert Bly and Marion Woodman, *Facing the Shadow In Men and Women*, Oral Traditions Archives, 1993

Deepak Chopra, *Quantum Healing Workshop*, Mystic Fire Audio, Sound Horizons Audio Video, 1990

Ken Cohen, *The Way of Chi Kung*, Sounds True Inc., 1993

James Hillman, Michael Meade and Meladoma Somez, *Images of Inititation*, Aural Traditions Archives, 1/24/92

John C. Lilly, *The Dolphin Experience*, Dolphin Tapes, 1969

Rollo May, *Violence and the Daimonic*, Dolphin Tapes, 1970

Fritz Perls, *Gestalt Therapy and How it Works*, Dolphin Tapes, 1966

Fritz Perls, *Dream Theory and Demonstration*, Dolphin Tapes, 1967–1968

Ram Dass, *Yoga of Daily Life*, Dolphin Tapes, 1970

William G. Sutherland:
*The Science of Osteopathy*
*The Hole in the Tree*
*The Reciprocal Tension Membrane*
*Cranial Articular Surfaces*
*The Primary Respiratory Mechanism*
*Types of Cranial Lesions*
(Audio Recordings made on to vinyl in 1953)

Marion Woodman, *Addiction and Sacred Emptiness*, c/o Inner City Books, Box 1271, Station Q, Toronto, Canada M4T 2P4

Shinzen Young, *The Red Road: A Review of Native American Spiritual Practices*, Insight Recordings

Shinzen Young, *Introduction to Vipassana: Where the Path Leads*, Insight Recordings

### Film

Documentary film on C.G. Jung, *Matter of Heart*, available from the Jung Foundation in Los Angeles. Telephone 310–556 1196

# Index of Techniques

# Index

This index contains entries for the ideas and treatments discussed in the text. Cultural references have not been indexed, generally. For an index of techniques, see page 474.

chemistry
  of bone, 8–9
  of connective tissue, 9
  of migraines, 230–231
*chi kung,* 45, 70, 223
childbirth
  belly dance and low back, 224
  bones affected by, 6, 11, 14, 39, 149, 159, 208–209
  cranial wave "jump-start" following, 40, 210
  techniques in preparation for, 82, 82–83
  trauma of, 89
  vestigial tail and, 67
  *see also* pregnancy
child development
  air sinus, 140–141
  auditory tubes, 126, 184
  bone deformation in, 6, 134
  concerns about, and craniosacral work, 209
  cranial, 11–12
  fontanels and sutures, 6, 10–12
  movement and joints, 6–7
  neurological, 50
  *see also* embryology
childrearing, 50
children
  craniosacral work with, 208–211
  deep-diving reflex of, 140–141
  ear infections in, 126
  repressed perception by, 43–45, 105
  time sense of, 209
  *see also* infants
chimpanzees, 50
chin, 189–190, 194
Chinese tradition
  acupuncture. *see* acupuncture
  complements in, 19, 39
    *see also* soul centers
  Taoist. *see* Taoism
chiropractic
  field acknowledged by, 39
Christ Consciousness, 103
Christianity
  pilgrimages of, and nomadic drive, 71

  *see also* religion
clients
  consciousness, clarity of, 45
  positioning of, 63, 65, 73
  preparations with. *see* preparations
  role in session, empowerments for, 63
  transference by. *see* transference and counter-transference
  *see also* healers; visionary work
cluster headaches. *see under* headaches
cocaine, 159
coccydynia, 68, 74
coccygeus muscle, *71*
  releasing, 78, *79*
coccyx
  articulation of, 68
  dysfunction of. *see* coccydynia
  movement of, 69
  root soul and, 70
  structure and location, 67, 68
  vestigial tail and, 67
coelacanths, 23
coma, cranial wave and, 36
compression head, 21, 35, 89, 126
  lesion pattern, *106–107,* 109–110
  treatment, 155, 201
  *see also* sphenobasilar lesion patterns
conditioning
  and headaches, 226
  and human development, 50
coning-in, 65
connective tissue, chemistry of, 9
consciousness
  anatomical location of, 51, 55–56
  defined, xvii
  quantum physics and, 45, 49
  techniques for altering, 95, 147, 243, 255, 257, 258–259
  *see also* glamour
constant-on engram, 27–28, 227–228
Continuum, 39, 214
core link, 18, 22
  diagnosis, 90
  and temporals, 126
  as term, 12
  treatment, 75, 90

deafness, 125

death

anatomical exit point for spirit, 133

cranial wave and, 36

of ego. *see* ecstatic consciousness

deep-diving reflex, 140–141

defibrillation, 36

denial,

*see also* repressed material

dental decay

beginning of, 26

and maxillary air sinus, 171

dental work

anesthesia, 22, 29, 190

cooperation between dentists and craniosacral therapists, 202

and cranial balance, 28–29, 172, 202

dura affected by, 22, 29

maxillae faulting through, 12, 171–172

and stomatognathic system problems, 28–29, 30, 31, 194

torsion lesion perpetuated by, 105

trauma of, as archaic wounds, 64, 172, 201

zygomae treatment and, 164

*see also* oral work; teeth

dentures, removing, 64

depression

sphenobasilar lesion patterns and, 109

treatment, 127, 130, 256–257

determination, 143, 192–193

diabetes, 62

lesion patterns as facilitating universal, 104

*see also* glamour; perception; treatment; *specific bones, body parts, or symptoms*

diencephalon, 55–56

diet

and auditory tubes, 184

and cancer, 236

and headaches, 230, *233*

and low-back pain, 219

and tinnitus, 126

directions and motion nomenclature defined, xvi-xvii

disc injuries. *see under* low-back pain

disease

three cardinal components in, 216, 252

*see also* trauma; *specific diseases*

dreambody

*see also* body; emotions; soul; spirit

dreams

of bone and tissue, and healing, 103

interpretation of, 103

treatments occuring in, 222

*see also* sleep

*Dryopithecus africanus. see* Proconsul

dura, 14–15

accessible to awareness, 15

assessment of, 90

elasticity of, 14, 22

endosteal, 14, *15*, 40

unwinding, 144

as layer of release, 113

slackening of, 41, 69, 88

*see also* reciprocal tension membrane; spinal dura

dural tube, 15

dyslexia

migraines and, 229

torsion lesions and, 105, 108

Ear Gate (Triple Warmer 21), 5, 57, 130, 258–259

ears, 123, 125, 126

ego

death of. *see* ecstatic consciousness

elbow nerve compression, and client position, 65

electromagnetic fields, and tumor formation, 235–236

embryology

brain development, 50, 54

cranial development, 10–11

drug and chemical exposure and, 235

eye development, 19

*see also under specific bones*

emotional abuse, treatment, 130

emotions

brain function and, 56–57, 143

breathing affected by, 36

and cancer formation, 234

of children, 210

client to report during treatment, 63

*body parts, symptoms, or diseases*

teeth

bite of, affected by torsion lesion, 105

bruxism, 32, 44

and evolution, 26, 27

and maxillae, 169–171

and stomatognathic system, 26–32 *passim*

unwinding, 31

*see also* dental work

telencephalon. *see* cerebral cortex

temperature reduction

of brain, 39, 55, 101

techniques for, 95, 101

temporalis muscle, 100, 197–198, 201, 243–244

temporal lobes, 52–53, 100

temporals, *120*

anatomy and musculature, 121–123

diagnostics, 124–126, 130

embryology and osteology, 121

energetics, 124–125, 126

etymology, 120

interconnectedness, 126

landmarks and location, 121

lateral pterygoids and, 201

and mandible, 123, 194

motion, 47, 102, 123–124

and sphenoid, 118, 123

sutures and articulations, 121

techniques, 126–131

treatment, 76, 126–131, 166

zygomae and, 164

temporomandibular joint

anatomy of, 27, *190, 194*

atlanto-occipital joint and, 28, 89

brain function and, 190

diagnostics, 194, 197, 198–200

dysfunction. *see* temporomandibular joint dysfunction

energetics of, 30

sphenoid and, 101

as stomatognathic system component, 23

torsion lesions and, 105

*see also* mandible; stomatognathic system

temporomandibular joint dysfunction

anatomy and, 27, 58

causes, 27–32 *passim*, 170, 173, 194, 203, 226, 227

questionaire to determine, 202–204

sexual trauma as, 32, 194, 203

considerations, 202–205

diagnostics, 194, 197, 198–200

headaches and, 226, 227

and ligament groups, 24, 27

occipital techniques and, 89

and sexual inhibition, 193

and talking, need for, 226, 227

treatment, 31–32, 76, 95, 178, 197, 198, 201, 202, 243–244

cautions, 200

client education, 32

considerations, 28

joint replacement surgery, 29

tentorium, 16, *19, 21,* 59

and occiput, 87

and parietals, 134

and sphenoid, 101, 102, 118

temporals and, 126

treatment, 94, 128, 129

thalamus, 55, 246

therapists. *see* healers

therapy

*see also* healing

third eye. *see* inner eye

third order wave. *see* cranial wave

thoracic outlet conditions, 127

thoracic pump, 253

thoracic spine, 222

thought

brain function and, 52

throat soul, *127,*

mandible and, 192

maxillae and, 171

stomatognathic system and, 30

temporals and, 124

treatment, 201, 255

vomer and, 158–160

time

brain function and, 55, 101, 103

children's sense of, 209, 210

duration of techniques, 64, 179
of headache onset, 143, 227
and healing, 220
and inner guidance, 37
tinnitus
causes, 125, 126, 201, 258
treatment, 126, 127, 130, 201
TMJ. *see* temporomandibular joint dysfunction
tongue, 24
and maxillae, 170
and meditation, 159
tonsillitis, 143
torus palatinus, 12, 158, 159, 160, 172, 178–179
touch
duration of, 64, 179
layers of tissue separation and, 113
palatines as testing skill in, 179
pressures exerted in, 63–64, 118
*see also* specific technique instructions
traction. *see* decompression
trance states, healing. *see* glamour
transverse sinus, 94
Traube-Hering Waves. *see* cranial wave
trauma
body's response to, 44
memory of
*see also* archaic wound
and prior wounds, 44–45
talking it out, and headaches, 226–227
techniques useful in, 83
to brain, 51, 53, 59
treatment of. *see* unwinding
*see also* repressed material; stress; *specific bones*
treatment, 45–46
closure of, 161, 244
of infants and children, 208–111
normal patterns of movement, determining, 45–46
opening techniques, 91, 146
*see also* unwinding
preparation for. *see* preparations
protocols, 238–239
cardinal eight, 243–244
familiarization, 240–241
headaches, 242, 243–244
lateral structures, 245–246
perineal session, 74

unwinding, 247–250
Windows to the Sky points, 251–261
zygomae in, as standard, 164
*see also* diagnosis; oral work; techniques; specific bones, body parts, symptoms, or diseases
tumors
brain, 234–236
cautions, 62, 129, 233, 236
treatment, 236
diagnosing, 90, 95
twins, 55

unconditional love, 49
unconscious, covert awareness and
archaic wounds arising in. *see* archaic wounds
with children, as technique of choice, 210
lesion pattern detection as passive, 103
protocols for, 247–250
*see also under specific bones or body parts*
uterus and pelvic diaphragm, *72*

Valsalva's maneuver, 184–185
venous sinuses, 15, 51, 140, 141
meningeal dura and, 14
straight sinus. *see* straight sinus
techniques, drainage, 94, 146
ventricles, 55
vertigo, 125, 127, 201
and migraines, 230
violence, domestic
viscerocranium, 2, *10*, 13, 43
CV4 diagnosis, 90, 93
protocols, 240–241, 245–246
sphenoid and, 142
treatment, 95, 115, 119, 154, 155, 172, 175, 243, 250
vishuddha. *see* throat soul
vision
brain function and, 53–55, 57–58
motor problems of, 105, 108
and parietals, 135
and sphenoid, 100, 102, 105, 108, 111
treatment, 172, 175
*see also* eyes
visualization
and quantum phenomena, 49

# About the Author

Hugh Milne is a third-generation Scottish osteopath. He spends most of his professional time teaching visionary craniosacral work in Germany, Italy, Japan, the United States, and Switzerland.

Hugh was born in 1948. He received his professional training at the British College of Naturopathy and Osteopathy in London. Repeated and startling clairvoyant revelations before and after graduation led to a determination to learn more about working with the inner eye. This search for higher teachings took him to India, where he lived for seven years. Hugh has spent the last fifteen years developing his teaching work.

He lives in Big Sur, California, where he is the director of the Milne Institute.

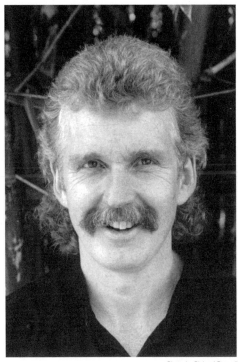

*Photo by Richard Russell*